# Wheelchair Selection and Configuration

# Wheelchair Selection and Configuration

## Rory A. Cooper, Ph.D.

DEPARTMENTS OF REHABILITATION SCIENCE
AND TECHNOLOGY AND BIOENGINEERING
Schools of Health and Rehabilitation Sciences, and Engineering
University of Pittsburgh
Pittsburgh, PA 15261

HUMAN ENGINEERING RESEARCH LABORATORIES
VA Pittsburgh Healthcare System
7180 Highland Drive, Pittsburgh, PA 15206

DIVISION OF PHYSICAL MEDICINE AND REHABILITATION
Department of Orthopaedic Surgery
University of Pittsburgh Medical Center
Pittsburgh, PA, 15261

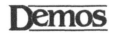

*Demos Medical Publishing, Inc., 386 Park Avenue South, New York, New York 10016*

**Library of Congress Cataloging-in-Publication Data**

Cooper, Rory A.
    Wheelchair selection and configuration / Rory A. Cooper.
       p.  cm.
    Includes bibliographical references and index.
    ISBN 1-888799-18-8
    1. Wheelchairs.  I. Title.
  RD757.W4C66  1998
  617′.03—dc21                        98-22858
                                          CIP

**Made in the United States of America**

# Dedication

Writing a book requires a significant amount of sacrifice on the part of the author's family and friends. I am indebted to my wife, Rosemarie Cooper, for encouraging me throughout the entire process of writing this book. I am also extremely grateful to my friends and colleagues for being supportive of this endeavor. I have learned a tremendous amount about wheelchairs and seating by working with students and people with disabilities. I thank them for challenging me to continue to learn and try to understand. I also thank my parents for instilling in me an unwavering desire to learn and teaching me many practical skills.

# Contents

# Preface

The audience for this book is undergraduate and graduate students who are studying occupational therapy, physical therapy, rehabilitation science, and rehabilitation engineering. The book also is a suitable reference for practicing professionals in engineering and the health professions. It provides comprehensive coverage of the key components of seating and wheelchair mobility. The book tries to provide the "why" in addition to the "how" of seating and mobility. It also was my intent to make this book a useful reference during preparation for the Rehabilitation Engineering and Assistive Technology Society of North America (RESNA) certification examinations. It is inherently difficult to write a book that serves different readers who come to the subject with various backgrounds and degrees of technical knowledge. The combination of technology and people with disabilities necessitates that rehabilitation be a markedly interdisciplinary field. Rehabilitation must focus on outcomes in the short term and over the long term. All people involved in the rehabilitation process must be knowledgeable about the potentials and limitations of assistive technology, whether available or pending.

This book reflects the current status of rehabilitation in that there is a lot of information on some topics and much less on others. This reflects the current status of the discipline and my personal biases. Because this book is intended for several audiences, some sections may appear simplistic to one reader and overwhelming to another. I have tried to place enough background and motivational material in the book to help readers learn what they need to understand the material or to have sufficient suggested readings to be able to develop that knowledge.

Students and professionals come to rehabilitation courses with a variety of backgrounds. Most therapy or bioengineering degree programs require that students take a course in assistive technology and sometimes specifically in seating and wheeled mobility. This book focuses on seating and wheelchair mobility, but provides concepts that are of much broader applicability. It assumes that the reader has taken a course in human anatomy, human physiology, and physics, or has working knowledge of these fields. Some exposure to clinical practice also is beneficial.

Rehabilitation is a humanistic profession. The context for the importance of selecting an appropriate wheelchair and seating system is developed in Chapter 1. In Chapter 1, I have attempted to describe some of the U.S. legislation related to assistive technology, and to put a human face on the disability rights movement. Rehabilitation professionals must be advocates for and partners with people with disabilities. This chapter addresses consumer concerns and provide an historical context.

Measurement of the user and wheelchair are critical to achieving maximum functional mobility. Chapter 2 describes how body measurements are made when selecting a wheelchair, as well as the critical wheelchair seating measurements that need to be specified. This chapter also addresses some basic human factors. The material should serve as a guide when measuring people for wheelchairs.

Wheelchairs are vehicles made from engineering materials. In order to assess wheelchair quality and understand the importance of different designs and features, Chapter 3 presents information about basic engineering as it relates to wheelchairs and seating. This material is presented at a level that should be suitable for non-engineers. Some basic mathematical concepts that are used in both seating and wheelchairs are developed. Mastery of this material will make it possible to understand many of the papers published on wheelchairs and seating in the professional literature and to better use the results from standardized testing.

Biomechanics and ergonomics provide the information necessary to understand many aspects of wheelchair use. These factors affect seating comfort and posture, propulsion efficiency, and pain. Chapter 4 provides basic to advanced information about wheelchair and seating biomechanics and ergonomics. The information provided in Chapter 3 provides the foundation for much of the material presented in Chapter 4.

In order to understand electric-powered wheelchairs, one must understand some of the basics of electronics. Chapter 5 presents some basic electronics that provide the foundation for understanding many of the design features of electric-powered wheelchairs and of seating systems with electronic controls. Some basic information about computers also is presented.

Wheelchair standards have been in development for nearly 20 years. Standards are designed to ensure a minimum level of quality and to provide a suitable means of comparing wheelchairs. Wheelchair standards have been a positive influence on the design and selection of wheelchairs. Chapter 6 describes the principles upon which the wheelchair standards are based. This chapter also provides an overview of the wheelchair standards and their application.

Many people with lower extremity impairments or cardiopulmonary limitations can benefit from manual wheelchairs. Manual wheelchairs are available in a wide variety of styles and include many options. Chapter 7 provides information about manual wheelchairs, their options, and assessing their performance.

Electric-powered wheelchairs provide increased mobility for some individuals. Electric-powered wheelchairs may be beneficial for people with upper and lower extremity impairments, people who have difficulty during exertion, or people with very limited endurance. Electric-powered mobility also may be the best choice for driving long distances or over taxing terrain. Chapter 8 explains the design of electric-powered wheelchairs, their design, and their important features.

Manual and electric-powered wheelchairs provide functional mobility to a large number of people. However, there are people who require more specialized wheelchairs to meet their needs. Chapter 9 addresses the design, selection and features of specialized wheelchairs. The focus is on reclining seats, tilt-in-space, adjustable seat heights, stand-up, and stair-climbing wheelchairs. Specialized wheelchairs can provide a person greater function, increased sitting tolerance, and more control.

Recreation and sports are an important part of life. For many people with physical disabilities, some form of adaptive sports equipment is required to participate in various sports or recreational activities. There seems to be a constant stream of new sports equipment and continuous improvements in sports/recreation devices. Chapter 10 covers some of the more common sports and recreational wheelchairs and related vehicles.

Proper seating also is an important aspect of wheelchair selection. Cushions provide pressure relief and some postural support. For many wheelchair users the cushion is an integral part of their mobility needs. Chapter 11 provides information about the basic theories of cushion design and cushion selection.

Most wheelchairs come with simple linear seating surfaces. However, some people need more support to accommodate or prevent postural deformities. The proper seating system can have a dramatic effect on a person's mobility, comfort, and ability to perform tasks from a wheelchair. Chapter 12 presents an overview of the specialized seating hardware available and describes the basic principles of specialized seating. There are other books that focus on specialized seating because this is a complex area that requires specific training.

Wheelchairs and their seating systems are more complex than they may appear at first glance. People spend years developing clinical expertise as seating and mobility specialists. Each consumer is unique and the seating and mobility team must work to meet the consumer's mobility goals. This requires instituting a process to ensure quality. Chapter 13 focuses on the assessment and intervention process within a seating and mobility clinic.

Wheelchairs often are used for up to 16 hours per day for almost 365 days per year. There are few devices that experience this much use. Moreover, the consequences for the user can be severe if the wheelchair is not properly maintained. Chapter 14 describes basic wheelchair maintenance. This information is designed to supplement the material developed by the manufacturer. Wheelchair users, therapists, rehabilitation engineers, and rehabilitation technologists all must be aware of wheelchair maintenance issues. Proper maintenance will yield better performance, longer wheelchair life, and greater reliability.

This book attempts to couch rehabilitation as a participatory process involving consumers, physicians, therapists, engineers, and manufacturers. It conveys a consumer-centered approach to rehabilitation. This approach assumes that the consumer sets the goals for the rehabilitation process. The rehabilitation team works with the consumer to attain the consumer's goals. There are many factors that influence the outcomes of the rehabilitation process. This book presents these issues using various examples.

This book is the result of 9 years of teaching and 18 years of research and design in rehabilitation and bioengineering. I have used portions of this book to teach students in physical therapy, occupational therapy, rehabilitation engineering, and rehabilitation science. It has been used to teach students at the University of Pittsburgh. The goal for this book was to develop a text suitable for teaching undergraduate and graduate students who were being trained in a rehabilitation profession. I also intended the book to be used by practicing professionals studying for the RESNA credentialing examinations. The book grew from lecture notes, seminar notes, laboratory exercises, and research projects related to rehabilitation science and technology. I have attempted to include material meaningful to engineers, physicians, therapists, and rehabilitation scientists.

I am very grateful to the University of Pittsburgh and to my colleagues for creating an environment for personal and professional growth, which enabled me to write this book. I also am thankful for having the opportunity to interact with diverse groups of students who challenge me to be a better professor and encourage me to continue to learn. I am indebted to a number of people in academic, government, and industrial circles who have contributed in different, but important, ways to the preparation of this book. In particular, I extend my appreciation to P. Axelson, G. Bardsley, J. Bollinger, M.L. Boninger, C.E. Brubaker, T. Capello, D. Counts, T. Detre, J. Feussner, J. Goldschmidt, D. Gray, K. Giacin, D. Hull, W.E. Langbein, S. Linnman, T.J. O'Connor, N. Pionati, N. Reinheimer, P. Stankovic, D.P. VanSickle. Special thanks go to Dr. Diana M. Schneider at Demos for her commitment to publishing this book. I also wish to acknowledge the individuals and organizations cited in the captions of numerous figures and photographs throughout the book for their generous permission to use that material. I thank the Paralyzed Veterans of America and its chapters for continuing to provide me with overwhelming support and opportunities.

# CHAPTER 1

# Wheelchairs as an Extension of Self

*Chapter Goals*

- ☑ To develop a basic understanding of the characteristics of wheelchair and seating in relation to users
- ☑ To understand basic relationships between wheelchair use and the environment
- ☑ To understand disability fundamentals sufficiently to be able to formulate and apply to wheelchairs
- ☑ To understand basic normal and abnormal development as related to wheelchairs
- ☑ To understand fundamental laws, regulations, and policies related to wheelchairs and seating

## 1.1 Introduction

The wheelchair has, for most of its history, been a design that segregated instead of integrated. People have had a long history of segregating other people based on appearance, language, religion, disability, and gender. Even in today's society, we have laws to address the needs of people with disabilities that seek to identify or categorize them. Although some of these laws provide invaluable services or protections, they also distinguish wheelchair users from other people. A long-standing struggle for people with disabilities and for individual wheelchair users is to be identified for who they are, and not for their wheelchair. John Hockenberry describes three types of jobs for people who use wheelchairs: jock jobs, disability jobs, and real jobs. People with jock jobs either make or attempt to make their profession from wheelchair sports. These people may work as representatives for wheelchair sports equipment companies or earn a living through prize moneys and endorsements. People with disability jobs work for agencies or organizations whose primary purpose is to promote or provide services to people with disabilities. Real jobs are those jobs that most any person would like to have. In other words, a real job is a job that you might hear a child with a disability talk about on career day.

The use of the wheelchair as a descriptor of people is also commonly used in the popular media. It is quite common to hear about how courageous a wheelchair user is for doing things that are not necessarily extraordinary. With such confused depictions of wheelchair users, it is difficult for the wheelchair user to bring personality to the forefront and be recognized for the person inside. The wheelchair must be thought of as an extension of self and as a means of self-expression. Some people may prefer a more subdued silver-and-black wheelchair, whereas others may prefer a brightly colored wheelchair with wildly stylish lines. In this way, a wheelchair is much like a person's clothing from a psychosocial perspective. We will try to blend many aspects of the wheelchair user in this chapter to bring a bit of color to the picture of wheelchair use.

## 1.2 History of Wheelchairs and Seating Systems

### 1.2.1 Development of the Wheelchair

Over the course of history, the progress of wheelchair design has been ploddingly slow. Most of the products currently in use were developed in the last fifteen years. Prior to that consumers used wheelchairs that more resembled hospital inventory than active mobility devices. Still, many people continue to use classic wheelchairs.

In ancient times, dependence characterized the lives of those who were disabled. Fortunate people relied on servants or family members to carry them on litters. Others went off to die. Being carried on a litter was not necessarily stigmatizing since it was the preferred mode of transportation for the wealthy and well-born. The earliest record of a wheelchair was incised in stone on a sixth century AD Chinese sarcophagus. By the European Middle Ages, the litter had been supplanted by the wheelbarrow. The wheelbarrow, while rather undignified and still requiring another's power, was convenient. The rolling chair was developed during the Renaissance as a heavy cushioned armchair with a reclining back and front legs equipped with casters. The rolling chair allowed people to rest anywhere in the house. In the sixteenth century, King Philip II of Spain had gout and used an elaborate rolling chair with horsehair upholstery and movable legrests and backrest. Later, Louis XIV used a *roulette* (a wheelchair of the period) while recovering from an operation. This popularized the roulette among the French court. In 1700, the palace of Versailles' inventory boasted 20 roulettes.

The wheelchair in its present form began developing in the early eighteenth century. During this time, wheelchairs were styled like an armchair equipped with two large wooden wheels in the front and one caster in the rear for balance. The early wheelchairs were ornate, heavy, difficult to operate, and provided little independence. With thousands of people with amputations left in the wake of the Civil War, lighter-weight wheelchairs appeared with caned seats and backs, and modern wheels of iron. These young veterans were typically shut away in state institutions or veterans' homes. Their wheelchairs only served to reinforce the notion that they were "invalids." World War I left legions of young men and women with disabilities. American veterans were given "advanced" 50-pound wheelchairs made almost entirely of India reed, still impractical for independent mobility. The British government, alerted to the risk of wasting the lives of thousands of young British veterans, revived spinner-knob tricycles (a wheel with a knob on it which when turned propelled the tricycle) and issued them to veterans with disabilities. A few years later the British Red Cross issued specialized motorized tricycles to these veterans with disabilities. Similar vehicles can be seen today in many developing countries.

In 1932, Herbert Everest along with his friend and fellow mining engineer Harry Jennings invented a sling-seat folding aircraft-steel wheelchair in Everest's quest for autonomy. This was a radical departure from previous designs and Everest, who had paraplegia from a mine collapse, became a rolling advertisement for their product. The E&J company continues to produce wheelchairs. This represents the "birth" of the modern folding wheelchair. During this same period, Franklin D. Roosevelt, who was affected by the 1931 polio epidemic, refused to be seen as anything but the vigorous man that he was. The White House respected his wishes and rarely showed his wheelchair in photographs. Roosevelt was unhappy with the image presented by the selections of wheelchairs available to him, and had several ordinary kitchen chairs equipped with wheels.

World War II led to improvements in medical care (e.g., rapid transport to a field hospital, widespread use) enabling many veterans with spinal cord injuries to live for the first time. However, veteran's hospitals were still equipped with wheelchairs from the Civil War. Toward the end of the war, many veterans were supplied with standard 18-inch seat width chrome Everest & Jennings model wheelchairs. It had not yet occurred to people that wheelchairs should fit the individual. They were, quite simply, chairs that provided users with some degree of mobility. However, many wheelchair users and rehabilitation clinicians were not satisfied with mere mobility; they wanted a means to be active and have an outlet for their energy.

Shortly after World War II, Sir Ludwig Guttmann and his colleagues originated wheelchair sports as a rehabilitation tool at Stoke Mandeville Hospital in England. Wheelchair sports developed out of the need to provide exercise and recreational outlets for the large number of young people recently injured in the war. News of Dr. Guttmann's success with the rehabilitation of his patients through the use of sports soon spread through Europe and to the United States. In 1948, he organized "Games" for British veterans with disabilities. In 1952, the Games developed into the first international wheelchair sporting competition for people with physical disabilities, with participants from the Netherlands, Germany, Sweden, Norway, and Israel.

The Vietnam conflict brought about dramatic changes in the lives of wheelchair users. Medical advances permitted great numbers of people with paraplegia and quadriplegia to live much longer and more active lives. Efforts began to restore a sense of self and enable people to be more mobile. Advocacy groups grew in popularity, the independent living center movement evolved, and greater civil rights for people with disabilities were also obtained.

Wheelchair sports also began to grow in popularity. During 1960 in Rome, Italy, athletes with disabilities competed for first time in the same venues as Olympic athletes. At the games of 1964 in Tokyo, Japan, the word "Paralympics" was coined. Since then the Paralympics have been held in conjunction with the Olympic games every four years, except 1980 and 1984.

In 1975, Bob Hall, a young man with paraplegia, became the first person to compete in the Boston Marathon in a wheelchair. This opened the door for many future road racers, prompting Dr. Caibre McCann, a leading physician, to say: "Running is natural, but propelling yourself in a wheelchair is an unnatural phenomenon. People never realize what a wheelchair athlete is capable of. This is a breakthrough in man's limits." Within a few years, several recognized U.S. road races initiated wheelchair divisions and more people with disabilities began to train for these races than had ever been anticipated. The movement became so effective that the government took notice and began to support research into how wheelchair users interact with their chair. Performance, durability, comfort, and appearance became factors in wheelchair design.

In 1985, George Murray became the first wheelchair racer to break the four-minute mile and to get his picture featured on a "Wheaties" box. In the years that followed, wheelchair racing continued to progress with improved equipment, training, and nutrition; consequently, world records were continuously being broken. Wheelchair racing began the path toward recognition as a legitimate Olympic sport in 1984 when the men's 1500-meter and the women's 800-meter wheelchair races were included as demonstration events in the Olympic Games held in Los Angeles. Over 5,000 athletes with disabilities participated in the 1992 Barcelona Paralympic Games.

Wheelchairs make a strong personal statement about the user that allows the individual to express his or her personality and not their disability. During the 1970s and 1980s many active wheelchair users began to develop a stronger sense of self. Physical activity and a strong desire for inclusion so empowered some wheelchair users that they started modifying their chairs with saws and welding tools to make the chairs better suited to their needs. This provided the catalyst for the manual wheelchair to evolve to less than 20 pounds. Some wheelchair users went on to form their own companies (e.g., Quickie, Top-End, Magic-in-Motion, Halls Wheels, Eagle Sportschairs), which were responsive to consumer's wishes and revolutionized the industry. The involvement of these consumers who began modifying and making wheelchairs in garages and went on to develop successful companies changed the character of life with a wheelchair.

The last ten years can be characterized as the decade of the power wheelchair. Although the electric wheelchair can trace its origins to the early twentieth century, its popularity was delayed because of the social and technical barriers facing people with mobility impairments. People with disabilities were thought of as frail and in need of protection; without communication among people with disabilities it was difficult to combat the stigma of disability. Therefore, people saw no need to pursue powered mobility. During the 1940s, automobile batteries and starter motors were used to make simple power wheelchairs. These early devices only operated at a single speed. Later, slip clutch mechanisms (i.e., a belt wrapped around a pulley which could be tightened or loosened to control speed) allowed some users to control the speed of their power wheelchairs. The mechanical relay (a type of electronic switch) was later used to provide limited electronic speed control. The 1950s saw development of the transistor, which led to electronic speed control of power wheelchairs.

The 1960s led to numerous improvements in medical care, which resulted in a virtual explosion in number of people survivors with quadriplegia due to accidents and disabling disease. This prompted the development of a wider variety of higher quality power wheelchairs. Electronic control permitted a variety of interface devices to be developed, providing many people with a greater degree of mobility. However, early electronically controlled power wheelchairs were unreliable. Maintenance was a nearly constant ordeal, and failures in the field were high. Improvements in electronic technology led to the development of digital controllers for power wheelchairs. Digital controllers provided improved reliability and increased the range of the power wheelchairs between battery charges.

Technical and clinical progress has led to the development of numerous interface (access) devices (e.g., joysticks, switch control, ultrasonic control), intelligent controllers (e.g., speed control, acceleration control, controllers that sense faults), and intelligent accessories (e.g., wireless links to computers, robotic arms, environmental control units). More people have independent mobility through manual and power wheelchair use than at any other time in history.

The wealthy have always been capable of obtaining conveyance, whereas the less fortunate have not. If the wheelchair could not go where the wealthy wished, servants could carry them. Some people had been fortunate to obtain wheelchairs through the government, charity, or insurance. As for the poor, many languished and died from whatever illness or accident created the disability. Unfortunately, from a global perspective little has changed. Some countries provide more than adequate access to wheelchairs, whereas in other countries they are virtually inaccessible without substantial financial means.

Wheelchairs have improved substantially during the twentieth century. Manual wheelchairs have become lighter, less intrusive, and more functional. Power wheelchairs provide independent mobility for many people with severe physical impairments. However, millions of people worldwide remain immobile or with limited mobility due to the lack of access to technology, outcome measures, and funding required for purchase.

### 1.2.2 Development of Wheelchair Seating

The concept of specialized seating is a recent development. For many years a simple blanket or pillow was thought to suffice for pressure relief. During the latter half of the twentieth century foam was used for cushion material. It took until the late 1970s and early 1980s to develop the techniques currently used for postural support. In the late 1960s, the state of the art of seating intervention was to provide cushions to people with insensitive tissue (i.e., the spinal cord–injured population). Choices were limited to a few manufacturers of air flotation, gel-filled, and foam cushions. The first systems especially designed for children with neuromotor deficits were the Mulholland and Gunnell systems. Nancy Mulholland, a physical therapist, proposed the theory that postural support system design can address tonal problems of children with cerebral palsy. This led to others examining the therapeutic effects of positioning systems. Anita Slominski investigated classroom seating and posture for children with disabilities. The combination of positioning in a wheeled base (e.g., wheelchair) and positioning as part of classroom furniture launched the field of specialized seating in the late 1960s.

Some of the first formal programs in seating were at the Assistive Devices Clinic at the Winnipeg Shriners Hospital and the Hugh MacMillan Rehabilitation Centre, formerly the Ontario Crippled Children's Center in Toronto. The motivation for these programs was partially provided by the thalidomide children crisis of the 1960s. The Canadian government, in an effort to deal with the complex and expensive technical needs of these children, established four centers where therapists, physicians, and engineers could work together with the children and their families to provide function through the application of technology. By the late 1960s, these technical teams had developed the expertise and received the mandate to examine the needs of the broader population of people with disabilities. The multidisciplinary composition of the seating clinics evolved in a similar fashion to the teams used throughout rehabilitation at that time.

Rehabilitation centers with broad-based teams of professional staff were the first to institute seating clinics. People would come to specialized clinics from all over the U.S. and Canada to be evaluated for their seating and mobility needs. Each seating system was individually designed and fit into the existing wheelchairs. Seating systems were made of plywood and foam with metal attachment hardware. Occasionally, plastics were used for planar seating bases, but the costs were higher. Head positioners and footrests were also custom-fabricated.

Seating was time consuming, as products were custom-made and required skilled upholsterers to make them aesthetically pleasing. The time from fitting to final delivery often took months. Unfortunately this is still true in some settings. Most of the seating systems were paid for through grants and contracts from government agencies or families who could afford to pay. Often these costs were not directly accountable and were covered under staff salaries and supplies. For example, a wheelchair would be purchased as a direct cost and the seating system was provided under the operating budget of the clinic through time-and-materials expenses. This funding structure discouraged innovation. Seating programs became heavily invested in salaries to provide plywood and foam seating, which made them reluctant to use other options as they became available. As commercial products became available, some clinics continued to fabricate seating systems rather than to purchase newer commercial systems or to use technologies that originated at other clinics. This was because some clinics had invested substantial resources in the development of personnel and facilities to fabricate seating systems.

As specialized seating evolved, researchers and clinicians began to notice that there were trends in the seating needs of children with disabilities. For example, children with mild-to-moderate tone and few orthopedic problems could be positioned with firm, planar components that could be made in several sizes. The rehabilitation engineering program at the University of Tennessee, Memphis, was one of the first clinics to use modular seating. There were also similarities in seating for more severely involved clients. Although the shape of the seating system was customized, the technology to produce it could be mass produced. The Desmo Project in Alabama made one of the first attempts to outline the body shape without the use of a direct cast of the child's body. This was accomplished using seating kits comprised of weather balloons, epoxy resin, and polystyrene beads. Kits were purchased from a distributor and molding was done in the clinic. This led to the development of custom-seating systems based on polystyrene beads and two component urethane foams, a commercial product that is still available today. In 1975, seating clinicians began to explore measuring the person in a seated posture rather than lying down to reproduce the effects of gravity on posture. The result was a measuring chair that had multiple length, height, and width adjustments. Measuring chairs (simulators) also incorporated the ability to alter the seating angle in space (i.e., tilt), and to reposition the backrest (i.e., recline).

Presently, there are so many seating systems and accessory components available that it has become challenging to stay abreast with the technology and to be competent in making appropriate selections. Clinicians and researchers must work together to transform the functional, physical, and environmental needs of the consumer into technical solutions.

## 1.3 Advocacy and Technology: Partners for a Better Life

Civil rights legislation for people with disabilities has been long in coming. The first major U.S. legislation providing services to Americans with disabilities was the Smith-Fess Vocational Rehabilitation Act, signed into law in 1920. Since that time people with disabilities have gradually won more recognition under the law. Some of the most critical pieces of legislation were introduced following major U.S. military conflicts. The Smith-Fess Act followed World War I, and Vocational Rehabilitation Act amendments followed World War II, the Korean Conflict, and the Vietnam Conflict. These acts laid the groundwork for the disability rights struggle of the 1970s and 1980s. Foremost in this movement was the desire and ability of diverse individuals with disabilities from a broad spectrum of arenas to work together, both formally and informally, toward the goal of full participation in world society for all people with disabilities. The strong desire for full participation and the conviction that this ideal is morally correct is undeniable, and is indeed the very foundation on which the freedom and opportunity of all citizens of the United States is based.

The first major success of the modern disability rights movement in America was the passage of the Rehabilitation Act of 1973 and the Education For All Handicapped Children Act of 1974. These acts did not come without struggle. The Rehabilitation Act of 1973 was passed in September of 1973 after two vetoes by President Nixon: in October of 1972 and March of 1973. Section 504 of this act contains the regulations for implementation. On April 28, 1977, Secretary Califano signed section 504 after extensive sit-ins at HEW offices in Washington and San Francisco, which garnered wide public and local political support . These laws prohibit discrimination on the basis of disability in local programs and activities benefiting from federal financial assistance. Enforcement has led to improved program accessibility for people with disabilities—to health care, social programs, recreation, housing, and transportation. Perhaps most important, these laws began to open educational opportunities at all levels for people with disabilities. The Education for All Handicapped Children Act of 1975 pushed further, requiring mainstreaming of children with disabilities into regular classrooms if appropriate, and the establishment of individualized educational programs.

Despite the advances of the 1970s, people with disabilities were far from fully integrated into society. In 1985, a poll conducted by the Louis Harris Company showed that the common thread of people with disabilities in America was unemployment. This poll showed that two-thirds of all Americans with disabilities between the ages of 16 and 64 were unemployed. These results confirmed those of the 1980 census, which found that nondisabled men participated in the labor force at 88% whereas men with disabilities participated at only 42%. Nondisabled women participated in the labor force at 64% whereas women with disabilities participated at only 24%. Although access to public-assisted programs had improved, employment, architectural, and technology-related access was not keeping pace.

The 1980s saw a legislative shift in policies relating to people with disabilities. Traditionally legislation had focused on employment; during the 1970s the emphasis expanded to include independence. In the 1980s, a period characterized by a conservative political climate, the emphasis shifted toward empowerment of consumers. Empowerment was supported in legislation through the encouragement of self-direction and personal dignity. The primary pieces of national legislation that promoted empowerment among people with disabilities are the 1986 amendments to the Rehabilitation Act (PL99-506) and the Education for Handicapped Children Act (PL99-457); the Employment Opportunity for Disabled Americans Act of 1986 (PL99-463); and the 1987 amendments to the Developmental Disabilities Assistance and Bill of Rights Act (PL100-146) and the Medicaid for Special Education Related Services (PL100-360). The Rehabilitation Act amendments of 1986 require state vocational rehabilitation agencies to include rehabilitation engineering services throughout the rehabilitation process. This change in the legislation demonstrated the intent of Congress for people with disabilities to have access to assistive technology devices and services. Another significant component of the amendments was the inclusion of access to electronic office equipment for federal employees. The 1986 amendments to the Education for Handicapped Children Act mandated the use of technology in education of students with disabilities. The amendments also provided for the design and adaptation of appropriate assistive technology for education. The amendments also changed the emphasis from research and development to assistive technology training for special education. The final regulations, issued in 1989, incorporated the use of assistive training to promote the acquisition of functional skills among children with disabilities who are three years of age or younger. The Employment Opportunity for Disabled Americans Act of 1986 provided programs to support employment through access to assistive technology. Beneficiaries of Supplemental Security Income (SSI) or Social Security Disability Income (SSDI) could obtain funds to support purchase of assistive technology to meet specific vocational goals on an approved timetable. The 1987 amendments to the Developmental Disabilities Assistance and Bill of Rights Act provide three value goals that embody the impact assistive technology can have on people with disabilities. The law sets independence, productivity, and integration as national priorities. *Independence* is defined by the extent to which people with developmental disabilities exert control over their own lives. *Productivity* is the metric of the individual's perception of his or her contribution to his or her community, while improving self-esteem in the process. *Integration* reflects the degree to which a person with a disability has access to services and establishments in the community, and the degree to which the person with a disability uses these services. Substantial foundation for this law was provided by surveys of people with disabilities, which was the beginning of a trend toward consumer participation in the development of legislation. The Medicaid amendments of 1988 ended the long-standing disagreement between school districts and Medicaid regarding payment for assistive technology and related services. Under these amendments, a broad range of assistive technology services are eligible for Medicaid reimbursement.

Legislative progress continued in 1988 and 1989. In 1988, the Technology Related Assistance for Individuals with Disabilities Act (PL100-407) increased the capacity of the states to provide assistive devices and services to people with disabilities. The primary purpose of this legislation was to provide awareness and coordination among agencies in the provision of assistive technology. This is believed to have the effect of increasing the probability that people with disabilities will be able to access and maintain appropriate assistive technology. The Medicaid Early and Periodic Screening, Diagnosis, and Treatment Amendments of 1989 (PL101-238) provide children under age 21 years with medically necessary diagnostic and treatment services under Medicaid for any physical or mental disability.

On July 26, 1990, President George Bush signed into law the "Americans with Disabilities Act" (ADA). This law (PL101-336) gives civil rights protection to persons with disabilities, similar to that provided to individuals on the basis of race, gender, national origin, and religion. The ADA provides equal opportunity for people with disabilities in the areas of employment, state and local government services, public transportation, privately operated transportation available to the public, places of public accommodation, and communication services offered to the public. The ADA arguably may be the most sweeping piece of civil rights legislation to date, because of the widespread physical and social barriers it could remove. The ADA attempts to promote integration of assistive technology as a civil right for persons with disabilities.

The Individuals with Disabilities Education Act of 1990 protects the rights of children with disabilities, and emphasizes the child rather than the disability as in previous legislation. The law also provides children the right to sue the state for not providing a free appropriate education, which removed the protection of states under the 11th Amendment of the Constitution. Assistive technology devices and services can be provided, as long as they are included in the child's individualized education program (IEP). Assistive technology can also be provided through the child's transition to work plan under the IEP. The Rehabilitation Act Amendments of 1992 (PL102-569) describe disability as "a natural part of the human experience" and clearly changes the focus of federal legislation. This legislation focuses on empowerment, informed choice, self-direction, inclusion, and full participation in society. The amendments require state agencies to provide a description of how rehabilitation technology will be provided through all stages of the rehabilitation process; provide for a broad range of assistive technology services statewide; provide a description of rehabilitation technology training to be provided; and to provide a description of the program for assessing the need for and providing assistive technology, as well as worksite assessments. Progress continues toward fully integrating people with disabilities into society, and assistive technology has an important role in facilitating integration.

Legislation does not change people's attitudes, it only provides a legal framework under which people must live. Changing behavior is a much more difficult task. Discrimination remains commonplace in the lives of persons with disabilities. Many people seem to believe that they know the limitations of a person with a disability. People with disabilities are just beginning to realize their potential. Opportunities for people with disabilities need to be created and nurtured. Some potential employers have learned what not to say on issues concerning persons with disabilities. Many people are politically correct while propagating a discrete discrimination process. Laws do not remove discrimination, they define the rules of ethical conduct. Hence discrimination post-ADA has become much more subtle. The primary issue of concern to persons with disabilities is access—access to gainful employment, access to training, access to promotion, access to health care, access to assistive technology, access to recreation, access to socialization, and most important, access to dignity.

The challenge to society is to open the doors and to permit persons with disabilities to maximize their potential. The challenge to rehabilitation engineering is to develop assistive technology to facilitate access. A major part of the problem within society is ignorance and fear—ignorance of the needs and desires of persons with disabilities and fear of the investment that may be required to give persons with disabilities access. Rehabilitation engineers need to learn to work with people with disabilities. Assistive technology is too often kluged together. People can become cyborgs swamped by intrusive technology, and are stripped of their dignity.

## 1.4 Disability and Wheelchair Users

Disability involves limitations in actions and activities because of mental or physical impairments. Over 14% of the U.S. population is limited in selected activities, with some of these limitations making wheelchair use necessary. Each year the National Center for Health Statistics conducts a National Health Interview Survey on Assistive Devices. This survey shows that there were 1,411,000 wheelchair users in the United States in 1992 (NCHS 1992). Arthritis is one of the leading causes of activity limitation in the United States and is second in prevalence to orthopedic impairments (LaPlante 1991). The quantity and epidemiology of wheelchair user etiology has changed over the past 40 years. Between 1980 and 1990 alone, the use of wheelchairs has increased 96.1% (McNeil 1993). Advances in the medical arena have led to numerous methods of prolonging life, thus increasing the demand for wheelchairs.

There are numerous reasons for a person to need wheelchair assistance. These causes fall into two major categories: traumatic injury and chronic degenerative disease. The table below presents data obtained in a survey conducted by the British Ministry of Health, which gave the diagnosis per hundred patients who obtained wheelchairs.

It is estimated that 5% of people over 70 years are wheelchair users (Sonn and Grimby 1994). This age-specific prevalence of disability is therefore higher for elderly persons and places them in a large subcategory of wheelchair users. For the elderly, the more common causes for wheelchair requirement are arthritis/rheumatism, hypertension, diabetes, cardiac and respiratory disease (Pickles and Topping 1994). The prevailing reason given for requesting a wheelchair was arthritis and unsteadiness (18.2%), with strokes and frequent falls ranking second

**TABLE 1.1  Percent of wheelchair users by disability etiology**

| | |
|---|---:|
| Arthritis | 28% |
| Organic nervous disease | 14% |
| Cerebral vascular disease | 13% |
| Other bone injuries and deformities | 11% |
| Lower limb amputations | 9% |
| Cerebral palsy | 8% |
| Traumatic paraplegia | 7% |
| Respiratory and cardiac disease | 3% |

and third respectively. Most of these people (54.5%) use their wheelchairs all of the time (Brooks 1994).

A common issue faced by the wheelchair user is the change in identity through transition from walking to mobility via a wheelchair. There are three processes that can be readily identified: sudden transition to using a wheelchair; gradual transition to using a wheelchair; and use of a wheelchair as part of the physical development process. Children who are born with a disability or who acquire one at very early age develop using assistive technology. Children who develop with a disability do not undergo an adjustment process from acquiring the disability, but must experience a process of realizing their abilities and the differences between their abilities and those of their peers. Parents, siblings, and rehabilitation professionals must work in concert with the child with a disability to maximize the child's abilities and anticipate the child's future needs. Children realize that they are different and will naturally ask why, and other children will also ask questions. A successful approach is to begin applying appropriate assistive technology early in the child's development. This can help the child develop emotionally, physically, and cognitively. The assistive technology should be made to be appealing to the child and the child's peers. This helps to facilitate acceptance by the child with a disability and acceptance by the child's peers. The child with a disability will benefit from socialization and exploration assisted through technology. At very early ages, commercial children's products and toys can be modified, and many communities have volunteer organizations that provide this assistance. In some cases, the modified toy or child mobility device is enticing to other children. For example, small children who use modified electric cars as mobility devices often interact better with their peers than when they are dependent on a parent or teacher for mobility. As the child ages, assistive technology can be used to encourage continued socialization and promote a solid education. Education must be provided in the least restrictive environment in order to have maximum benefit for the child with a disability. The least restrictive environment often benefits other students as well, through diversifying the classroom and introducing applications of technology.

Sudden transition to a wheelchair can come from trauma or the rapid progression of disease. In such cases, the person has little time to adjust to the change in mobility from walking to a wheelchair. The person often undergoes a dramatic change in the sense of self and autonomy. Many new skills or those once second nature must be learned or relearned. This can be a significant source of aggravation and possible depression. Typically, people undergo several changes during the rehabilitation process. They will often experience a phase of denial where they believe they will not benefit from a wheelchair and will return to the same type and level of activity as prior to the accident or onset of the disease. During this phase, clinicians must provide them with a realistic prognosis and be supportive. This is a good time to provide these persons with some literature on their disability and the activities that can be performed. The family of the person with the disability should also be provided with information, and solicited to provide reassurance.

After the denial phase, people often develop a sense of depression and feel overwhelmed by the challenges that face them. The sense of being overwhelmed can be alleviated by peer counseling and introduction to support groups that share common interests. The person may not be receptive at first and may express anger. However, exposure to healthy activities and to people who have adjusted well to their disability can have a positive effect even several months postexposure. Peer counseling can also involve identifying another person with nearly the same disability who is of comparable age and has similar interests as the person with the newly acquired disability. Peer counseling can be very effective in providing coping strategies, and in teaching activities of daily living skills to the person with a newly acquired disability. Peer counseling provides concrete examples for the training provided by therapists and other rehabilitation professionals. Eventually, most people develop a sense of acceptance of their disability. Once they have accepted the disability, they tend to be much happier and progress toward self-direction becomes more rapid. Some people progress to a point where they can provide support to other people with disabilities or become advocates for disability issues of personal interest. Ultimately, the best measure of successful adaptation is a satisfying work or school, home, and recreational life.

The gradual development of a disability follows a similar process, but often the process does not occur in acute rehabilitation. When a person gradually develops a disability, the process is a slow deterioration of some body functions, which at first may be nearly unnoticeable. Often, the initial focus is on preserving as much function as possible or in prolonging the need for a wheelchair. For many people, the use of a wheelchair is viewed as a significant step toward their acquiescence to the disease or disabling condition, even though many people would obtain increased mobility and function through the use of a wheelchair. The initial transition to a wheelchair is often emotionally painful, but if the person is encouraged to remain active he/she will often be relieved by the increased level of activity which they are able to sustain, and by their increased interaction with family and friends.

For a person with a newly acquired disability, adaptation to the realities of a new life is the first step, usually, toward reentry into mainstream society. During this exploration period, people express two factors that can make transition easier: the will to remain as active as possible, and the availability of expert advice on both coping strategies and the specific equipment and accessories available to meet the person's goals. Much of this phase is experienced during the person's acute rehabilitation. During this time it is critical that therapists, psychiatrists, counselors, and rehabilitation engineers provide meaningful and useful advice. The assistive technology provider must use experience and training to anticipate the technology demands to meet the user's rehabilitation goals. The will of the client comes from within, but it can be intensified by interaction with positive role models. The advice and expertise comes from many sources including therapists, doctors, rehabilitation engineers, equipment dealers, and other users. When informative assistance and adaptive equipment are available, people with disabilities find the physical aspects of returning to work, school, home, and social activities less formidable than many initially expect.

## 1.5 Maximizing Abilities

### 1.5.1 Development and Socialization

Exploring the environment plays an important role in the cognitive development of people. Our ability to move within the environment influences our learning ability. Exploration of the environment is also important for people with disabilities, and must be supported and encouraged with assistive technology.

Parents of children with disabilities often do not recognize the need for mobility in their child's cognitive development. It becomes too easy to transport the child, and have the child remain dependent on the parents for mobility until the child is school-aged. This can be detrimental for both the child and the family. This can lead to children entering school without having learned necessary social and daily living skills. Research has shown that children as young as two years can be independently mobile with the appropriate manual or power wheelchair. The ability of children to be independently mobile can lead to easier acceptance by peers and better performance in school. Learning and socialization may be improved through the encouragement of independent mobility at an early age.

### 1.5.2 Recreation and Play

Recreation and play have important roles in maintaining health. It is important for people to recreate alone or in groups, be it through sports, play, or other healthful activities. Wheelchair sports are an important modality in the rehabilitation of people with physical impairments, and influence their successful return to society. One must be cautious to avoid emphasizing wheelchair sports for people with paraplegia to the neglect of people with more severe impairments, especially people who use powered mobility. Through sports and recreation, people learn cooperation and develop relationships. It is important to develop and support activities that promote recreation involving people with and without disabilities. Wheelchair designers and manufacturers have discovered the desire for recreation among both manual and power wheelchair users, and have developed sporty wheelchairs suitable for many recreational activities.

### 1.5.3 Learning and Working

The most secure path to success is to obtain a good education, especially for people with disabilities. In many cases people with disabilities have reduced occupational possibilities. In order to expand the employment horizon, people with disabilities should pursue specific learning objectives. People with severe physical impairments require assistive technology in order to attain their occupational goals. The challenge for rehabilitation professionals and people with disabilities is to select or design the proper assistive technology.

The number of people with severe physical impairments who are unemployed or underemployed hovers around 60% in industrialized countries. Unemployment is much higher in nonindustrialized countries. Three reasons can be identified for the high rate of unemployment: the education and training of many people with disabilities is insufficient to obtain or maintain employment; employers believe that costs associated with making jobs accessible are excessive; and the employment expectations of society for people with disabilities, and of people with disabilities for themselves, are too low. Much of the unemployment problem could be overcome through improved primary school education for children with disabilities, and through improved job retraining for adults with disabilities. People with disabilities should be encouraged and supported to pursue careers in engineering, medicine, and business.

## 1.6 Building Coalitions: The Concept of Interdependence

Independence is often set as the ultimate goal for rehabilitation. However, this goal may be unattainable for many people and may be harmful. People with severe disabilities should not be overburdened with technical and medical assistance in order to obtain greater independence. People without a disability do not consciously strive for independence; they more often strive for a sense of belonging. People work together nearly every day and they help each other attain common goals.

The goal of rehabilitation should not be independence, rather it should be *interdependence* and *self-direction*. Rehabilitation should focus on helping people to recognize and emphasize their strengths. Concentration should no longer focus on the identification of weaknesses, but on building on one's strengths. Interdependence is based on the concept that everyone is a member of society. The success of society depends on its ability to profit from the strengths of each of its members. People with disabilities also possess strengths that make important contributions to society. People must recognize that society is strengthened through its diversity. Everyone must also have the ability to exercise self-direction. The importance of self-direction, apart from independence, is sometimes neglected in rehabilitation and in society. People must have the opportunity to choose their own path based on their strengths and interests. Through the recognition of the importance of interdependence people with disabilities can hope to be fully integrated into society.

Assistive technology should emphasize a person's strengths and suppress a person's weaknesses. The proper application of assistive technology can expand the horizons of people with disabilities and encourage their full integration into society. However, problems faced by people with disabilities cannot be solved by technology alone. People with various backgrounds and occupations must work together.

## 1.7 Get Out There

Life for wheelchair users is changing rapidly. Once wheelchair users were provided no options except the wheelchair that was provided for them, and became resigned to survive a totally dependent life. Often the humiliation and mental anguish that accompanied physical disability was of only short duration, as people passed on. As with most things, the quality of life of people who use wheelchairs gradually moved forward with advances in medical care, social mores, and technology. Early pioneers of wheelchair living returned to work and were active in their community. The opportunities for people with disabilities have grown tremendously during the twentieth century, and promise to continue to grow into the next century. People with disabilities have come from being patients who needed constant care to leaders in many fields.

For example, President Franklin D. Roosevelt used a wheelchair for personal mobility due to his physical disability from polio. President Roosevelt was a vibrant and active man who was a very capable leader. His mobility impairment was no impairment to his ability to lead the United States. However, the social and political climate of his time made it desirable for President Roosevelt to hide his wheelchair and conceal his mobility impairment. Today, things are changing. In 1988,

George Covington became the first White House adviser for disability issues. Mr. Covington, who is visually impaired, worked with then Vice President Quayle to bring disability issues to the forefront of American politics, and promote opportunities for people with disabilities. During Mr. Covington's tenure in the White House, the ADA and several other important pieces of disability legislation were passed, the official residence of the vice president was made accessible, and the vice president met with more people with disabilities than during any previous administration. When President Clinton was elected, he continued to advocate for the rights of people with disabilities. One of President Clinton's most significant appointments was Judith Huemann, a wheelchair user, as Assistant Secretary for the Office of Special Education and Rehabilitation Services within the U.S. Department of Education. Ms. Huemann is one of the founders of the independent living center movement, a leader in employment opportunities, and one of the founders of the World Institute on Disability (WID). WID is an international think tank on disability rights issues, operated for and by people with disabilities.

Wheelchair users are making significant contributions to other areas besides the political arena. The design of wheelchairs has been revolutionized by several wheelchair users. Herbert Everest was the first of the notable wheelchair users to impact the design of wheelchairs in the modern era. Mr. Everest developed an international business out of his desire for greater personal mobility. He revolutionized the design and distribution of wheelchairs and brought increased mobility to millions of other wheelchair users. He also became a business leader. However, his company became complacent after being successful for many years. Some wheelchair users saw the complacency of E&J as an opportunity for them to capitalize on the growing demand among wheelchair users for greater mobility and better wheelchairs. Many people started small wheelchair companies during the late 1970s and early 1980s. Marilyn Hamilton emerged as the undisputed winner of the ultralight wheelchair revolution. Although she was not the first person to start building ultralight wheelchairs, and some may argue that her company did not produce the best product, Ms. Hamilton's and her partners' company, Quickie, is by any measure the most successful of the ultralight wheelchair companies started during this time. Marilyn Hamilton is a well-educated, highly intelligent, and extremely motivated person, who by some intervention of fate had an accident and became a wheelchair user. Fortunately, for many wheelchair users, Ms. Hamilton channeled her energy, knowledge, and enthusiasm into building and selling a better wheelchair. As she and her colleagues became more successful, they worked on building a better and more humane wheelchair industry. Her company has had impact on nearly every aspect of the lives of people who use wheelchairs, and has gone a long way to change the public image of wheelchair users.

Bobby Hall is to racing wheelchairs what Quickie is to ultralight wheelchairs. Although Hall's Wheels is not as well known, and not nearly as large, it has had no less impact. Arguably, Bobby Hall created the business opportunity that Marilyn Hamilton was able to exploit. Bobby Hall is the first person to complete a marathon in a wheelchair, and he had the genius to select his hometown Boston Athletic Association Marathon (the Boston Marathon). Mr. Hall went on to promote wheelchair road racing around the country, and to establish the wheelchair division of the Boston Marathon. While promoting the sport of wheelchair road racing, Bobby Hall worked to constantly improve racing wheelchairs. His efforts led to the development of an entirely new sports activity and an entirely new type of wheelchair, the racing wheelchair. Wheelchair road racing was the vehicle for the disability rights movement in the 1980s. Wheelchair road racers were mostly young, educated, articulate, brash, bold, daring, and demanding. The road racing pioneers of the early 1980s became the symbol of wheelchair users in the public image. They were capturing national media attention in a positive and sometimes controversial way. The public image of a wheelchair user began to transform from a sickly person in a conventional "hospital type" wheelchair to a muscular, healthy person in a flashy, sleek racing wheelchair. In 1984, wheelchair racing had progressed to the point where it was introduced as an Olympic exhibition sport, and televised worldwide as a sporting event. Wheelchair racing is now big business for manufacturers, and for athletes who vie for prize money and commercial endorsements.

Other sports have had significant impact on wheelchair users as well, most notably skiing. Wheelchair racing was successful because people who use wheelchairs could train and compete alongside runners. Eventually, wheelchair racers became faster than runners, which garnered mutual respect. Skiing followed a similar path. In the United States, Peter Axelson is widely considered the founding father of skiing for wheelchair users. Mr. Axelson is a Stanford University–trained engineer who uses a wheelchair and has a passion for skiing. Peter Axelson started his skiing revolution with the Arroya sit-ski, and then went on to develop the mono-ski. The Arroya sit-ski formed the basis for Mr. Axelson's company, Beneficial Designs. The mono-ski allows wheelchair users to ski alongside stand-up counterparts, and to enjoy even the most difficult ski slopes. The mono-ski created a new business of skiing for people with disabilities.

One should not get the impression that wheelchair users can only make their mark through politics, wheelchair manufacturing, or recreation. There are some great scientists and humanitarians who are wheelchair users. Ralf Hotchkiss is a professor at San Francisco State University in California, and a wheelchair user. Professor Hotchkiss has spent much of his adult life assisting people with disabilities in developing countries to build and produce wheelchairs. Professor Hotchkiss has built teams in many countries and has successfully developed factories for his Whirlwind wheelchair, which provides mobility to tens of thousands of people who would otherwise have been immobile. Professor Hotchkiss has brought international recognition to the issue that personal mobility is a human rights concern which must be addressed by the United Nations and the World Health Organization. Professor Hotchkiss has been awarded an honorary doctorate, and is a MacArthur Foundation fellow because of his efforts and genius.

Others have followed more traditional paths in science. Dr. David Gray, who is a wheelchair user due to quadriplegia, is a professor at Washington University in St. Louis. Dr. Gray is a former director of the National Institute on Disability and Rehabilitation Research, U.S. Department of Education, and of the National Center for Medical Rehabilitation Research, National Institutes of Health. Dr. Gray has been a driving force for promoting science and engineering education for people with disabilities, and for developing research that examines the impact of disability on all aspects of life. Dr. Gray was instrumental in developing many of the programs that help young scientists and engineers with disabilities to develop research careers. Professor Gray continues his work in promoting science and engineering education for people with disabilities, and in understanding the physical, social, and psychological impact of disability.

Journalism is not without its reporters who use wheelchairs. A fair number of wheelchair users have had modest roles in reporting sporting events or disability related events. However, John Hockenberry is undoubtedly the most recognized, and likely most successful, journalist who by chance uses a wheelchair. Mr. Hockenberry is a reporter for National Public Radio (NPR) and the National Broadcasting Corporation (NBC). He was interviewed to be the first journalist in space, reported on the Persian Gulf War (Operation Desert Storm), and covered numerous other stories both in the United States and abroad. He is also the author of a very successful book. Mr. Hockenberry has been awarded two Peabody awards and an Emmy for his work. Through his skill and spirit of adventure, he has been able to demonstrate that he is an excellent journalist who happens to use a wheelchair.

The fields of medicine, entertainment, law, and engineering have all been influenced by people who use wheelchairs. The opportunities continue to grow, and the outlook for people who use wheelchairs is good.

## 1.8 Summary

Wheelchair users are forcing people to face old stereotypes. Wheelchairs have become a tool to enhance lives and change perceptions. People with disabilities are also searching for their collective identity. In a quest for unity amidst diversity a few "leaders" have defined the terminology and goals of people with disabilities. Facing the differences among people with disabilities is often avoided. However, without open discussion and critical thinking persons with disabilities may be limiting their future. Too often society develops impressions of disability handed down from television and politics. Many people still insist "disabled" is an acceptable umbrella for all people with impairments. However, disabled is often defined as "without abilities." Some people are satisfied that disabled is different from "handicapped." Some people have coined names like "physically challenged" or "differently abled" to be politically correct. It is important to embrace diversity and encourage greater inclusion of people with disabilities.

Issues of cultural and ethnic diversity among people with disabilities must also be addressed. Sociocultural, environmental, and economic factors are all important considerations in the assessment and intervention process. Professionals need to be sensitive to issues important to persons with a disability and to the communities in which they live.

## References and Further Reading

Bartolucci M. (1992) Making a chair able by design. *Metropolis*, 12(4):29–33.

Brooks L. (1994) Use of devices for mobility by the elderly. *Wisconsin Medical Journal*, January.

Cantore J. A. (1993) Reading between the lines. *CAREERS & the disABLED*, 9(2):45–46.

Cooper R. A. (1995) *Rehabilitation Engineering Applied to Mobility and Manipulation*. London, UK, Adam Hilger Institute of Physics Publishing.

Cornes P. (1984) *The Future of Work for People with Disabilities: A View from Great Britain.* New York International Exchange of Experts and Information in Rehabilitation, World Rehabilitation Fund, Inc.

Deptula D. L. (1993) In the spirit of the law. *CAREERS & the disABLED*, 9(2):37–38.

Enders A. (1989) Funding for assistive technology and related services: An annotated bibliography. *Physical and Occupational Therapy in Pediatrics*, 10(2):147–173.

Erlanger H., Roth W. (1985) Disability policy: The parts and the whole. *American Behavioral Scientist*, 28(3):319–346.

Flippo K. F. (1995) *Assistive Technology: A Resource for School, Work, and Community.* Baltimore, MD, Paul H. Brookes Publishing Company.

Fricke R. C. (1992) *Digest of Data on Persons with Disabilities.* Washington, DC, National Institute on Disability and Rehabilitation Research, U.S. Department of Education.

Hockenberry J. (1995) *Moving Violations.* New York, NY, Hyperion.

Hough S., Kisseloff L. (1994) Crossing cultures. *Team Rehab Report*, 5(3):14–18.

LaPlante M. (1991) The demographics of disability. *Milbank Quarterly*, 69 (Suppl 1–2):55–77.

Kamenetz H. (1969) *The Wheelchair Book: Mobility for the Disabled.* Springfield, IL, C.C. Thomas.

McNeil J. M. (1993) *Americans with Disabilities: 1991–92.* Data from the Survey of Income and Program Participation, P70–33.

National Center for Health Statistics. (1992) *Public Use Data Documentation, National Health Interview Survey of Assistive Devices, 1990.* Hyattsville, MD.

Oliver J., Brown L. B. (1988) The development and implementation of a minority recruitment plan: Process, strategy and results. *J Social Work Education*, 24:175–185.

Paralyzed Veterans of America. (1993) *The Americans with Disabilities Act: Your Personal Guide to the Law.* Washington, DC.

Pickles B., Topping A. (1994) Community care for Canadian seniors: An exercise in educational planning. *Disability and Rehabilitation*, 16(3):181–189.

Prevalence of disabilities and associated health conditions, United States, 1991–1992. *The On-line Journal of Current Clinical Trials.* 4(164), 950105 MMWR 43(40), Oct. 14, 1994.

Rioux M. H. (1992) A culture of diversity. *Abilities*, 11 (Spring): 60–61.

Robinson C. J. (1993) What is "rehabilitation engineering?" *IEEE Transactions on Rehabilitation Engineering*, 1(1):1.

Roessler R. (1986) Technology utilization in rehabilitation. *Rehabilitation Literature*, 47(7/8):170–173.

Schneider J. (1993) The Prudential looks for the best. *CAREERS & the disABLED*, 9(2):40–43.

Sonn U., Grimby G. (1994) Assistive devices in an elderly population studied at 70–76 years of age. *Disability and Rehabilitation*, 16(2):85–93.

Thompson D. L., Thomas K. R., Fernandez M. S. (1994) The Americans with Disabilities Act: Social policy and worldwide implications for practice. *International Journal of Rehabilitation Research*, 17:109–121.

U.S. Equal Employment Opportunity Commission. (1991) *The Americans with Disabilities Act: Your Responsibilities as an Employer.* Washington, DC.

U.S. Equal Employment Opportunity Commission and U.S. Department of Justice Civil Rights Division. (1992) *The Americans with Disabilities Act: Questions and Answers.* Washington, DC.

Watson G. F., DiTomaso N., Farris G. F., Barclay D., Batten E., Richards S., Smith T. J. (1992) Diversity in the high-tech workforce. *IEEE Spectrum*, 29(6):20–32.

Weaver C. L. (1990) The ADA: Another mandated benefits program? *The American Enterprise*, May/June:81–84.

Wilkerson M. B. (1982) The masks of meritocracy and egalitarianism. *Educational Record*, 63(1):4–11.

Williams J. M. (1993) A clouded crystal ball. *CAREERS & the disABLED*, 9(2):54–56.

Wilson D. L. (1992) New federal regulations on rights of the handicapped may force colleges to provide better access to technology. *The Chronicle of Higher Education*, 38(21):A1, A21–22.

Yanok J. (1986) Free appropriate public education for handicapped children: Congressional intent and judicial interpretation. *RASE*, 7:49–53.

Zola I. K. (1982) Denial of emotional needs to people with handicaps. *Archives of Physical Medicine and Rehabilitation*, 63:63–67.

# CHAPTER 2

# Wheelchair Measurement

*Chapter Goals*

- ☑ To understand basic person-to-wheelchair interface
- ☑ To understand the characteristics of wheelchairs in relation to users
- ☑ To appreciate basic principles of human factors/ergonomics as applied to wheelchairs

## 2.1 Introduction

Attaining a properly fitting wheelchair requires several important measurements and an understanding of how these measurements relate to performance. Wheelchairs are not "one-size-fits-all," and require knowledge of how a person is fitted with the proper size wheelchair. At one time, wheelchair measurement was quite simple because all wheelchairs were basically of the same design and only a few limited sizes were available. Commonly, wheelchairs are specified by their seat width and seat depth. However, the trend is toward greater design flexibility and greater customization. Nearly all wheelchair manufacturers will customize their products for an individual. Therefore, if the consumer's measurements cannot be accommodated by catalog items, it is worthwhile to contact various wheelchair manufacturers and ask them about availability and cost of custom products. This chapter presents information related to collecting body measurements, the use of wheelchair seating standards, and concepts related to wheelchair seating ergonomics.

## 2.2 Body Measurements

For many people a few simple measurements can be used to determine the proper dimensions for a wheelchair. Body measurements are typically made with the consumer in the seated position. However, some therapists prefer to make body measurements on a mat. Both methods will work well, provided the therapist is familiar with the measurements to be made and has adequate experience. Body measurements are best made with a steel or nylon tape measure designed specifically for taking body measurements. Such a tape measure is called an *anthropometric tape measure,* and it incorporates a spring attached to the end that limits the amount of force applied to soft tissue. This helps reduce error created by one person applying a small amount of force and causing small distortion of soft tissue, and another person applying larger force and causing larger distortion of soft tissue, resulting in different measurements for the same consumer. Calipers can also be used to get more accurate breadth and depth measurements. However, calipers are primarily used by specialized seating clinics and research laboratories.

Probably the most obvious body measurements are the consumer's height and weight. The consumer's weight is critical to obtaining a wheelchair that is suitably strong to accommodate the user's weight. For example, most wheelchairs are tested with 100 kilogram (220 pound) test dummies. The test dummies are made of wood or aluminum and are stiffer than a real person, but nevertheless the wheelchair needs to be rated for the end user's weight. Many manufacturers claim in their owner's and service manuals that their wheelchairs are rated for 250 pounds. When selecting a wheelchair for someone who weighs more than 220 pounds, it is best to inform the wheelchair manufacturer. The wheelchair provider should also verify that the wheelchair has been tested for a weight greater than the actual weight of the client.

The height of the wheelchair user provides information about the person's size, and can be used to check the final wheelchair measurements. For example, the sum of the sitting height, sitting depth, and lower leg length should be close to the person's supine height. Height and weight also provide information about a person's stature. This is helpful for people building the wheelchair who may never see the client, and for future use by therapists who can use stature as a quick measure of whether the client's status has changed substantially since the previous wheelchair was selected.

The measurements required to select the proper wheelchair for an individual are illustrated in Figure 2.1. Additional measurements and definitions are used when specialized seating and postural support systems are required. Some of these additional measurements will be defined in Chapter 12. The critical body width measurements are shoulder width, chest width, waist width, and pelvic width. The shoulder width is important when the wheelchair user requires shoulder supports or a shoulder harness. The chest width is important for determining the width of the backrest and backrest supports. The more severely impaired an individual is, the higher the backrest must be to provide adequate sitting balance. However, if the backrest is too narrow, it will cause discomfort. If the backrest is too wide, it can interfere with the individual's ability to propel the wheelchair. For manual wheelchair users, the backrest width is more critical than for power wheelchair users. The backrest width should be about 2 centimeters wider than chest width at the highest point on the backrest.

The waist width is important in order to accommodate armrests, side guards, and the wheels on some wheelchairs. Typically, armrests and side guards (devices used to keep clothing from touching the wheels) are at waist width. The distance between the armrests and waist width should be between 5 and 10 centimeters. The dimension becomes more critical for manual wheelchair users. If the armrests are too far apart, the wheelchair user will have to place the arms in forward flexion to reach the pushrims. This is often described as "chicken winging," because the propulsion stroke resembles a person imitating a chicken.

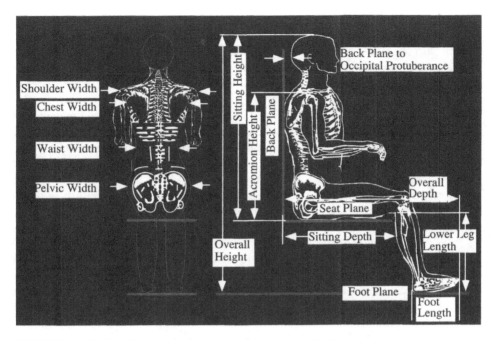

**FIGURE 2.1** Critical body measurements for wheelchair users

The pelvic width is used to determine the seat width of the wheelchair. The seat width of the wheelchair should be as close as possible to the pelvic width for manual wheelchairs. This allows the wheelchair user to reach the pushrims most easily, and places the arms in a position of greater leverage. Active wheelchair users prefer the seat width to be about 1 centimeter greater then the pelvic width. However, other wheelchair users prefer greater space to accommodate a coat or sweater, or to allow some room to adjust seating position. With manual wheelchairs more than about 3 centimeters difference between seat width and pelvic width can have a negative impact on stroke biomechanics. Power wheelchair seat width measurements are also important to maintaining postural support needed to control the wheelchair.

Several important seated measurements are made with respect to the sagittal plane (side view). When viewing the sagittal plane, the edges from three seat position planes are used as references for defining an individual's wheelchair seating. The back plane is a vertical plane that contacts the posterior-most part of the individual's back (see Figure 2.1). Typically, the person being measured is placed in as close as possible a vertical torso posture. When the individual being measured can assume a normal erect sitting posture, the back plane will contact the spine in the thoracic region. The seat plane is a horizontal plane that intersects the back plane and contacts the inferior-most portion of the individual's seated surface during seated weight bearing. Typically, the point of contact for the seat plane will be the ischial tuberosities. The foot plane is also a horizontal plane defined by the point of contact with the base of the feet. It is important to remember that the back plane, seat plane, and foot plane are imaginary planes, used as references. The actual wheelchair seat may vary substantially from these planes, depending on the functional anatomy of the individual.

The overall height of the individual in the seated position is the distance between the foot plane and the top of the person's head. This measurement is important when considering a person's interaction with the environment. For example, the seated overall height of an individual is going to define whether the roof of a van will need to be elevated, and by how much. The overall height also defines how low a person can sit properly in a wheelchair without having the feet contact the ground. The sitting height is defined as the distance between the seat plane and the top of the head. The sitting height combined with the seat height provides information about how high a person sits. This helps to define the minimum and maximum reach. The sitting depth is the distance between the back plane and the popliteal fossa (hamstring tendons). The sitting depth is used to determine the depth of the wheelchair seat. The lower leg length is measured from the popliteal fossa to the foot plane. The lower leg length is used to select and adjust the legrest length.

Wheelchair footrests come in various sizes, depending on the size of the individual's foot and the flexibility of the foot and ankle. The foot length is the maximum length of the foot with shoe. The overall depth for a seated person is defined as the distance between the tips of the toes and the back plane. This distance is important when determining the depth of a table top or desk top required to accommodate a wheelchair user. The overall depth also affects the maneuverability of the wheelchair user. Some people require more support than can be provided by a simple linear seating system. Headrests are often used to provide support for the head and neck for people with higher levels of impairment. The headrest height is related to the seated height and acromion height. The acromion height is measured from each acromion to the seat plane. The measurement to each acromion provides information about postural asymmetry. The distance between the occipital protuberance and the back plane is used to specify the range of the headrest fore-and-aft adjustment.

Experienced clinicians can make the required measurements with the individual either seated or lying on a mat. Most therapists prefer to make seating measurements with the individual in the seated position because it accounts for the effects of gravity on posture. It is also important to determine the individual's range of motion and postural asymmetries.

## 2.3 Standardized Wheelchair Seating Measurements

Wheelchair manufacturers have used different ways to define the seating dimensions of wheelchairs. This has led to confusion among some people when ordering wheelchairs, and has caused some clinicians to rely on manufacturer representatives to provide guidance in selecting the properly configured wheelchair. Part of the problem was nonstandard ways of directly relating an individual's anatomical measurements to the appropriate wheelchair dimensions. Several people realized that standardizing wheelchair measurements could improve wheelchair service delivery. Through many years of continuous effort, the American National Standards Institute (ANSI) and the Rehabilitation Engineering and Assistive Technology Society of North America (RESNA) developed a standard for seating and wheel dimension within the United States. The development of an international standard paralleled the work in the United States, and culminated in the International Standards Organization (ISO) standard for seating and wheel dimensions.

When specifying a wheelchair there are several critical seating dimensions which if specified improperly can have substantial negative impact on performance, and in some cases can lead to pain and injury. Some wheelchair dimensions are fixed upon manufacture and, therefore, cannot be adjusted by the clinic or durable medical equipment dealer. Fixed wheelchair dimensions must be specified properly when ordering or the wheelchair will not provide the user optimal fit. Seat width and seat depth are the most common fixed critical dimensions. For most of the history of wheelchairs, these were the only measurements that could be used to customize a wheelchair; all other dimensions were set by the manufacturer. Today, this is no longer true, and specifying a wheelchair requires much more knowledge.

### 2.3.1 Defining the Wheelchair Seat

The standardized definition for seat width is illustrated in Figure 2.2. Wheelchairs are produced in a variety of seat widths. Many manufacturers use seat widths in increments of 25 millimeters (1 inch). Seat width is measured as the width of the seating surface. For a common tubular-frame wheelchair, the seat width would be defined by the outside edges of the seat tubes. If the wheelchair were to be ordered with armrests, and if they protrude into the area of the seating surface, then that would narrow the seat width. Following the procedures outlined in the ANSI/RESNA standard, the seat width is the crosswise dimension of the seating surface of the wheelchair with a seated occupant. Measurement with a seated occupant is important, as many wheelchairs use upholstery for the seat material. The upholstery may sag or stretch and reduce the effective seat width. The ANSI/RESNA standard calls for using a dummy to load the seat in order to pro-

**FIGURE 2.2**    Illustration of wheelchair seat width definition

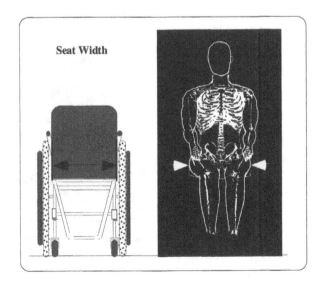

vide an accurate measurement of the seat width for an actual user. Use of the standard will help to minimize the problem of the wheelchair pulling in and becoming too small for the user. Seat width is measured at the height above the seat plane where the trochanters are expected to reside. Therefore, the clinician measures the distance between the trochanters and adds the desired amount of clearance to obtain the desired seat width.

Most wheelchair users prefer a narrow wheelchair seat. A narrow wheelchair seat width can be used to obtain a narrow overall width for the wheelchair. A narrow wheelchair can provide enhanced access to buildings and enclosed spaces. A narrow seat width also places the rear wheels in a better position for the arms when pushing, leading to greater propulsion efficiency and possibly reduced risk of pain and injury associated with prolonged wheelchair use. However, most wheelchair users prefer some clearance between the seat width and the distance between their trochanters. Clearance is required to accommodate clothing and to allow for some motion and weight shifting. For example, if the trochanter width of the individual is 325 millimeters (13 inches), then a seat width of 350 millimeters (14 inches) would be appropriate.

The depth of the seat is also important. The seat depth must be specified prior to purchasing the wheelchair. When applying the ANSI/RESNA seating standard, the seat depth is determined as the distance between the intersection of the backrest with the seat plane, and the intersection of the seat plane with the leg reference plane (see Figure 2.3). The leg reference plane is defined as a line extending upwards at a right angle from the footrests, starting at the heel loop or calf support.

The seat depth should be about 50 millimeters less than the person's sitting depth. This helps to prevent placing excessive pressure on the popliteal fossa (hamstring tendons). The proper seat depth creates better weight distribution over the seating surface. If the seat depth is too short, insufficient weight will be borne by the

**FIGURE 2.3**    Illustration of the definition of the seat depth from the ANSI/RESNA seating standard

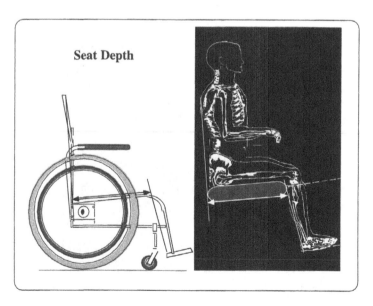

thighs, increasing the pressure on the bony prominences (e.g., ischial tuberosities, greater trochanters). Wheelchair seat depth is measured with a dummy in place. This is because the backrest may bend or stretch when an individual sits in the wheelchair. In many cases the seat depth is greater than the distance between the intersection of the backrest canes with the seat plane and the front edge of the seat upholstery. It is also important to note that calf supports may increase the effective seat depth of the wheelchair. If the effect of calf supports is not accounted for, the wheelchair user may be unable to sit upright in the wheelchair without some modifications.

The seat plane to leg reference plane angle is often used to define the front of the wheelchair frame. The leg reference plane is at a right angle from the footrest, and intersects the footrest at the point where the person's heels would be (i.e., up against the heel loops or calf supports). This is illustrated in Figure 2.4. The seat plane to leg reference plane angle is similar to the angle between the femur and tibia. Some wheelchair manufacturers require specifying the seat plane to leg reference plane angle when ordering. The seat plane to leg reference plane angle is called the rake angle on some order forms. It is often desirable to have the seat plane to leg reference plane angle equal 90 degrees. However, some people do not have the flexibility to obtain 90 degrees or require less of an angle to promote blood flow. Angles less than or greater than 90 degrees are quite common. Smaller angles tend to make the wheelchair shorter and more maneuverable in confined spaces. Larger angles may provide greater heel clearance for the casters to swivel, and can be used to provide a longer wheelbase, making it easier to negotiate some obstacles. The seat plane angle may be selected at the time of manufacture or in some cases it is adjustable. The seat plane angle is illustrated in Figure 2.5.

The seat plane angle is the angle with respect to horizontal made by the seat with the dummy in it. Some people refer to the seat plane angle as pinch. The seat

**FIGURE 2.4**  Depiction of seat plane to leg reference plane angle as defined in ANSI/RESNA seating standard

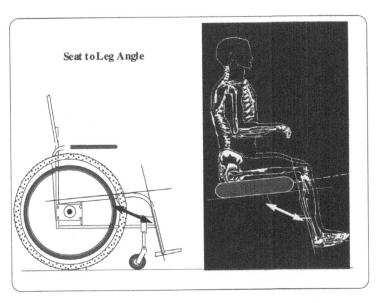

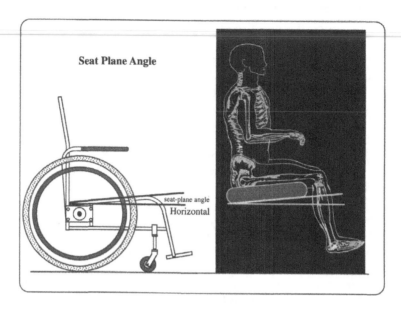

**FIGURE 2.5**   Illustration of the definition of seat plane angle

plane angle is typically between zero and five degrees. However, some active wheelchair users prefer to have as much as 20 degrees. The larger seat plane angle encourages the user's body to settle firmly at the back of the seat. This helps to improve performance during sports like basketball, tennis, and slalom. For some people it helps to improve their sitting balance. A greater seat plane angle tends to place more pressure over the ischial tuberosities and trochanters. Therefore, one must carefully weigh the benefits and risks for each individual prior to selecting a fixed seat plane angle. With an adjustable seat plane angle, the user and clinician can apply some experimentation prior to settling on an angle.

### 2.3.2 Defining the Wheelchair Backrest

The backrest angle may be either fixed or adjustable. Most wheelchairs designed for long-term use by an individual (i.e., wheelchairs that are often classified as rehabilitation wheelchairs) usually incorporate adjustable backrest angles. The backrest angle is determined with a dummy in the wheelchair. The backrest angle is the angle that the back of the dummy makes with respect to vertical, as illustrated in Figure 2.6. The backrest angle is typically set between 90 and 95 degrees. In some wheelchairs the backrest angle can be altered by adjusting rear wheel position or front caster position. When setting or selecting the seat plane and backrest angles, consideration must be given to the individual's flexibility.

The height of the backrest is very important when selecting a wheelchair. Backrest heights vary considerably. Typically the backrest height is similar to the seat depth, and adjustable over a range of about 150 millimeters (6 inches). Figure 2.7 shows how backrest height is measured. Higher backrests are used by people who are more severely mobility-impaired. A person with paraplegia would likely use a lower backrest height than a person with quadriplegia. Furthermore, a person who uses an active-duty manual wheelchair is likely to require a lower back-

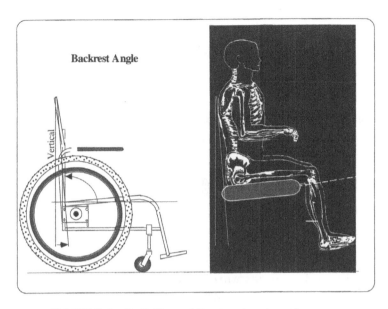

**FIGURE 2.6**  Definition of the backrest angle

rest than a person who uses an electrically powered wheelchair. An effective method for determining a suitable backrest height is to assess the individual's unsupported seating balance. Foam pillows can be used to determine the amount of support required to obtain functional sitting balance. Many clinics have individuals try several wheelchairs and adjust them until the person feels comfortable and can adequately drive the wheelchair.

**FIGURE 2.7**  Measurement of wheelchair backrest height

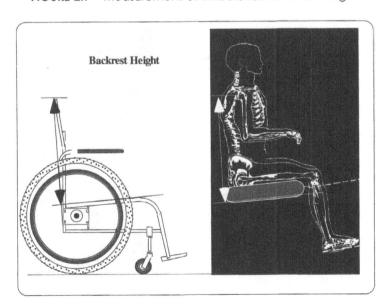

For some individuals a backrest alone provides insufficient support. In such cases, a headrest can provide the additional support necessary for functional mobility. Headrests are typically required by people who have very severe mobility impairments. Headrests can be used on either manual or electric-powered wheelchairs. However, they are used most often with manually powered wheelchairs driven by an assistant, or with electric-powered wheelchairs. Headrest height is measured from the intersection of the seat and backrest planes to the individual's occipital protuberance (see Figure 2.8). Many types and styles of headrests are available depending on each individual's needs.

### 2.3.3 Measuring for Legrests and Armrests

Most wheelchairs have adjustable legrest lengths. This is because the legrest length is dependent not only on the length of the individual's lower leg, but also on the type and thickness of the cushion the person uses. The wheelchair manufacturer will measure the range of adjustability for its legrest using a dummy without a cushion in the wheelchair. The appropriate legrest length is best measured with the individual in a wheelchair with the size and type of cushion to be used and the type of shoes to be worn. The legrest length measured this way should be used to select a legrest with a midrange value similar to that of the particular individual. Footrests are available is a variety of styles. The styles of legrests are described in Chapter 7. In some cases, persons may be limited in their choices due to personal legrest length requirements. For very tall people, the seat height or the seat angle may need to be increased. Figure 2.9 describes how legrest length is measured.

Once all the fixed seating parameters and the range of variable seating parameters have been selected, the seat height can be determined. The min-

**FIGURE 2.8**    Definition of wheelchair headrest height

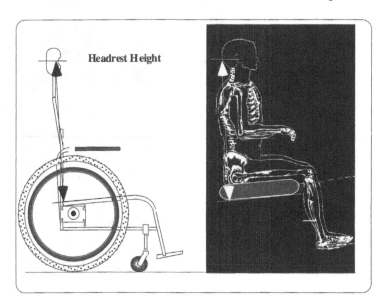

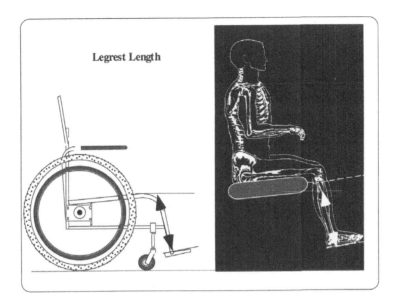

**FIGURE 2.9**   Measurement of legrest length

imum seat height is limited by the height of the person, especially the individual's leg length. Most wheelchairs require a footrest clearance of about 50 millimeters (2 inches) to be functional. Lower foot clearance can present problems at ramp transitions, or when negotiating common obstacles like door thresholds. The maximum seat height for manual wheelchairs is limited by the user's reach to the drive wheels. Ideally, an elbow angle of about 120 degrees will be maintained when the hands grasp the tops of the pushrims with the user sitting fully upright. For both manual and electric-powered wheelchairs, the seat height influences the stability of the wheelchair. If the wheelchair becomes too tall, it will tip over during some common activities (e.g., negotiating ramps, curbcuts). Also, the ability of the individual to transfer in and out of the wheelchair is influenced by the wheelchair's seat height. Wheelchair seat height is measured to the front edge of the seat when the wheelchair is loaded with a test dummy (see Figure 2.10). The overall sitting height of the individual is going to be influenced by the seat height and the seat angle.

Some wheelchair users prefer to use armrests. Armrests provide a place to rest the arms when sitting, being pushed, or when driving a power wheelchair. Armrests function as handles when transferring to or from the wheelchair, when leaning to grab something from the floor. Armrests are also used as handles for performing a push-up for pressure relief or to reach objects that would normally be out of reach. Armrests come in many styles. This is to accommodate the interests and activities of the wheelchair user. To determine the appropriate armrests, two dimensions are required: armrest height and armrest length. Armrest height is referenced to the front edge of the seat plane with a test dummy (see Figure 2.11). This method is used to ensure that the armrests will comfortably fit the user. The armrest height and seat height must be viewed in combination when evaluating whether the armrests will interfere with the individual's ability to approach a table or desk.

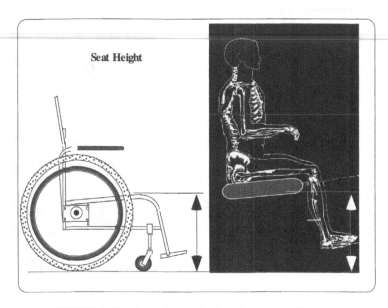

**FIGURE 2.10**   Definition of wheelchair seat height

The armrest length affects the function of the armrest as well as the ability of the user to approach desks and tables. Armrests are available in various lengths and styles in order to accommodate the activities performed by the user. Armrest length is determined from the back plane to the tip of the supporting surface of the armrest (see Figure 2.12). The armrest length should be long enough to support the arms comfortably, and short enough not to interfere with activities. In some cases armrests are used to hold an access device (e.g., a joystick for a power

**FIGURE 2.11**   Measurement of armrest height

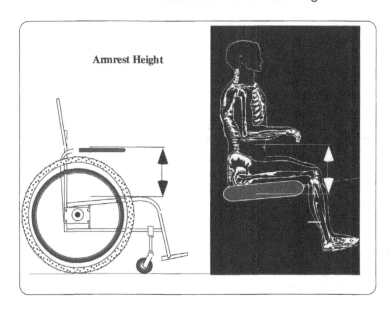

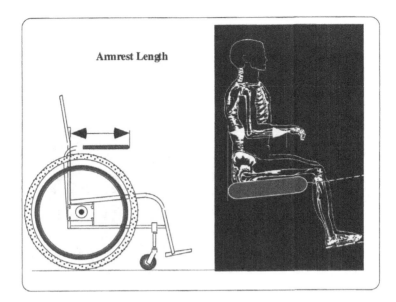

Armrest Length

**FIGURE 2.12**   Measurement of functional armrest length

wheelchair) and must allow the access device to be positioned comfortably. Some people use lap trays with the wheelchairs. In such cases the armrests must be sufficiently long and sturdy to support the lap tray and the items that may be set upon it.

In some cases, armrests may make the seating area narrower. This is because the armrests may protrude into the space occupied by the wheelchair user. If the armrests are fixed, then this may cause the wheelchair user difficulty when transferring into or out of the wheelchair. The armrests may constrain the user and become restrictive or uncomfortable. The armrest width provides information on the minimum amount of space between the armrests (see Figure 2.13). This information can be used to ensure that the armrests perform their necessary functions without interfering with the comfort or function of the wheelchair user. Armrests can be removable or flip/fold out of the way. This allows the armrest width to be optimal for the user while sitting in the chair, yet prevents interference with transferring in or out of the wheelchair. Some armrests add to the overall width of the wheelchair. This sometimes happens because the brackets mounting the armrests require the spacing between the drive wheels and the frame to be increased. If the placement of the rear wheels or the overall width of the wheelchair is critical to the user's mobility, then armrests that do not affect drive-wheel position should be used.

Standardized means of measuring wheelchairs reduces the need to be familiar with every make and model of wheelchair. In the past, each wheelchair manufacturer used unique measurement definitions. This created some concern among people specifying wheelchairs because the measurements from each individual had to be translated into the measurements required for a specific wheelchair. By using standardized measurements, an individual's measurements can be used to choose from a variety of wheelchairs and their custom options. It is also important to realize that most manufacturers will customize nearly all aspects of

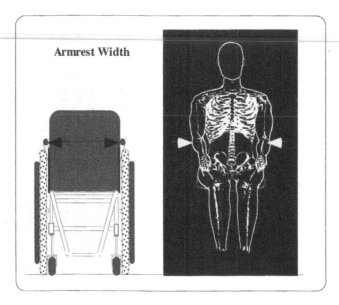

**FIGURE 2.13**   Functional width between armrests

their wheelchairs to suit an individual's specific needs. However, extensive customization requires substantial knowledge of wheelchair design and of the needs of the consumer. Some wheelchair companies specialize in custom fabrication of wheelchairs, and in some cases will allow the customer to come to the factory for a fitting.

## 2.4 Basic Wheelchair Human Factors

While determining the correct wheelchair dimensions in relation to each individual's body is of the utmost importance, consideration for the environment in which the wheelchair will be used is also of substantial importance. If a wheelchair fits an individual, but is incapable of maneuvering within the user's environment, it is not very effective as a mobility device. In most cases, if the wheelchair can be small it will provide the greatest maneuverability. However, smaller wheelchairs often require greater skill on the part of the user to perform some activities.

### 2.4.1 Importance of Overall Dimensions

The size of a wheelchair can be grossly described by four variables: overall length; overall height; overall width; and overall weight (mass) (see Figure 2.14). The weight of a wheelchair influences the mobility of its user. In general, the lighter the wheelchair the better. Ingenious consumers, clinicians, and engineers have worked diligently to reduce the weight of wheelchairs without compromising safety, comfort, or durability. Light weight makes a wheelchair easier to push, to load into a motor vehicle, and to negotiate obstacles. Even electric-powered wheelchairs benefit from being lighter. Lightweight power wheelchairs can drive farther with smaller batteries, are easier to transport, and can negotiate more

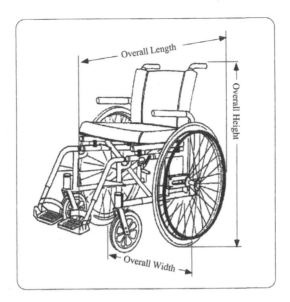

**FIGURE 2.14** Definitions of overall width, overall length, and overall height

obstacles. However, weight alone does not determine the performance of a wheelchair, especially power wheelchairs. The design of the wheelchair also determines performance.

The overall length and overall width of the wheelchair help to determine its maneuverability, ease of transport, and storage requirements. The overall width determines the minimum door width required for the wheelchair to pass through. In typical residential houses, interior doorways range from 600 to 800 millimeters (24 to 32 inches). The door itself effectively reduces the door width by about 37 millimeters (1.5 inches), unless it is a pocket door. Most people use wheelchairs with seat widths of 400 to 450 millimeters (16 to 18 inches). This usually results in an overall width of 600 to 650 millimeters (24 to 26 inches). Since bathrooms have the smallest doors, and are typically located off a hallway, they tend to cause the most difficulties for wheelchair users. If a wheelchair becomes too narrow, it may become unstable on side slopes.

The overall length of a wheelchair influences maneuverability. For example, if a bathroom is located along a 900 millimeter (36 inch) hallway, the wheelchair user may not be able to make the turn into the bathroom if the overall length is too long. It is not uncommon for a wheelchair to have an overall length of 1200 millimeters (48 inches). If the hallway is wide enough and the wheelchair short enough, the wheelchair may be able to do a simple turn (see Figure 2.15). In some cases, the wheelchair user will be able to do a three-point turn. In other cases, the wheelchair may not be able to turn. Electric-powered wheelchairs tend to be longer than manual wheelchairs. Because of the difficulty in getting into rooms along hallways, many drivers of powered wheelchairs will remove the legrests and let their legs dangle while maneuvering in narrow hallways. This effectively reduces the overall length of the wheelchair, but it also places the user in a potentially unstable situation. If the wheelchair stops abruptly, the user may slide forward out of the wheelchair. Moreover, the legrests are not available to protect the

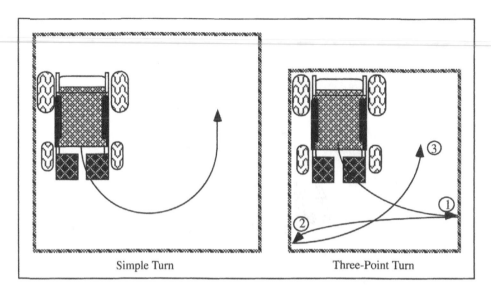

Simple Turn　　　　　　　　　　　Three-Point Turn

**FIGURE 2.15**　Diagram illustrating how the turning space affects maneuvering

user's legs in the event of inadvertently hitting a wall or fixture. In many homes, the user has no choice but to remove the legrests. In such cases, a seat belt should be used while driving to help prevent the user from sliding out of the seat, the speed control should be set to minimum, and extreme caution should be used.

The overall dimensions have a strong influence on the transportability of a wheelchair. When the wheelchair is reduced to its smallest size through either folding or simple disassembly, it must fit into some storage compartment in a motor vehicle. Manual wheelchairs are commonly stored in the front passenger seat or in the foot well of the rear seat behind the front passenger seat. Common folding wheelchairs become narrower, but do not change their overall height or overall length when folded. Therefore, the automobile must have a space accessible by the user (ideally) or a companion, which is of a size large enough to fit the folded wheelchair. Most lightweight wheelchairs incorporate removable legrests to reduce their overall length, and removable "quick-release" rear wheels to reduce overall height and width. Nearly all rigid-frame wheelchairs incorporate removable rear wheels to facilitate transport.

Electric-powered wheelchairs and scooters must also be transported. Scooters are often made to disassemble into components that can be placed in the rear storage compartment of many vehicles. Ideally, people would be required to lift no more than 10 kilograms (about 25 pounds) to transport a wheelchair or scooter. In most cases, this weight limit is not attained—the batteries are often the limiting factor. Some batteries weigh over 18 kilograms (40 pounds). When the batteries are heavy, the scooter or wheelchair frame must also be made heavier, which makes transport even more difficult. A method to improve transportability is to use removable battery containers. Quickie, a division of Sunrise Medical, developed the concept of "click-&-zoom" technology for electric-powered wheelchairs. The "click-&-zoom" concept integrates the controller, drive train, and batteries into a single unit that can be easily removed without the use of tools. This makes the wheelchair simpler to transport on an aircraft, and makes the batteries easily accessible for removal from the "click-&-zoom" package. Most electric-powered wheelchairs and scooters provide means of removing the batteries without the use of tools. The design of individual models dictates how easy this task is to accomplish. International wheelchair standards require that the connectors for wheelchair batteries do not permit improper connection.

Electric-powered wheelchairs and scooters are a vital source of mobility for many people. Electric-powered wheelchairs are primarily used by people who have severe mobility impairments such as high quadriplegia or severe cerebral palsy. Electric-powered wheelchairs might be more popular among people with less involved physical impairments if it were not for the increased size, increased weight, and reduced performance during many activities of daily living. Powered wheelchairs allow people to travel greater distances without fatigue, and their mobility is less influenced by the addition of specialized seating and postural support hardware. The use of an electric-powered wheelchair often restricts the user to a van for personal transportation or to using public transportation services.

Scooters are used by a wider variety of people for whom mobility with a manual wheelchair is too strenuous or impossible. Scooters are generally lighter in weight and smaller in size than electric-powered wheelchairs, and also incorporate simpler designs. This combination makes them attractive to a large consumer market. It also provides greater options for transporting scooters in motor vehicles. Many scooters employ modular designs that permit them to be partially disassembled by the consumer for transport in a motor vehicle. Scooters may be lifted into an automobile with a hatchback either by hand or by using a simple vehicle-mounted hoist. Devices have also been designed to place scooters on the roof of an automobile using a lifting and storage system.

Overall dimensions are thus important because they influence driving performance, contribute to the maneuverability of the product, and define the transportation needs. Therefore, the user's mobility needs, the characteristics of the product, and their combined effect on the individual's mobility must be considered in concert.

### 2.4.2 Wheel Position and Performance

Most manual wheelchairs provide some degree of adjustment in wheel position with respect to the seating position of the user. This is less common among electric-powered wheelchairs and scooters. More details about specific adjustments will be provided in subsequent chapters. In this section, two fundamental concepts will be examined. The contact points of the wheelchair's wheels with the ground significantly contribute to the driving behavior of the wheelchair or scooter. The wheel contact points are largely described by two variables: track width and wheelbase (see Figure 2.16).

The *track width* of a wheelchair is defined as the distance between the points of contact with the rolling surface (i.e., ground) of the wheels. Two values may be reported for the track width: one for the width across the casters and one for the width across the drive wheels. Perhaps the simplest method for measuring track width is to push the wheelchair through a puddle of water onto a smooth dry surface like a cement floor. The distance between the water marks represents the track width. Track width helps to define the stability of the wheelchair, especially

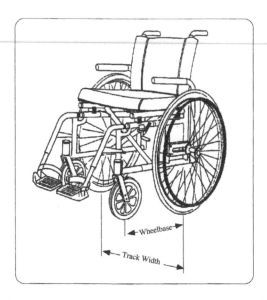

**FIGURE 2.16**   Illustration of wheelchair wheelbase and track width

its *lateral stability* (i.e., side-to-side stability). For example, if the track width becomes zero, than the wheelchair becomes like a bicycle. Track width also determines the minimum path required to push the wheelchair, and it influences maneuverability. As the track width is increased, the lateral stability increases, but the chair tends to require greater turning space. It also becomes more difficult to reach objects. The track width is determined by the width of the frame, the spacing between the wheels and the frame, and the amount of camber in the wheels. *Camber* is the angle at which the wheels are tilted or slanted.

The *wheelbase* is used to describe the distance between the front wheels and rear wheels. Wheelbase is measured along a line parallel to the centerline of the wheelchair or scooter, between where the front and rear wheels touch the rolling surface. Wheelbase can be measured by rolling the wheelchair through a puddle of water onto a clean, dry cement surface. A piece of chalk, marking pen, or pencil can be used to connect the contact points for each of the wheels. The distance along the water marks between the chalk lines for the front and rear wheels is the wheelbase. Wheelbase affects the stability and maneuverability of the wheelchair. The longer the wheelbase, the more stable the wheelchair can be made against tipping forwards or backwards. However, as the wheelbase is lengthened more turning space is required. Lengthening the wheelbase can also make it easier to climb over curbs or other obstacles. The angle over which the individual's and wheelchair's center of gravity must be lifted is related to the height of the object and the wheelbase. The object height represents the rise, and the wheelbase represents the run. The longer the wheelbase the lower the angle. Wheelbase is determined by the length of the wheelchair, the size of the individual's body, and the positioning of the wheels and caster along the frame. A short wheelbase often makes the wheelchair more responsive, but poorer at negotiating obstacles.

The abilities of the user largely dictate the dimensions of the wheelchair within the adjustable or selectable limits. The more highly skilled an individual is or becomes, the wheelchair can be set up to be more responsive and maneuverable. The environment within which the wheelchair is driven is also important. For environments that include many obstacles a longer wheelbase and wider track width may be desirable; in a school setting a shorter wheelbase and narrower track width may be desirable.

### 2.4.3 Wheelchair Seated Reach

When selecting or specifying a wheelchair one cannot neglect the environment in which the wheelchair will be used. The environmental information is obtained partially through home, worksite, and school evaluations. This provides useful information about the requirements for the wheelchair, possible modifications to the environment, and insight into the skills asked of the wheelchair user. A question that must be asked is "What tasks will the wheelchair user be performing?" A follow-up question is "How can the proper wheelchair and appropriate modifications to the user's environment make performing the tasks possible?" These and other questions will be explored in greater detail in the chapter on service delivery (Chapter 13). However, some basic concepts will be presented here. Most tasks in a wheelchair are performed while seated, although standing wheelchairs exist. While seated, one's perspective and reach are different from those of an individual who may stand. In addition, people who have no physical impairment have many more motions at their command to perform a given task. Engineers sometimes refer to this as having more degrees of freedom. For example, an unimpaired person may use a stepladder to reach an object that is 2 meters above the floor. The stepladder effectively increases the person's reach, and is considered by some to be an assistive device. For a wheelchair user who desires to reach the same object, a stepladder is insufficient for performing the task; an elevating wheelchair, a stand-up wheelchair, or a "reacher" may be needed. A reacher is a device that allows a person to extend his or her grasp via something similar to a very long pair of pliers. This example illustrates the concept of reachable space.

We define that area in which a person performs a task as the *workspace*. The workspace can be divided into more precise areas that reflect the degree of flexibility an individual has within certain areas of the workspace. For simplicity, we will assume that the person remains stationary and seated in the wheelchair. Within this framework, reachable space, functional space, and flexible space can be defined. *Reachable space* describes the entire space that a person can reach using the entire range of motion. Reachable space is defined by the area swept out by the arms while bending the trunk (see Figures 2.17 and 2.18). *Functional space* is defined by the volume in which a task or set of tasks may be performed. By definition, functional space may require a task to be performed only one way; however, it does not preclude some tasks from being performed in more than one way. *Flexible space* requires that all tasks performed within this volume can be performed in multiple ways. Using these definitions, reachable space encompasses the largest volume, functional space the next largest volume, and flexible space defines the smallest volume.

For example, if someone wished to drink a glass of water, and all that was known about the position of the glass in the person's workspace was that the glass was in the reachable workspace, then all that could be said is that the person can touch the glass, but may not be able to drink the water. If the glass were known to be in the functional workspace for this task, then it could be said that the person can drink the water. If the glass were known to be in the flexible workspace, then it

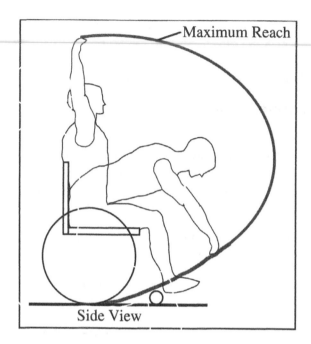

**FIGURE 2.17**   Side view depicting reachable space while seated in a wheelchair

**FIGURE 2.18**   Front view depicting reachable space while seated in a wheelchair

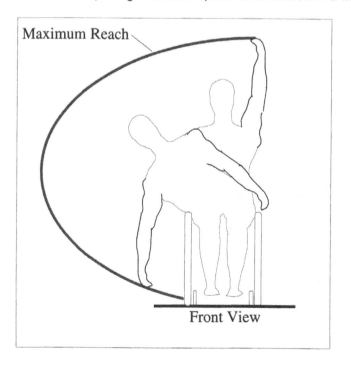

would be known that the person could drink the water in more than one way. The concept of flexible workspace is important because the world is a dynamic place and things change. Being within a flexible workspace allows adaptation of the task to changes in the environment. For example, if more objects were placed in the workspace, then the manner in which the water is drunk may need to be changed.

Because people perform a variety of tasks and each person has distinct abilities, there are different types of wheelchairs and various options for most wheelchairs. For example, armrests come in a variety of styles to accommodate desks, to protect loose-fitting clothing from the wheels, or to provide handles for reaching or transferring. Legrests come in a variety of styles as well. Some are fixed in place, while others flip-up, and still others swing away. All styles have their strengths and weaknesses, and some features influence the workspace. For example, swing-away legrests allow the person to swing the legrests to the side and move closer to objects. This helps in transfer onto other seats, or in performing some tasks like working at a countertop.

Some wheelchairs are specifically designed to expand the reachable workspace. Stand-up wheelchairs provide support in the standing position to allow people to grasp higher objects or to provide greater flexibility in performing tasks at countertops designed for people who stand. Elevating wheelchairs permit the user to change the seat height while seated in the wheelchair. This permits reaching items placed higher in the workspace, and in some cases lower as well.

Reachable, functional, and flexible workspace are by definition functions of the user's abilities and the tasks to be performed. The degree of impairment and the person's adaptation to it will influence the ability to perform tasks. During a thorough assessment the reachable, functional, and flexible workspace should be determined, and devices should be placed in the appropriate locations within the workspace. For example, the joystick used to drive an electric-powered wheelchair should be placed within the flexible workspace. Placement in the reachable workspace is required, otherwise the user could not even touch the joystick, and that would make driving extremely difficult. In order to drive the wheelchair, the joystick must be placed at least within the functional workspace. However, if the joystick arm rattles loose the joystick may move outside the user's workspace and prevent the person from driving the wheelchair. If placed in the flexible workspace, the user could adapt the method or position of operating the joystick in response to the change in location or orientation of the joystick arm.

## 2.5 Summary

Selection of the proper wheelchair is critical to the mobility and self-image of the user. Each wheelchair must be selected and configured based on the person's individual measurements, abilities, and desired activities. Proper selection requires knowledge of disability, anthropometry, ergonomics, and wheelchairs. The following case illustrates the impact the proper wheelchair can have on an individual. Larry developed multiple sclerosis when he was in his forties. Larry led an active lifestyle, was considered quite stylish and careful in maintaining his appearance. The multiple sclerosis progressed to the point where Larry could benefit from the use of a manual wheelchair to increase his personal mobility. Larry was aware only of the chrome hospital-type wheelchair and was quite apprehensive about relying on a wheelchair for his mobility. Eventually, Larry required a wheelchair and much to his dismay he was provided a "chrome hospital-type" wheelchair. The wheelchair was provided from hospital stock, because it was available and relatively inexpensive. Larry's wheelchair was much too large for him, and difficult to propel. Larry's mobility did not increase as he had expected. He began to spend much of his time at home, until he met another man who used a wheelchair and who invited him to come to a meeting of other wheelchair users. Larry was reluctant at first, but the man (who was about Larry's age) had a colorful wheelchair that appeared lightweight, and the man seemed to get around quite well. So, eventually Larry went to a meeting, where other people in wheelchairs showed and talked about all of the things that they could do, and Larry became exposed to a variety of wheelchair options and designs. The group worked with Larry to get an appointment at a specialized wheelchair and seating clinic. Larry was fitted for a new, much smaller wheelchair. Larry chose a lightweight folding model that was bright red. He worked with the clinic to get all of the features that he needed, to help him present a more stylish image. Larry was very happy with his new wheelchair, and went on to help other people visit the clinic. He began to participate in sports again, and went on to become active with his friends again. Larry told his new friends at the wheelchair user's meeting that he "felt like a new man."

## References and Further Reading

Axelson P., Minkel J., Chesney D. (1994) *A Guide to Wheelchair Selection: How to Use the ANSI/RESNA Wheelchair Standards to Buy a Wheelchair*. Washington, DC, Paralyzed Veterans of America.

Cook A. M., Hussey S. M. (1995) *Assistive Technologies: Principles and Practice*. St. Louis, MO, Mosby-Year Book, Inc.

Cooper R. A. (1995) *Rehabilitation Engineering Applied to Mobility and Manipulation*. London, UK, Adam Hilger Institute of Physics Publishing.

Davies T. D., Beasley K. A. (1988) *Design for Hospitality: Planning for Accessible Hotels and Motels*. New York, NY, Nichols Publishing.

Davies T. D., Beasley K. A. (1992) *Fair Housing Design Guide for Accessibility*. Washington, DC, Paralyzed Veterans of America.

Jacobs K., Bettencourt C. M. (1995) *Ergonomics for Therapists*. Boston, MA, Butterworth-Heinemann.

Kapit W., Elson L. M. (1977) *The Anatomy Coloring Book*. New York, NY, Harper & Row, Publishers.

Trefler E., Hobson D. A., Taylor S.J., Monahan L. C., Shaw C. G. (1993) *Seating and Mobility for Persons with Physical Disabilities*. Tuscon, AZ, Therapy Skill Builders.

Wilson A. B. (1992) *Wheelchairs: A Prescription Guide*. New York, NY, Demos.

# CHAPTER 3

# Wheelchair Engineering Fundamentals

*Chapter Goals*

- ☑ To understand mechanical and material properties
- ☑ To understand the relationship between technology and its environment
- ☑ To know how to problem-solve and integrate technical and functional information
- ☑ To understand the roles, constraints, and perspectives of designers and fabricators

## 3.1 Introduction

A thorough understanding of wheelchairs requires some knowledge of engineering principles and concepts. Engineering requires a rigorous mathematical foundation. In this chapter, a few important mechanical and electrical concepts will be introduced. Mastery of these concepts provides an opportunity to understand not only the "how" of wheelchair function, but also the "why" of wheelchair function. The concepts described in this chapter also provide the background necessary to understand the basics of wheelchair seating and propulsion biomechanics. Once this material is thoroughly understood, the reader should be able to communicate effectively with rehabilitation engineers, better understand engineering test results, and apply engineering concepts to the analysis of wheelchair use.

## 3.2 Fundamental Mathematics of Engineering

This book is not designed as an engineering or mathematics book, but rather to give health professionals sufficient appreciation and understanding of mathematical and engineering fundamentals to select and configure wheelchairs as professional assistive technology service providers. The fundamental mathematics of engineering can be divided into several areas. The basic principles are quantities like length, time, and mass. Based on these and other basic principles, other important concepts can be developed such as force, velocity, work, energy, and power. The basic principles must be understood prior to learning derived concepts.

### 3.2.1 Basic Properties and Definitions

Basic properties denote the nature of quantities. Every measurable quantity has properties and corresponding units associated with it. A property is a description of a quantity, whereas a unit is associated with a set of international definitions. The System International (SI) standard is most commonly accepted throughout the world. For example, a ruler has a property of length associated with it, and has units of inches or centimeters. Most people are familiar with measuring many basic properties. The basic properties of length, time, and mass will be used most when describing the use of wheelchairs. The basic properties of length, time, and mass are represented using SI convention as follows:

$$l = \text{length (meters)}$$
$$t = \text{time (seconds)}$$
$$m = \text{mass (kilograms)}$$

Length can simply be measured using a rule or tape. Time is simply measured with a stopwatch. Mass is simply measured with a scale. Mass is usually determined by measuring weight (a secondary property), and applying knowledge about the relationship between mass and weight on earth. Charge is also an important basic property which will be described in the section on electric circuits. Secondary dimensions are derived from dependent basic concepts. For example, the area of a square is calculated by multiplying the lengths of two adjacent sides. Therefore, the secondary dimension is area (A), and the secondary units are meters squared. For a cube, the volume is determined by multiplying the length of three adjacent sides. Area and volume are important secondary dimensions:

$$A = \text{area} = l \bullet l = l^2 \ (\text{meters}^2)$$
$$V = \text{volume} = l^3 \ (\text{meters}^3)$$

Other secondary properties are not as obvious, but are equally important. To describe the behavior of a wheelchair and the motion of its user, time-motion analysis is required. This leads to the concept of a derivative. The derivative is a fundamental concept of calculus, but one need not understand calculus to understand the basic principle. Speed is a derivative of displacement and time. For example, when traveling in a car the speedometer measures the amount of time required to drive a certain distance (length). Speed is distance divided by time and has dimensions of length divided by time, and units of meters per second. Speed provides no indication of direction. Velocity is the term used to describe speed with a specific direction. Acceleration is a derivative of speed or velocity. To calculate acceleration the change in speed at two times is divided by the difference in the two times:

$$a = \frac{v_{finish} - v_{start}}{t_{finish} - v_{start}} \tag{3.1}$$

In this equation, the speeds (velocities) are expressed in meters per second, and the times are expressed in seconds. Therefore, the units of acceleration are meters per second squared. Acceleration is one of the most important secondary properties that will be used in this book. For example, the rate at which an object falls to earth is defined as an acceleration. The acceleration towards earth due to its gravity is a constant for any object, and has the value 9.81 meters per second squared ($m/s^2$).

$$v = velocity = 1/t \text{ (meters/second)}$$
$$a = acceleration = 1/t^2 \text{ (meters/seconds}^2)$$

Some secondary properties have special names associated with their units. Often these names are of great scientists through history. Sir Isaac Newton, a British physicist and mathematician in the 1700s, developed fundamental theories of calculus and mechanics. The unit of force bears his name. Force can be defined in many ways. Force can be defined as the action of one object against another. It can also be defined as a mechanical disturbance or load. It is force that causes objects (bodies) to move or deform. Twisting, bending, and rotational movements are caused by moments or torques. Forces and moments can be related by a distance called a moment arm (which will be defined in a later section). Force and torque can be defined using basic units:

$$F = force = m \cdot 1/t^2 \text{ (kilograms} \cdot \text{meters/seconds}^2) = Newton \text{ (N)}$$
$$\tau = moment \text{ (torque)} = ml^2/t^2 \text{ (kilograms} \cdot \text{meters}^2/\text{seconds}^2) = N \cdot m$$

Power is also a secondary property that can be derived from other secondary properties or from basic properties. Power is the rate at which work is done over time. Power is an important factor in determining the capabilities of electric powered wheelchairs, and the ability to negotiate terrain in a manual wheelchair. Power can be calculated by multiplying force times linear velocity or moment times angular velocity. The units of power are watts, named after the British inventor and scientist James Watt, who investigated steam and water power during the 1800s.

$$p = power = ml^2/t^3 \text{ (kilograms} \cdot \text{meters}^2/\text{seconds}^3) = N \cdot m/t = watts \text{ (W)}$$

Secondary properties can also be combined based on natural laws. The rule that governs the combination of units is called the "law of dimensional homogeneity." This important law will be described in greater detail in the following section.

### 3.2.2 Law of Dimensional Homogeneity

When properties are added together they must follow specific rules. Secondary properties are combined as a consequence of certain natural laws. The validity of an equation relating several physical quantities can be verified by analyzing the individual terms forming the equation. The *law of dimensional homogeneity* imposes restrictions on the formulation of such equations. If three variables, made up of primary or secondary properties, are combined using a linear equation, then each term in the equation must have the same resultant units. If a variable Z is a result of combining W, X, and Y, then aW, bX, and cY must have the same units.

$$Z = aW + bX + cY \tag{3.2}$$

If Z has units of N • m, then aW, bX, and cY must also have units of N • m. ~~This type of unit equality must hold true for all combinations of properties. This~~ is helpful when solving problems and checking solutions.

### 3.2.3 Newton's Laws

The motion and biomechanics of wheelchairs can largely be understood by the understanding and application of a few basic laws. The most important among the basic laws are the laws of Newtonian mechanics, put forth by Sir Isaac Newton. These laws form the basis for statics and dynamics. Newton proposed three fundamental laws:

1. Newton's First Law: A body originally at rest will remain at rest, or a body in motion will move in a straight line with constant velocity (speed), if the net force acting upon it is zero.
2. Newton's Second Law: A body with a net force acting on it will accelerate in the direction of that force, and the magnitude of the acceleration will be proportional to the magnitude of the net force.
3. Newton's Third Law: For every action there is always an equal and opposite reaction, and the forces of action and reaction between interacting bodies are equal in magnitude, opposite in direction, and have the same line of action (i.e., if you push on a body it will push back).

Newton's first law introduces the concept of equilibrium to mechanics. The concept of equilibrium provides an explanation for why an object stays put once we set it on a table top. Equilibrium also helps to explain why a ball flies through the air when we throw it. Newton's second law explains why the ball eventually falls to the ground. This happens because the ball has some mass, therefore, the earth is pulling down on it. Since nothing is holding the ball in the air, gravity will eventually pull it down to the ground. In outer space, outside the earth's atmosphere an object will fly for a very long time before striking another object or being pulled into another planet's atmosphere by its gravity. Newton's third law explains why, when you throw a ball, you feel it pushing against you. The harder you try to throw the ball, the harder the ball pushes against you. Newton's third law also forms the basis for the "free-body diagram," which is a useful tool for solving problems in statics and dynamics.

Assume that an assistant is pushing a wheelchair. The application of Newton's laws can be used to determine the relationship between the amount of force applied by the assistant (i.e., how hard the assistant pushes), and the acceleration of the wheelchair. The force applied by the assistant will be denoted by $F$, the mass of the wheelchair will be denoted by $m$, and the acceleration of the wheelchair will be denoted by $a$.

Before the wheelchair moves it has an acceleration of zero (0). From Newton's first law, both the wheelchair and the assistant are in equilibrium. Once the assistant applies force, Newton's second and third laws come into action. Newton's second law says that the acceleration of the wheelchair will be proportional to the applied force.

$$F \propto ma \tag{3.3}$$

Newton's third law says that the force on the wheelchair will be opposite the force applied to the attendant, and have the same magnitude. From this, we can determine the relationship between the force applied to the wheelchair by the attendant, and the acceleration of the wheelchair.

$$F - ma = 0 \qquad (3.4)$$

Equation (3.4) can be thought of as "the sum of all forces must be zero." Equation (3.4) can be rearranged to a more familiar form:

$$F = ma \qquad (3.5)$$

Some additional knowledge is required to solve more complex problems using Newton's laws. Many practical problems can be solved by properly understanding and applying Newton's laws.

### 3.2.4 Basic Vector Mathematics

Most problems cannot be solved without the use of vectors. To understand vectors, one must first master some basic concepts. Most people are familiar with using numbers, and understand that a number may have a value. Some values are larger than others, whereas some are smaller. These are familiar basic concepts. In engineering terms the value of a basic number or variable is its magnitude. If a variable has only magnitude, then it is called a *scalar*. Concepts like mass, time, energy, temperature, and power are scalar quantities. Knowing that ten minutes has elapsed is enough to understand how long it has taken to get to where you are. Some concepts are more complex. Force, distance, velocity, and acceleration require more than just a magnitude to describe them, and are samples of *vector* quantities.

Various notations are used to refer to vector quantities. Throughout this book, the use of bold lower-case letters will be used. For example, **v** will refer to a vector, and $v$ will refer to a scalar. In illustrations, vectors will be represented by arrows. The length of the arrow is typically shown to be proportional to the magnitude of the vector. The direction that the arrow points provides the direction of the *line of action* of the vector. The arrowhead demonstrates the *sense* of the vector. The end of the arrow opposite the arrowhead represents the *point of application* of the vector. Figure 3.1 illustrates the force vector (**f**) applied by a person's hand to the pushrim of a wheelchair.

Vectors do not follow the same rules for addition and multiplication as scalars. To understand basic vector mathematics, some fundamental principles must be understood. A critical theorem related to vector mathematics is the Pythagorean theorem, developed by the Greek mathematician Pythagoras. The Pythagorean theorem states that the square of the length of the hypotenuse of a right triangle is equal to the sum of the squares of the other two sides. This is illustrated in Figure 3.2; note that the $\pi/2$ angle is marked with a square in its corner.

The angles made by the adjacent sides of the triangle are related by trigonometric functions. The most commonly used functions are the sine, cosine, and tangent. The definitions of the sine, cosine, and tangent for the triangle illustrated in Figure 3.2 are

$$\sin\alpha = a/c \qquad \cos\alpha = b/c \qquad \tan\alpha = a/b$$

and

$$\sin\beta = b/c \qquad \cos\beta = a/c \qquad \tan\beta = b/a$$

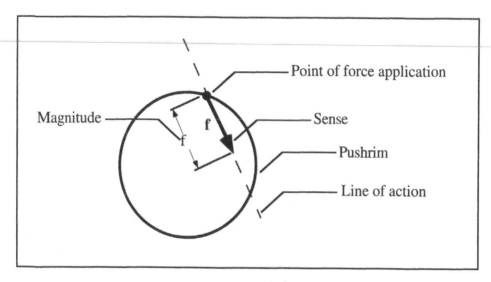

**FIGURE 3.1**   Definition of a vector in the context of a force vector applied by a person's hand to a wheelchair pushrim

Sine and cosine are always less than or equal to one. The tangent function may be greater than one. The sine and cosine function are related to one another through a simple formula,

$$\sin \alpha^2 + \cos \alpha^2 = 1 \tag{3.6}$$

Equation (3.6) is true for any angle. The Pythagorean theorem and the trigonometric relations that follow provide the foundation for many vector operations. Scientists and engineers often define the space in which we live in terms of coordinates. Coordinates are simply positions on a map, much like an address on a street map. A vector defined within a coordinate system will have components along the axes of the coordinate system. The most commonly used coordinate system for wheelchair engi-

**FIGURE 3.2**   Illustration of the Pythagorean theorem relating the lengths of the sides of a right triangle

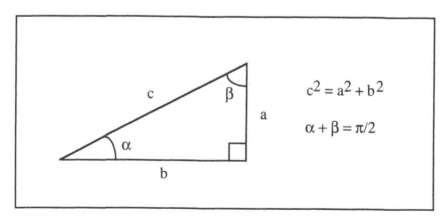

neering is the Cartesian coordinate system, which uses the familiar x, y, and z axes. The x axis is commonly defined along the line of progression (i.e., posterior-anterior), the z axis is defined side to side (i.e., medial-laterally), and the y axis is defined along a line vertical from earth (i.e., inferior-superior). We will examine the example of the force vector applied by the hand onto a pushrim (see Figure 3.3). In this case, the force vector will be examined in the x-y plane. We will ignore the z axis for the moment.

The force vector (**f**) can be examined in terms of its components along the x axis and y axis. The x and y components of **f** can be viewed as sides to a right triangle with **f** as the hypotenuse (see Figure 3.4). This method is commonly used to evaluate mechanical problems.

The components of **f** are determined by using the known direction of **f** with respect to one of the axes, either x or y. In this case, we have assumed that the angle ($\theta$) between **f** and the x axis is known. Therefore, the components of **f** are

$$f_x = f\cos\theta \qquad f_y = f\sin\theta \qquad (3.7)$$

Note that the magnitude of **f** is used to calculate the components $f_x$ and $f_y$. Representing a vector by its components plays an integral role in solving many engineering problems. Therefore, a special notation has been developed to represent vectors using their components in Cartesian coordinates. This representation is based on the concept of a unit vector. A unit vector is called such because it has a magnitude of one. Each of the x, y, and z axes are represented by a unique unit vector **i**, **j**, and **k**, respectively. The unit vector **i** has magnitude of one, and direction along the positive x axis. The unit vectors **j** and **k** are defined similarly, but with regard to their respective axes. Using conventional unit vector notation, the force vector (**f**) applied by a hand on a pushrim is

$$\mathbf{f} = f_x\mathbf{i} + f_y\mathbf{j} \qquad (3.8)$$

**FIGURE 3.3** Illustration of the force vector applied by a hand on the pushrim of a wheelchair in the x-y plane

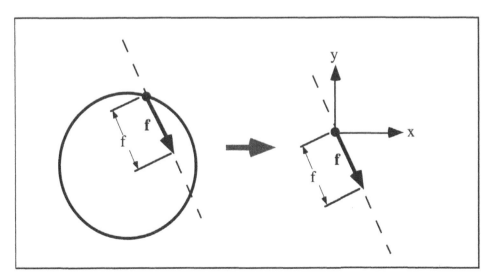

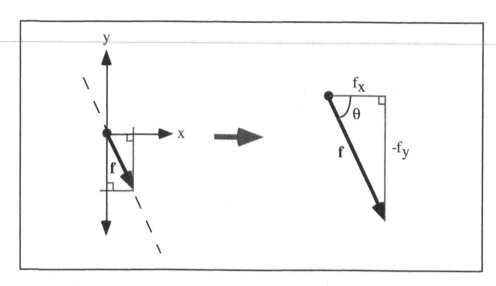

**FIGURE 3.4**   Triangle illustrating the components of **f** along the x and y axes

Note that **i** and **j** are in bold because they are vectors.

Based on the Pythagorean theorem, the magnitude of any vector represented by its components can be calculated. For the specific example of the vector **f**, its magnitude squared is

$$f^2 = f_x^2 + f_y^2 \qquad (3.9)$$

Any vector can also be converted to a unit vector by dividing by its magnitude. This is sometimes useful when attempting to find the angle between two vectors. The example of the force vector applied by a hand on the pushrim yields the unit vector

$$\mathbf{f}/f = f_x/f\,\mathbf{i} + f_y/f\,\mathbf{j} \qquad (3.10)$$

Note that although **f**/f has magnitude of one it has components along both the x and y axes. The use of unit vector and the concept of components of a vector greatly simplifies vector algebra. The addition of two vectors is simply the addition of their components, provided they are both described in the same coordinate system. Vectors **a** and **b** in Cartesian coordinates are added as follows:

$$\mathbf{a} = a_x\mathbf{i} + a_y\mathbf{j} \qquad \mathbf{b} = b_x\mathbf{i} + b_y\mathbf{j}$$
$$\mathbf{c} = \mathbf{a} + \mathbf{b} = (a_x + b_x)\mathbf{i} + (a_y + b_y)\mathbf{j} = c_x\mathbf{i} + c_y\mathbf{j} \qquad (3.11)$$

The magnitude of c is simply

$$c = \sqrt{c_x^2 + c_y^2}$$

Multiplication of two vectors is not simply defined. However, there are two very important products of vectors which are often very useful. We will attempt to clarify these products and to provide illustrations of their application and meaning. The dot product is a scalar quantity that is the product of two vector quantities. For example, force and displacement (i.e., distance along a specified direction) are vector quantities. Force over a distance produces work. Work can be calculated as a dot product between a force vector and a displacement vector. Work is a scalar quantity. The dot product of any two vectors is a scalar with magnitude equal to the product of the magnitude of the two vectors times the angle between the two vectors (see Figure 3.5).

The dot product is given by equation (3.12), using the same definitions for **a** and **b** as above.

$$\mathbf{a} \cdot \mathbf{b} = ab\cos\theta_{ab} = a_x b_x + a_y b_y = \begin{bmatrix} a_x a_y \end{bmatrix} \begin{bmatrix} b_x \\ b_y \end{bmatrix} = \mathbf{a}^T \mathbf{b} \tag{3.12}$$

The dot product may result in either positive or negative quantities, depending on the angle between the two vectors. The notation $\mathbf{a}^T\mathbf{b}$ is often called the inner product of two vectors, and is equivalent to the dot product. The notation $\mathbf{a}^T\mathbf{b}$ is presented here because it is commonly used in mathematics software packages. Equation (3.12) shows that the dot product is calculated by multiplying the like components together (i.e., multiplying $a_x$ and $b_x$, then multiplying $a_y$ and $b_y$) and then adding all of the products together. This pattern holds true for three-dimensional vectors as well. Examination of the definition of the dot product between unit vectors may help to illustrate how the dot product is calculated in general. Remember that all of the unit vectors are orthogonal to one another; mathematicians say that they form an orthonormal basis, which means that the angle between each of the unit vectors (**i**, **j**, **k**) is $\pi/2$. This means that the cosine of the angle between any unit vector and another unit vector is going to equal zero. Therefore their dot product will be equal to zero (see equation (3.13)).

**FIGURE 3.5** Graphic representation of the vector dot product

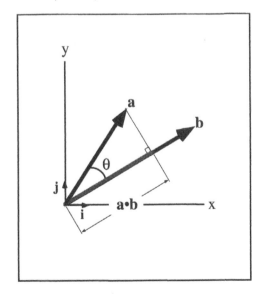

$$i \bullet j = j \bullet k = k \bullet i = 0 \qquad (3.13)$$

However, the angle between any like unit vector is zero. Therefore their dot product will be equal to one (see equation (3.14)).

$$i \bullet i = j \bullet j = k \bullet k = 1 \qquad (3.14)$$

Using our knowledge about the results of the dot products between the three unit vectors ($i$, $j$, $k$), we can show the results of the three-dimensional dot product in equation (3.15).

$$
\begin{aligned}
a \bullet b &= (a_x i + a_y j + a_z k) \bullet (b_x i + b_y j \, b_z k) \\
&= (a_x b_x)(i \bullet i) + (a_x b_y)(i \bullet j) + (a_x b_z)(i \bullet k) + (a_y b_x)(j \bullet i) + \\
&\quad (a_y b_y)(j \bullet j) + (a_y b_z)(j \bullet k) + (a_z b_x)(k \bullet i) + (a_z b_y)(k \bullet j) + (a_z b_z)(k \bullet k) \\
&= a_x b_x + a_y b_y + a_z b_z
\end{aligned}
\qquad (3.15)
$$

Some quantities relating vectors result in new vectors. A common example of this is torque, which is the cross product of the applied force and the distance to the center of rotation. For example, examine the force vector applied by a hand to a pushrim in Figure 3.6.

The torque ($\tau$) that drives the wheelchair forward is the cross product of the force vector and the distance vector. The distance vector in this case would be the radius of the pushrim ($r$).

$$\tau = f \times r = (f_x i + f_y j) \times (r\cos\phi \, i + r\sin\phi \, j) = (f_x r\sin\phi - f_y r\cos\phi)k \qquad (3.16)$$

**FIGURE 3.6** Schematic of the cross product between the force vector applied by a hand to a pushrim and the distance vector between the center of the wheel hub and the point of force application. The cross product results in the wheel propulsion torque

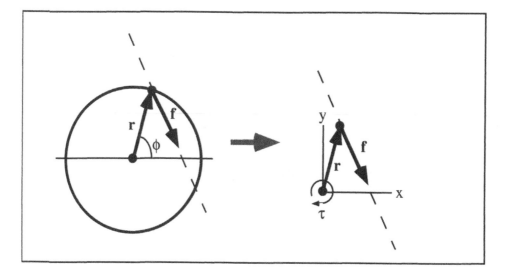

In this example, $\phi$ is the angle between the horizontal and a line connecting the center of the wheel hub (i.e., the wheel axle) to the point of application of the force vector. The cross product shows that torque is dependent on the x and y components of the force vector applied by the hand onto the pushrim, the point where the hand applies force to the pushrim, and the radius of the pushrim. This basic example demonstrates the power of the cross product to provide information about wheelchair propulsion biomechanics. The cross product has many other useful applications.

The cross product can be interpreted graphically similar to the dot product discussed earlier. The cross product can be viewed as the product of the magnitude of the two vectors times the sine of the angle between them (see Figure 3.7).

The cross product follows a known pattern. In this book, we will only deal with two- and three-component cross products.

$$\mathbf{a} \times \mathbf{b} = ab\sin\theta_{ab} = (a_x\mathbf{i} + a_y\mathbf{j}) \times (b_x\mathbf{i} + b_y\mathbf{j}) = (a_xb_y - a_yb_x)\mathbf{k} \qquad (3.17)$$

The cross product of two vectors in the x-y plane results in a vector along the z axis. This is helpful when checking results, as the results of any cross product of two vectors represented in a single plane will yield a vector along the remaining axis. Let us revisit the example of the force vector applied by a hand to the pushrim of a manual wheelchair. The torque about the wheel was shown to be related to the cross product of the radius and the applied force vector. Another approach can be used to examine this problem (see Figure 3.8).

**FIGURE 3.7** Graphic illustration of cross product between two vectors

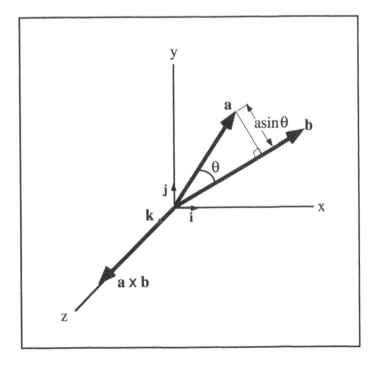

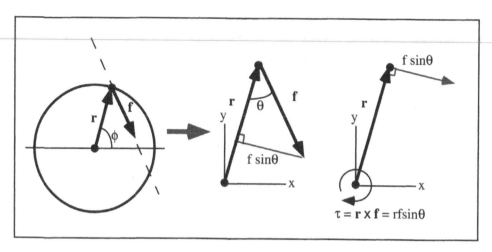

**FIGURE 3.8** Cross product between the force vector applied by the hand and the distance vector between the center of the hub and the point of force application

The cross product between the force vector applied by the hand to the pushrim and the distance vector between the hand and the point of force application yields the wheel propulsion torque. Torque is also equal to the force times the moment arm. The moment arm for a wheelchair pushrim is simply its radius. The action force is the component of the force vector which is tangential ($f_t$) to the pushrim (see equation (3.18)).

$$f_t = f\sin\theta(-\sin\phi\,\mathbf{i} + \cos\phi\,\mathbf{j})$$
$$\mathbf{r} = r(\cos\phi\,\mathbf{i} + \sin\phi\,\mathbf{j}) \tag{3.18}$$
$$\mathbf{r} \times \mathbf{f} = r(\cos\phi\,\mathbf{i} + \sin\phi\,\mathbf{j}) \times f\sin\theta(\sin\phi\,\mathbf{i} - \cos\phi\,\mathbf{j}) = rf\sin\theta\,\mathbf{k}$$

The magnitude of $f_t$ is simply f, and the magnitude of $\mathbf{r}$ is r; the magnitude of $\tau$ is simply the magnitude of $f_t$ times the magnitude of $\mathbf{r}$. This shows that only the component of $\mathbf{f}$ which is perpendicular to $\mathbf{r}$ in the x-y plane will contribute to the wheel propulsion torque. The radial force ($f_r$), the component of $\mathbf{f}$ along $\mathbf{r}$, helps to generate friction between the hand and pushrim. However, excessive $f_r$ contributes to inefficiency.

The three-dimensional case is a bit more complex than the two-dimensional cross product. The three-dimensional cross product yields a three-dimensional vector.

$$\mathbf{a} \times \mathbf{b} = (a_x\mathbf{i} + a_y\mathbf{j} + a_z\mathbf{k}) \times (b_x\mathbf{i} + b_y\mathbf{j} + b_z\mathbf{k})$$
$$= (a_y b_z - a_z b_y)\mathbf{i} + (a_z b_x - a_x b_z)\mathbf{j} + (a_x b_y - a_y b_x)\mathbf{k} \tag{3.19}$$

Close examination of equation (3.19) shows that the $\mathbf{i}$ component of the cross product does not include any x terms, the $\mathbf{j}$ component does not include any y terms, and the $\mathbf{k}$ component does not include any z terms. There is also a symmetry to each of the terms (components) of the results from a cross product of two vectors.

## 3.3 Mechanics of Motion

Mechanics of motion involves understanding two fundamental areas in mechanics: statics and dynamics. Statics is the study of a body or bodies at rest or in equilibrium. Dynamics is the study of a body or bodies in motion. Dynamics involves kinematics and kinetics. Kinematics examines the relationships between displacement, velocity, and acceleration in translational or rotational motion. Kinetics examines moving bodies and the external and internal forces that produce motion.

### 3.3.1 Kinematics

Kinematics involves the combination of translation and rotation. Translation describes motion along a line or curve. Rotation describes motion about a point. For example, as a wheelchair rolls down a ramp the axle of the rear wheel translates down the ramp from top to bottom (see Figure 3.9). At the same time the wheel rotates about its axle. Hence, the wheel is translating and rotating. As the wheelchair goes down the ramp, the frame undergoes pure translation (i.e., it is not rotating). If one were to remove a rear wheel from the same wheelchair, hold it by the axle, and spin the wheel, then the wheel would exemplify pure rotation.

Translation is defined by three primary properties: position, velocity, and acceleration. Position, velocity, and acceleration are vector quantities. They are all related via differential or integral relationships. Position defines the direction and distance of a body. Velocity defines the direction in which the position is changing and the rate at which a body is traveling. Acceleration defines the direction in which the velocity is changing, and the rate at which the velocity is changing. For example, let us assume a wheelchair user is driving his electric-powered wheelchair around a standard 400-meter running track. The driver starts in the middle of the front stretch (i.e., the side with the start-finish line) and drives to the backstretch at full speed. We start our stopwatches as soon as our driver enters the backstretch (i.e., the straight on the opposite side of the track). We stop our stopwatches when the driver has gone 50 meters. The elapsed time is 18.6 seconds. We will determine the position vector and the velocity vector for the wheelchair, given the origin is at the start point.

**FIGURE 3.9** Illustration of translation and rotation for a wheelchair going down a ramp

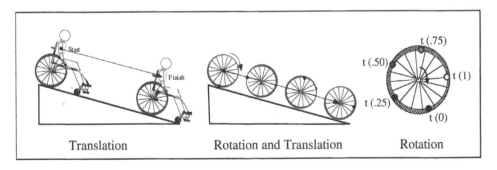

Translation          Rotation and Translation          Rotation

First, we will determine the driver's position. Since the track is oval and the driver ends at a 50-meter mark of the backstretch, the driver has x position of zero (0). However, he drives around the first and second curves before entering the backstretch. If we assume that the distance around the curve is 50 meters and has constant radius (r), we can determine the y distance traveled. The circumference of the turn is 50 meters, which is equal to

$$c = 50 \text{ meters} = \pi r$$
$$r = c/\pi = 50/\pi = 15.9 \text{ meters}$$

To get to the other side of the track, the driver must drive $2r = 31.8$ meters in the y direction. Therefore, the position of the driver is

$$\mathbf{p} = 0 \, \mathbf{i} + 31.8 \, \mathbf{j}$$

The position of the driver ($\mathbf{p}$) is a vector quantity giving the location of the driver in the track. To determine the speed, we must know the direction the driver is heading, and time elapsed for a given distance. For this example, the speed of the driver is

$$v = d/\Delta t = 50/18.6 = 2.7 \text{ meters per second (about 6 mph)}.$$

Speed is a scalar quantity representing the magnitude of the velocity. The velocity of the driver is

$$\mathbf{v} = -2.7 \, \mathbf{i} + 0 \, \mathbf{j}$$

The position and the velocity of the driver tell us the driver's location and heading. One must be cautious to be consistent in the use of units when solving position and velocity problems. The position vector (p) is generally the x, y and z coordinates of the body,

$$\mathbf{p} = x \, \mathbf{i} + y \, \mathbf{j} + z \, \mathbf{k} \tag{3.20}$$

The velocity of the body is the derivative of the change in position versus the change in time. In most real problems the derivative is solved numerically using the finite difference method. Given the position ($\mathbf{p}_0$) at time zero ($t_0$) and the position ($\mathbf{p}_1$) at some known time later ($t_1$),

$$\begin{aligned} \mathbf{p}_0 &= x_0 \, \mathbf{i} + y_0 \, \mathbf{j} + z_0 \, \mathbf{k} \\ \mathbf{p}_1 &= x_1 \, \mathbf{i} + y_1 \, \mathbf{j} + z_1 \, \mathbf{k} \end{aligned} \tag{3.21}$$

the velocity is calculated by taking the difference between the two position vectors and dividing by the elapsed time ($\Delta t$),

$$\mathbf{v}_{1-0} = \frac{\mathbf{p}_1 - \mathbf{p}_0}{t_1 - t_0} = \frac{\mathbf{p}_1 - \mathbf{p}_0}{\Delta t} = \frac{x_1 - x_0}{\Delta t} \mathbf{i} + \frac{y_1 - y_0}{\Delta t} \mathbf{j} + \frac{z_1 - z_0}{\Delta t} \mathbf{k}$$

$$\mathbf{v}_{1-0} = v_{x,1-0}\mathbf{i} + v_{y,1-0}\mathbf{j} + v_{v,1-0}\mathbf{k} \tag{3.22}$$

Acceleration is also a vector quantity, and it is calculated in a manner similar to that of the velocity vector. Given the velocity ($v_0$) at time zero ($t_0$) and the velocity ($v_1$) at some known time later ($t_1$),

$$
\begin{aligned}
\mathbf{v}_0 &= v_{x0}\,\mathbf{i} + v_{y0}\,\mathbf{j} + v_{z0}\,\mathbf{k} \\
\mathbf{v}_1 &= v_{x1}\,\mathbf{i} + v_{y1}\,\mathbf{j} + v_{z1}\,\mathbf{k}
\end{aligned}
\tag{3.23}
$$

the acceleration is calculated by taking the difference between the two velocity vectors and dividing by the elapsed time ($\Delta t$),

$$
\mathbf{a}_{1-0} = \frac{\mathbf{v}_1 - \mathbf{v}_0}{t_1 - t_0} = \frac{\mathbf{v}_1 - \mathbf{v}_0}{\Delta t} = \frac{v_{x1} - v_{x0}}{\Delta t}\,\mathbf{i} + \frac{v_{y1} - v_{y0}}{\Delta t}\,\mathbf{j} + \frac{v_{z1} - v_{z0}}{\Delta t}\,\mathbf{k}
\tag{3.24}
$$

$$
\mathbf{a}_{1-0} = a_{x,1-0}\mathbf{i} + a_{y,1-0}\mathbf{j} + a_{z,1-0}\mathbf{k}
$$

Sometimes, position is represented as a function. For many functions the derivative can be determined explicitly, and then the velocity and acceleration can be determined using analytical derivatives rather than numerical derivatives. We will examine the common case of the spline function. The cubic spline is often used to describe kinematic data. The x data can be represented as,

$$
x(t) = at^3 + bt^2 + ct + d
\tag{3.25}
$$

and the y data can be represented by,

$$
y(t) = et^3 + ft^2 + gt + h
\tag{3.26}
$$

The coefficients of the $x(t)$ and $y(t)$ polynomials (i.e, cubic splines) are a, b, c, d, e, f, g, and h. The coefficients can assume positive or negative values. Regression can be used to fit experimental data about cubic spline. The analytical derivative is based on assuming that $\Delta t$ becomes infinitely small (i.e., we take the limit as $\Delta t$ approaches zero). Velocity is the first derivative of position,

$$
v_x(t) = 3at^2 + 2bt + c
$$

$$
v_y(t) = 3et^2 + 2ft + g
\tag{3.27}
$$

Acceleration is the first derivative of velocity or the second derivative of position, and both are equivalent,

$$
a_x(t) = 6at + 2b
$$

$$
a_y(t) = 6et + 2f
\tag{3.28}
$$

The derivative exists for numerous functions, and several textbooks have been written to guide interested readers in calculating derivatives. Some of these books are listed at the end of this chapter.

Rotation is a very important form of motion when studying kinematics. The vector's position, velocity, and acceleration for translational motion have dual properties of angular position, angular velocity, and angular acceleration for rotational motion. Rotation appears for many types of activities. With a manually propelled wheelchair the drive wheels are rotated to cause motion. With electric-powered wheelchairs the motors turn the drive wheels with rotary motion. Even the seats and/or backrests of some wheelchairs rotate. When propelling a manual wheelchair, the user's arm segments rotate about joints to provide movement. We will use $\theta$ to represent angular position, $\omega$ to represent angular velocity, and $\alpha$ to represent angular acceleration. Angular position is referenced to horizontal and increases in the counterclockwise direction.

We again examine the case of the wheelchair pushrim. The position of a point on the pushrim can be defined in a cylindrical coordinate system with coordinates ($\theta$, r) or in Cartesian coordinates with (rcos$\theta$, rsin$\theta$) (see Figure 3.10).

Vectors in cylindrical coordinates are represented in a unique form, often referred to as phasor form,

$$\mathbf{p} = r \angle \theta \tag{3.29}$$

In Cartesian coordinates, the same position vector p has the form,

$$\mathbf{p} = r\cos\theta\mathbf{i} + r\sin\theta\mathbf{j} \tag{3.30}$$

The angular velocity of point **p** can be determined by taking the derivative of its position as a function of time,

$$\omega = \frac{d\theta(t)}{dt} \cong \frac{\Delta\theta(t)}{\Delta t} = \frac{\theta(t_f) - \theta(t_0)}{t_f - t_0} \tag{3.31}$$

**FIGURE 3.10**   Schematic of the angular and linear position, and angular velocity and linear velocity of a point on a pushrim

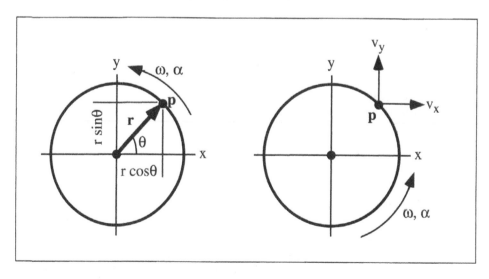

Angular velocity is positive for increasing angular position. The linear velocity of the same point can be calculated by taking the derivative, time rate of change, in the linear position,

$$\mathbf{v} = \frac{d\mathbf{p}(t)}{dt} \cong \frac{\Delta\mathbf{p}(t)}{\Delta t} = \frac{\mathbf{p}(t_f) - \mathbf{p}(t_0)}{t_f - t_0}$$

$$= \left( \frac{r\cos\theta(t_f) - r\cos\theta(t_0)}{t_f - t_0} \right)\mathbf{i} + \left( \frac{r\sin\theta(t_f) - r\sin\theta(t_0)}{t_f - t_0} \right) \tag{3.32}$$

The angular and linear velocity are related to each another, as one might expect. The functional relationship between linear and angular velocity for rotation of a rigid body with a constant radius, like a wheelchair pushrim or wheel, can be found using derivatives,

$$\mathbf{v} = \frac{dr\cos\theta(t)}{dt}\mathbf{i} + \frac{dr\sin\theta(t)}{dt}\mathbf{j} = -r\frac{d\theta(t)}{dt}\sin\theta(t)\mathbf{i} + r\frac{d\theta(t)}{dt}\cos\theta(t)\mathbf{j} \tag{3.33}$$

The derivative of $\mathbf{v}$ requires use of the chain rule, which is a fundamental theorem in calculus. Readers who are not well versed in derivatives should review the appropriate material in one of the books among the reading list at the end of the chapter. However, it should suffice to know that the derivative of the $\sin\theta$ is $\cos\theta$, and the derivative of $\cos\theta$ is $-\sin\theta$. The time derivative of angular position ($d\theta/dt$) is equal to angular velocity ($\omega$). This can be used to equate linear velocity to angular velocity,

$$\omega(t) = \frac{d\theta(t)}{dt} \qquad \mathbf{v} = -r\omega(t)\sin\theta(t)\mathbf{i} + r\omega(t)\cos\theta(t)\mathbf{j} \tag{3.34}$$

The magnitude of the velocity vector (v) is related to the angular velocity ($\theta$) by a simple but useful function,

$$v^2(t) = r^2\,\omega^2(t)\sin^2\theta(t) + r^2\,\omega^2(t)\cos^2\theta(t)$$
$$= r^2\,\omega^2(t)\left[\sin^2\theta(t) + \cos^2\theta(t)\right] = r^2\,\omega^2(t) \tag{3.35}$$

$$\omega^2(t) = \frac{v^2(t)}{r^2} \qquad \omega(t) = \frac{v(t)}{r}$$

Equation (3.35) provides a useful formula for converting between linear and angular velocity. The pushrim and wheel have the same angular velocity because they are attached to one another, but they do not have the same linear velocity because they have different radii. For example, if a rehabilitation engineer reported that the angular velocity of the pushrim was 3.28 radian/second (2 $\pi$ radians = 360 degrees), and that the wheel had a radius of 0.3048 meters (12 inches), what would be the speed of the wheelchair? The speed of the wheelchair is identical to the speed of the wheel, if we can assume no slip. Therefore, the speed of the wheelchair is

$$v = \omega r = (3.28 \text{ radians / s})(0.3048 \text{ meters}) = 1 \text{ m / s} \tag{3.36}$$

Note that the radians do not transfer to the final units. Radians are one of the few units that have no dimensions, and therefore are not reflected in the final dimensions. We have examined angular position and velocity, but angular acceleration remains to be examined. Angular acceleration is important since torque is related to angular acceleration as force is related to linear acceleration. Angular acceleration ($\alpha$) is the time derivative of angular velocity ($\omega$),

$$\alpha = \frac{d\omega(t)}{dt} \cong \frac{\Delta\omega(t)}{\Delta t} = \frac{\omega(t_f) - \omega(t_0)}{t_f - t_0} \tag{3.37}$$

Angular acceleration is positive for increasing angular velocity. The linear acceleration of the same point can be calculated by taking the derivative, time rate of change, in the linear velocity,

$$\begin{aligned}
\mathbf{a} &= \frac{d\mathbf{v}(t)}{dt} \cong \frac{\Delta\mathbf{v}(t)}{\Delta t} = \frac{\mathbf{v}(t_f) - \mathbf{v}(t_0)}{t_f - t_0} \\
&= \left(\frac{-r\omega(t)\sin\theta(t_f) + r\omega(t)\sin\theta(t_0)}{t_f - t_0}\right)\mathbf{i} + \left(\frac{-r\omega(t)\cos\theta(t_f) - r\omega(t)\cos\theta(t_0)}{t_f - t_0}\right)\mathbf{j}
\end{aligned} \tag{3.38}$$

The angular and linear acceleration are also related to one another. The functional relationship between linear and angular acceleration for rotation of a rigid body with a constant radius, like a wheelchair pushrim or wheel, can be found using derivatives and the product rule,

$$\begin{aligned}
\mathbf{a} &= \frac{d}{dt}r\omega(t)\sin\theta(t)\mathbf{i} + \frac{d}{dt}r\omega(t)\cos\theta(t)\mathbf{j} \\
&= -r\left[\omega\frac{d\theta}{dt}\cos\theta + \frac{d\omega}{dt}\sin\theta\right]\mathbf{i} + r\left[-\omega\frac{d\theta}{dt}\sin\theta + \frac{d\omega}{dt}\cos\theta\right]\mathbf{j}
\end{aligned} \tag{3.39}$$

From our previous calculation of the angular velocity as a function of linear velocity, we know that

$$\omega(t) = \frac{d\theta(t)}{dt} \tag{3.40}$$

and by definition

$$\alpha \equiv \frac{d\omega(t)}{dt} \tag{3.41}$$

Therefore,

$$\begin{aligned}
\mathbf{a} &= -r\left[\omega\frac{d\theta}{dt}\cos\theta + \frac{d\omega}{dt}\sin\theta\right]\mathbf{i} + r\left[-\omega\frac{d\theta}{dt}\sin\theta + \frac{d\omega}{dt}\cos\theta\right]\mathbf{j} \\
&= -r\left[\omega^2\cos\theta + \alpha\sin\theta\right]\mathbf{i} + r\left[-\omega^2\sin + \alpha\cos\theta\right]\mathbf{j}
\end{aligned} \tag{3.42}$$

We have shown

$$\omega^2 = \frac{v^2}{r^2} \tag{3.43}$$

Therefore,

$$\mathbf{a} == -r\left[\omega^2\cos\theta + \alpha\sin\theta\right]\mathbf{i} + r\left[-\omega^2\sin\theta + \alpha\cos\theta\right]\mathbf{j}$$
$$= -r\left[\frac{v^2}{r^2}\cos\theta + \alpha\sin\theta\right]\mathbf{i} + r\left[-\frac{v^2}{r^2}\sin\theta + \alpha\cos\theta\right]\mathbf{j} \tag{3.44}$$

The radius of the pushrim (r) can be brought within the brackets to simplify the linear acceleration equation,

$$\mathbf{a} = -r\left[\frac{v^2}{r^2}\cos\theta + \alpha\sin\theta\right]\mathbf{i} + r\left[-\frac{v^2}{r^2}\sin\theta + \alpha\cos\theta\right]\mathbf{j}$$
$$= -r\left[\frac{v^2}{r^2}\cos\theta + r\alpha\sin\theta\right]\mathbf{i} + \left[-\frac{v^2}{r}\sin\theta + r\alpha\cos\theta\right]\mathbf{j} \tag{3.45}$$

Close examination of equation (3.45) reveals a symmetry that can be exploited to yield additional information about the linear acceleration,

$$\mathbf{a} = -\left[\frac{v^2}{r}\cos\theta + r\alpha\sin\theta\right]\mathbf{i} + r\left[-\frac{v^2}{r}\sin\theta + r\alpha\cos\theta\right]\mathbf{j}$$
$$= -\frac{v^2}{r}\left[\cos\theta\mathbf{i} + \sin\theta\mathbf{j}\right] + r\alpha\left[\sin\theta\mathbf{i} + \cos\theta\mathbf{j}\right] \tag{3.46}$$
$$= \mathbf{a}_n + \mathbf{a}_t$$

where $\mathbf{a}_n$ and $\mathbf{a}_t$ are the normal (radial) and tangential acceleration components of the linear acceleration. The normal acceleration is related to the change in direction of the linear velocity vector and has magnitude,

$$a_n = \frac{v^2}{r} \tag{3.47}$$

The tangential acceleration is related to the change in magnitude of the linear velocity vector and has magnitude,

$$a_t = r\alpha \tag{3.48}$$

The magnitude of the acceleration of the pushrim is equal to the magnitude of the vector sum of the normal and tangential linear acceleration components,

$$a = \sqrt{a_n^2 + a_t^2} \tag{3.49}$$

The techniques and definitions described in this section provide much of the foundation required to understand basic wheelchair biomechanics, mechanics of multi-configuration wheelchairs (e.g., tilt-in-space, recliner, stand-up), and basic power wheelchair operation. These concepts are also used extensively in wheelchair standards. Engineers and scientists use more complex analysis tools and methods, but this section should provide the material necessary to communicate and provide background for further learning in this area.

### 3.3.2 Kinetics

Forces are classified as either *internal* or *external*. Internal forces are either those that result from external forces or forces generated within the body. When muscles contract they generate force. Muscle forces are considered internal forces. When a person stretches a rubber band, an external force is being applied. However, forces internal to the rubber band are felt by the person as the rubber band stretches. Forces are also considered passive or active. Passive forces do not require an energy source. For example, a spring supplies a passive force. In other words, a spring responds to an external force. Active forces are generated by an *actuator*. An actuator is a device that converts energy from a source (e.g., electricity, magnetism, hydraulics, water) and converts it to mechanical energy. An electric motor is an example of an actuator as it converts electricity to torque or mechanical power. An active force can be used to drive or move an object. Muscle forces are active forces. Muscles convert metabolic energy through glycolysis to mechanical energy through muscle contraction across a joint or joints.

Two or more forces acting on a single body constitute a force system. Both manual and powered wheelchairs involve force systems. Manual wheelchairs interact with forces applied by the user's hands to the pushrims, to the user's body against the seat, to the user's legs against the legrests, to the ground through the wheels and casters, and to assistants against the canes. Electric-powered wheelchairs also experience multiple forces, many of which are similar to those of manual wheelchairs, but they also experience the forces exerted by the motors, arms against armrests, and vehicle tie-downs against the frame.

Forces are further classified according to their orientation or line of action with respect to the body that they are acting on. We will address a few of the more common classifications of forces, which will be used to describe actions and reactions during wheelchair use. The concepts of tangential and normal forces have already been introduced. A normal force is applied perpendicular to the contact surface. When a wheelchair sits on or rolls along the floor it applies a normal force to the floor (see Figure 3.11). This normal force is what contributes to compression of the tires, and friction between the tires and the ground. The friction between the floor and the tires is a tangential force which retards the motion of the wheelchair. In reality, some friction is required to drive the wheelchair forward, otherwise the drive wheels would spin (e.g., when driving on ice the friction is reduced and the tendency for the wheels to spin is increased). Similarly, the hand applies a force vector to the pushrim of a manual wheelchair that has both a normal and tangential component. The normal component helps to generate friction between the hand and pushrim, whereas the tangential force turns the wheel to drive the wheelchair.

Coplanar and collinear forces have similar definitions. Collinear forces act along a common line of action. The magnitude of the resultant force for collinear forces requires only simple addition or subtraction, depending on how the forces interact. The forces acting on a rope used to pull a wheelchair would be collinear

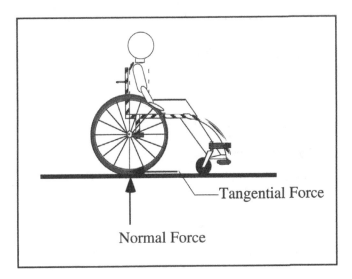

Tangential Force

Normal Force

**FIGURE 3.11** Illustration of normal and tangential forces acting on a wheelchair

(see Figure 3.12). Coplanar forces act in a common plane. Coplanar forces are sometimes referred to as two-dimensional forces, because the appropriate choice of coordinates makes one of the direction components zero for both force vectors. For example, all forces that act only in the sagittal plane are coplanar forces.

Concurrent force systems have lines of action that intersect at a common point. For example, the force applied by the hands of a scooter driver to the tiller of a scooter are concurrent forces (see Figure 3.13). If the angles and magnitudes of concurrent forces are known, the geometry of the concurrent force system can be used to conduct a more in-depth analysis. For example, the forces applied by an assistant to the push handles on the canes of a wheelchair form a concurrent force system. Knowledge of the force system can be used to analyze the backrest forces.

Tensile forces tend to stretch or elongate a body. Tensile forces are applied to the rope in Figure 3.12, or to a rubber band when stretched. Compressive forces

**FIGURE 3.12** Illustration of collinear forces

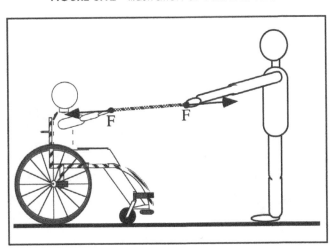

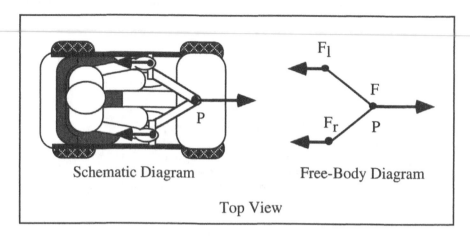

Schematic Diagram          Free-Body Diagram

Top View

**FIGURE 3.13**  Concurrent forces applied by the driver's hands to the tiller of a scooter

tend to push an object together. Compressive forces are in action when a wheelchair tire drives over a tack. The tack compresses the tire through the force of the weight of the wheelchair and rider upon the tires, and the tack pushes upward with the reaction force of the same magnitude. If the forces are high enough, the tack punctures the tire (see Figure 3.14).

Parallel forces have lines of action parallel to each another. The propulsive force of the wheel against the ground acts parallel to the friction force which retards the motion of the wheelchair. If a person holds the upper arm vertical and forearm horizontal (the humerus vertical and ulna horizontal) with a weight in the hand, then the force of gravity acting on the weight will be parallel to the force applied by the biceps, and the reaction force through the humerus.

Gravitational forces have an important role in the study of wheelchair use. Gravitational forces are always proportional to the mass of an object. This is because

**FIGURE 3.14**  Illustration of compressive forces experienced when a wheelchair tires rolls over a tack

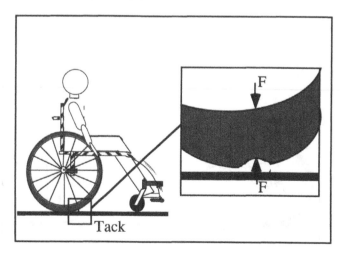

earth has a constant acceleration due to gravity. All objects are pulled toward the earth at the same rate of acceleration. This rate of acceleration is denoted by the symbol g, for gravity. The earth's gravitational acceleration (g) has a constant value of 9.81 m/s² (32 ft/s²). The force due to gravity is commonly called the weight of an object and can be found by the formula

$$W = m \bullet g \text{ (Newtons)} \qquad g = 9.81 \text{ m/s}^2 \qquad (3.50)$$

Gravity is always in the direction of the earth's center. Hence the force of gravity always points toward the earth's center, regardless of the orientation of the object. The fact that the direction of the gravitational force remains constant is important in the analysis of many problems.

### 3.3.3 Distributed Force Systems and Pressure

For most problems involving wheelchairs, the wheelchair and user can be assumed to be made of rigid members that are interconnected. Several forces may act on a rigid member simultaneously. When a force or set of forces is applied over an area, we call it or them a distributed force. When a person's hand grasps a pushrim, it applies a distributed force over the palmar surface of the hand in contact with the pushrim. However, for analysis it is convenient to represent a distributed force by a single force. A distributed force applied over an area can be represented by an equivalent force or concentrated load. The magnitude of the equivalent force is equal to the sum of all applied force vectors.

Gravity acting on a body acts as a distributed force, but is often treated as a single equivalent force (see Figure 3.15). When the distributed force of gravity is applied, the line of action for the equivalent force passes through the center of mass (center of gravity). The center of mass is the point about which an object will balance in three-planes. A simple way to measure center of mass is to hang an object by three different points, and to determine the point of intersection of the three lines (see Figure 3.16).

**FIGURE 3.15** Illustration of distributed force due to gravity acting on a body

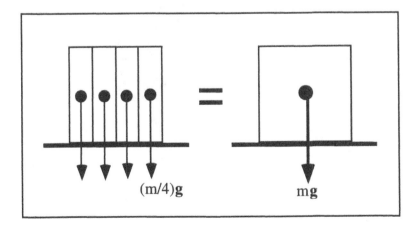

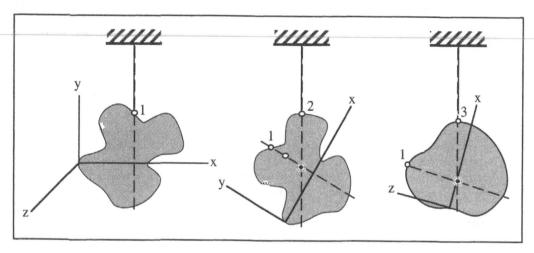

**FIGURE 3.16**  Illustration of three-point method for determining the center of gravity for an arbitrary body. The three points must be in two different planes. The intersection of the three vertical lines passing through the different hanging points provides the center of gravity. The use of x, y, and z axes attached to the body help to locate the center of gravity.

The center of gravity for homogeneous objects (i.e., objects made of the same material or same distribution of material) can be found using the geometric center of the body (see Figure 3.17). This method can be used to estimate the center of mass using simple geometric shapes.

**FIGURE 3.17**  The center of gravity (c.o.g. = • ) is located at the geometric center of homogeneous objects

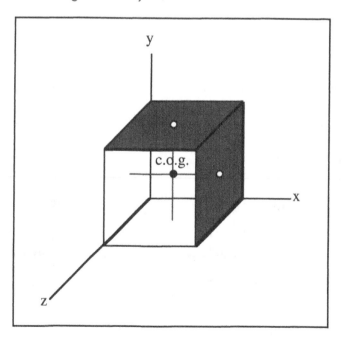

The center of gravity can also be determined for bodies of multiple geometric shapes. The center of gravity is determined for the x, y, and z planes for each geometric shape. The center of gravity for the entire body (x, y, z) times the total (m) is equal to the sum of the masses of each of the elements times the center of gravity location for each of the masses,

$$mx = m_1\,x_1 + m_2\,x_2 + m_3\,x_3 \ldots + m_k\,x_k$$
$$my = m_1\,y_1 + m_2\,y_2 + m_3\,y_3 \ldots + m_k\,y_k$$
$$mz = m_1\,z_1 + m_2\,z_2 + m_3\,z_3 \ldots + m_k\,z_k \qquad (3.51)$$
$$m = m_1 + m_2 + m_3 \ldots + m_k$$

The composite center of mass is illustrated in Figure 3.18. The square in this figure is made up of five smaller squares. Each of the smaller squares has a center of mass represented by $x_1$, $x_2$, $x_3$, $x_4$, and $x_5$ along the horizontal axis. Each of the five smaller squares also has a mass of $m_1$, $m_2$, $m_3$, $m_4$, and $m_5$, respectively. Mass is a scalar, therefore the total mass (m) is simply the sum of the masses of each of the parts. The composite center of mass is related to the individual centers of mass by equation (3.51).

Pressure is a metric of the intensity of distributed loads. Pressure is defined as the total applied force divided by the area over which the force is applied.

$$p = pressure = F/A \ (m/lt^2) \qquad (3.52)$$

Pressure is reported in $N/m^2$ or Pascals (Pa). An important property of pressure is that it increases as the surface area decreases, and vice versa. Pressure is con-

**FIGURE 3.18**   Example of center of mass for a composite mass

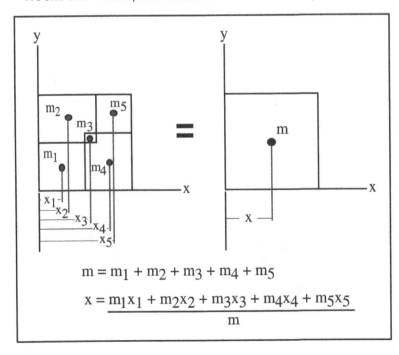

sidered clinically important when evaluating seating or cushion systems for people with disabilities. Decubitus ulcers (also known as pressure sores) form from occluded blood flow to soft tissue. Prolonged sitting causes decubitus ulcers to form over the ischial tuberosities or greater trochanters. This is believed to happen because these bony prominences carry a substantial portion of the body's weight while seated. The force due to body weight can be considered constant while sitting, thus the pressure can be lowered by increasing the amount of area supporting the seating surface (see Figure 3.19).

Pressure also plays an important role in the selection of casters and tires. We will examine pressure further in the context of seating.

### 3.3.4 Moments

A force can be applied to bend and/or rotate an object, depending on how the force is applied and the object is situated. A moment is associated with the bending or rotating action of the applied force. Previously, we showed that the moment is related to the vector cross product. A moment is also a vector quantity. Let us revisit the example of the force vector applied to the pushrim by a user's hand. The

**FIGURE 3.19**  Seating force pressure is affected by the contouring of the cushion. For a foam cushion, contouring increases the contact area, which reduces the pressure.

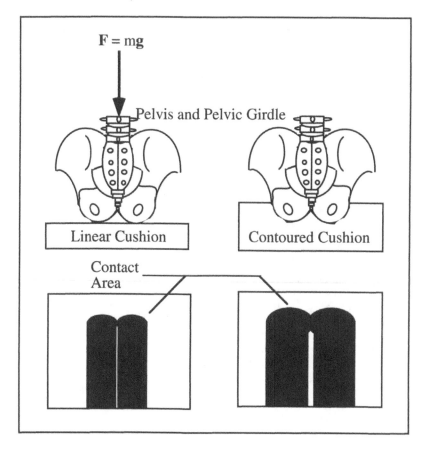

moment is the cross product between the pushrim radius vector and the force vector applied by the hand,

$$\mathbf{f}_t = f\sin\theta(-\sin\phi\ \mathbf{i} + \cos\phi\ \mathbf{j})$$
$$\mathbf{r} = r(\cos\phi\ \mathbf{i} + \sin\phi\ \mathbf{j})$$

$$\mathbf{r}\ \mathrm{x}\ \mathbf{f} = r(\cos\phi\ \mathbf{i} + \sin\phi\ \mathbf{j})\ \mathrm{x}\ f\sin\theta(\sin\phi\ \mathbf{i} - \cos\phi\ \mathbf{j}) = rf\sin\theta\ \mathbf{k}$$

$$(3.53)$$

The equations above describe the applied moment by using the concept of the tangential force times the radius to determine the moment about the wheel's hub. Another approach is to use the concept of the moment arm. The magnitude of a moment is equal to the applied force times the moment arm.

$$M = df \tag{3.54}$$

The right-hand rule is used to define a positive moment. The moment arm is the perpendicular distance between the point of force application and the center of rotation. The moment arm is useful when examining how forces are applied. Figure 3.20 examines the case of the pushrim. As the force vector applied by the hand to the pushrim becomes more tangential, the moment arm becomes closer to the radius of the pushrim. The moment arm is often easier to visualize than the vector cross product, and provides a means for estimating how forces are going to affect a body.

Moments are vectors and as such are subject to the rules of vector mathematics. Moments are important when assessing the strength of wheelchair components, examining wheelchair propulsion, evaluating power wheelchair drive train components, and in understanding the biomechanics of multi-configuration wheelchairs.

**FIGURE 3.20**  Schematic of the concept of a moment arm when examining moments produced by a force

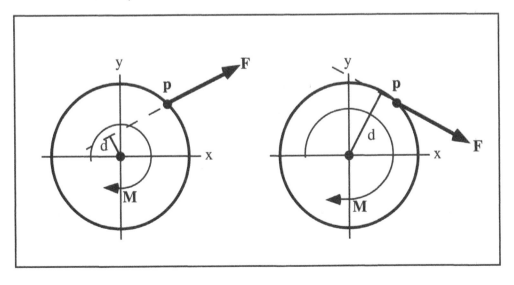

### 3.3.5 Dynamics of Motion

The biomechanics and analysis of motion of wheelchairs requires the use of forces as well as vectors which describe motion (e.g., position, velocity, acceleration). Combining such information provides greater insight into the workings of the body, and provides information about the use of wheelchairs and the effect on the wheelchair. We will introduce four important dynamics properties in this section: inertia, momentum, energy, and power. These properties will reappear in subsequent chapters related to specific aspects of wheelchairs.

*Mass moment of inertia* (I) behaves similar to mass in rotational systems. Inertia in the general sense means resistance to change. In mechanics, mass moment of inertia is the resistance to angular acceleration, much the same way mass can be viewed as the resistance to linear acceleration. The mass moment of inertia of a rigid body is proportional to its mass and volume. Therefore, when determining the mass moment of inertia, consider the mass, geometry, and location. The distribution of the body's mass about the axis of rotation affects the body's resistance to angular acceleration. The mass moment of inertia for most wheelchair systems and their associated biomechanics can be defined using simple geometry and an axis of symmetry (called a *centroid axis*) (see Figure 3.21). The mass moment of inertia is a scalar quantity that has units of kg • m².

The mass moment of inertia about a centroid axis would be of limited use for many applications. In realistic situations, rotations may be about arbitrary axes. However, rotations can be described about the three orthogonal axes x, y, and z. Hence, rotations can be viewed as axes parallel to the centroid axes. The *parallel axis theorem* states that if the mass moment of inertia of a body is known about a centroid axis, then the mass moment of inertia about any other axis parallel to that centroid axis can be determined by the relation

$$I = I_0 + m\delta^2 \tag{3.54}$$

where I is the mass moment of inertia about the parallel axis, $I_0$ is the mass moment of inertia about a centroid axis through the center of mass, m is the total mass of the body, and $\delta$ is the perpendicular distance between the two axes. The parallel axis theorem is important in studying the biomechanics of wheelchair propulsion. Most published tables present the mass moment of inertia for limb segments (e.g., forearm, upper arm, torso) about their centers of mass. However, most limbs rotate about joints that are not located at their centers of mass. The parallel axis theorem provides a tool for finding the mass moment of inertia about a joint from the mass moment of inertia about the center of mass.

Newton's second law states that force (f) is proportional to acceleration,

$$\mathbf{f} = \mathbf{ma} \tag{3.55}$$

We have shown that acceleration is equal to the time rate of change of velocity (i.e., acceleration is the time derivative of velocity),

$$\mathbf{a} = d\mathbf{v}/dt \tag{3.56}$$

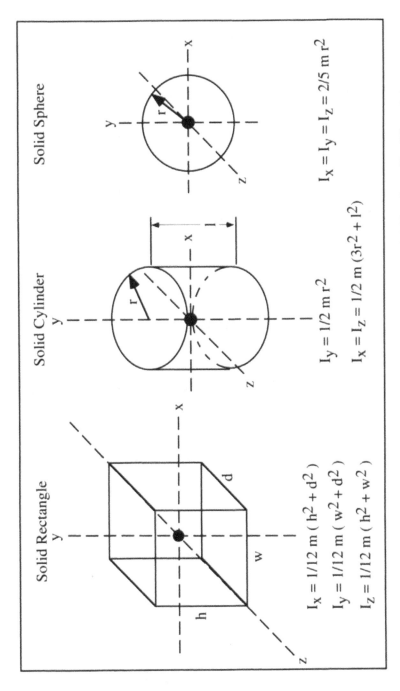

**FIGURE 3.21** Mass moments of inertia for common homogeneous rigid bodies with different shapes

Solid Rectangle

$I_x = 1/12 \, m \, (h^2 + d^2)$
$I_y = 1/12 \, m \, (w^2 + d^2)$
$I_z = 1/12 \, m \, (h^2 + w^2)$

Solid Cylinder

$I_y = 1/2 \, m \, r^2$
$I_x = I_z = 1/2 \, m \, (3r^2 + l^2)$

Solid Sphere

$I_x = I_y = I_z = 2/5 \, m \, r^2$

The resultant force on an object is equal to the time rate of change in the momentum of the object,

$$f = \frac{d}{dt}(mv) \qquad (3.57)$$

Momentum is a vector quantity; the mv term is called the *linear momentum.* The line of action of the linear momentum vector is the same as the velocity vector. The magnitude of the velocity vector is equal to the mass times the speed of the object. Momentum is an important property when solving many wheelchair and biomechanics problems. Momentum is used to analyze problems that involve rapid changes in velocity. For example, the dynamics of a wheelchair during a vehicle accident can be analyzed using momentum methods. Rotational systems may also contain momentum. For example, a flywheel stores energy based on its momentum. Linear momentum is the product of the object's mass and its velocity. Similarly, *angular momentum* is the product of an object's inertia, which we have learned behaves like an object's mass in rotational systems, and its angular velocity,

$$\text{angular momentum} = I\omega \qquad (3.58)$$

The angular velocity and angular momentum of an object will increase if a torque is applied in the direction of motion. We must define a few other important properties before moving to an illustrative example. Work is a concept that most people are familiar with, but in engineering it has a very specific meaning. *Work* is the product of force and displacement. Work is a scalar quantity. When a person pushes a wheelchair he or she is performing work. An important concept related to

**FIGURE 3.22**  Example of tangential pushrim force applied to the pushrim of a manual wheelchair from 100 degrees to 15 degrees. Only the tangential component of the force contributes to work, because that is the direction of motion.

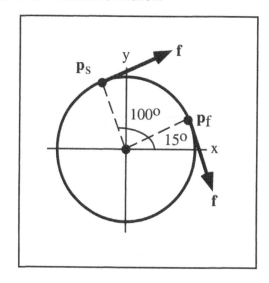

work is that without motion no work can be performed. Let's examine the case of pushing the pushrim of a wheelchair (see Figure 3.22).

If a person applies a constant tangential force of 70 Newtons on a pushrim of 0.26 meters radius from 100 degrees to 15 degrees, then the amount of work done is

$$W = fs \text{ Joules (J)} \tag{3.57}$$

We must calculate the distance over which the force is applied. In this case, the distance is the arc length of the pushrim from the starting angle (100 degrees) to the finishing angle (15 degrees). The arc length (s) is equal to the difference in the angle in radians times the radius of the pushrim,

$$100 \text{ degrees} = 1.74 \text{ radians}$$
$$15 \text{ degrees} = 0.26 \text{ radians}$$

$$s = (1.74 - 0.26)r = 1.48r = 1.48(0.26) = 0.38 \text{ m}$$

Therefore, the work done on the pushrim is

$$W = fs = 70(0.38) = 26.6 \text{ N} \bullet \text{m} = 26.6 \text{ J}$$

Work is important when evaluating manual wheelchair propulsion because it is related to efficiency of the stroke biomechanics. A person can increase the amount of work done on the pushrim either by increasing the amount of force or by extending the arc length over which the force is applied. Because it may be impossible for some wheelchair users to generate higher forces, and in some cases higher forces may lead to repetitive strain injuries, mobility specialists often try to optimize positioning to increase stroke length. This is exaggerated in wheelchair racing, as we shall demonstrate later.

We will work with two basic forms of energy throughout this book: electrical and mechanical. This chapter focuses on mechanical energy. Electrical energy will be dealt with in subsequent chapters. *Energy* describes the capacity of a system of bodies or elements to do work. Energy is a scalar quantity. Mechanical energy can be divided into potential energy and kinetic energy. *Potential energy* is related to the position of a body or element. Wheelchairs experience two types of potential energy. Gravitational potential energy is a function of the body's position with respect to the earth's surface. The higher an object is from the earth, but still within the earth's strong gravitational field, the greater its potential energy. Previously, we showed that the earth's gravity can act on a body to create a force. If the body is elevated above the earth, then the force has a greater distance over which to perform work. Therefore, gravitational potential energy (P.E.) is a function of the body's mass (m), the earth's gravitational acceleration (g), and the height of the object above the earth (h),

$$\text{P.E.} = mgh \tag{3.58}$$

Potential energy is used extensively in the analysis of wheelchairs, and, as anyone who has pushed a wheelchair up a ramp will tell you, potential energy has a definite effect on wheelchair use. In the wheelchair standards, various wheelchair components are dropped from a specific height to determine if they will retain their function after impact. The heights specified are based on the potential energy of the wheelchair component.

Springs also provide an important source of potential energy. The potential energy from a spring is called *elastic potential energy*. Many materials used in wheelchairs have elastic properties: foam cushions, wheelchair frames, wheels, casters, and upholstery. We will concentrate on analyzing the elastic potential energy of wheelchairs and wheelchair use through the application of the *theory of springs* (also known as Hooke's Law), proposed by Robert Hooke in 1642. There are many types of springs, and some of them will be introduced throughout the text as they relate to specific applications. However, an important property of springs that we will use is: the force (f) applied by a spring is proportional to the displacement of the spring (x),

$$f = kx \qquad (3.59)$$

Once a spring is either compressed or stretched, it has the ability to perform work. This property is exploited by the spring suspension system. When a person in a wheelchair drives off a curb, the foam cushion compresses upon impact and the cushion gains elastic potential energy. The foam then performs work on the person's body, returning it to the same seating position. The elastic potential energy is equal to the integral of the spring force over the displacement of the spring,

$$P.\,E._{\text{spring}} = \int_0^{x_f} f dx = \int_0^{x_f} kx dx = \frac{1}{2} kx_f^2 \qquad (3.60)$$

Wheelchairs often experience potential energy and kinetic energy. Potential energy is associated with position, whereas *kinetic energy* is associated with motion. Kinetic energy is a function of an object's mass (m) and speed (v),

$$K.E. = 1/2\, mv^2 \qquad (3.61)$$

Kinetic energy is a scalar quantity. Kinetic energy and work are related. The *work-energy theorem* states that the net work done on an object is equal to the change in kinetic energy. In the example of the work done on the pushrim from 100 degrees to 15 degrees, we found the net work to be 26.6 Joules. If the starting (initial) speed is 1 m/s and the wheelchair and rider have a mass of 100 kilograms, we can use the work-energy theorem to find the final speed of the wheelchair as the hand reaches 15 degrees,

$$W_{100°-15°} = \tfrac{1}{2} mv_f^2 - \tfrac{1}{2} mv_s^2$$

$$26.6\,\mathbf{J} = \tfrac{1}{2}(100)v_f^2 - \tfrac{1}{2}(100)(1)^2 \qquad (3.62)$$

We must use some algebra to rearrange the above equation to solve for $v_f$,

$$26.6 + \tfrac{1}{2}(100)(1)^2 = \tfrac{1}{2}(100)v_f^2$$

$$v_f^2 = \frac{26.6 + \tfrac{1}{2}(100)(1)^2}{\tfrac{1}{2}(100)} = 1.53$$

$$v_f = \sqrt{1.53} = 1.2 \ \mathbf{m/s}$$

This example shows that as work is performed on the pushrim, the speed of the wheelchair and rider increases. Because of the cyclic nature of wheelchair propulsion (i.e., the arms push the pushrims, and then let go for the next stroke), the wheelchair is nearly always changing speed. First the wheelchair accelerates as the hands begin to apply force, and then it decelerates as the hands release the pushrim in preparation for the next stroke. The amount of force required to maintain a desired speed is related to the design of the wheelchair, wheelchair user interaction, and the abilities of the user. We will examine these factors throughout various chapters in this book.

When assessing both manual and power wheelchairs, power is a useful metric. *Power* is the time rate of change of work,

$$P = \frac{dW}{dt} \approx \frac{\Delta W}{\Delta t} = \frac{W_f - W_s}{t_f - t_s} \tag{3.63}$$

Power is more commonly determined as the dot product between force and velocity,

$$P = \mathbf{f} \bullet \mathbf{v} \tag{3.64}$$

In rotational systems, power is the dot product of moment and angular velocity,

$$P = \mathbf{m} \bullet \omega \tag{3.65}$$

Power is a scalar and has units of watts. Power can be related to energy expenditure of the body during manual wheelchair ergonomic studies and is an important part of measuring gross mechanical efficiency. Gross mechanical efficiency (G.M.E.) is the ratio of mechanical power to metabolic-power,

$$\text{G.M.E.} = \frac{P_{\text{mechanical}}}{P_{\text{metabolic}}} \tag{3.66}$$

Power is also important in selecting the appropriate size of the motors and batteries required for electric-powered wheelchairs. Power can also be used to estimate the type of power wheelchair required for a particular user. For example, the power required to push a manual wheelchair during various types of activities can be compared to a person's fitness (i.e., ability to convert metabolic power) to assist in selecting a wheelchair, or when considering whether an electric-powered wheelchair may be more appropriate for an activity than a manual wheelchair. Power measurements can also be used to determine the type of power wheelchair required for various activities.

Momentum and energy methods can be used to solve important wheelchair design and fitting questions. The world is full of obstacles for wheelchair users. During rehabilitation, clinicians attempt to teach neophyte wheelchair users to negotiate curbs, doors and door thresholds, ramps, and curb cuts, among other things. It is important when prescribing and evaluating the use of a wheelchair to assess the user's ability to negotiate common obstacles in the environment. Tips and falls are among the most common causes of injury among wheelchair users.

The proper design and prescription of a wheelchair is not a trivial matter. Prescribing wheelchairs for children can be particularly challenging, because few wheelchairs are designed specifically for children. A common compromise clinicians make is to use smaller components on an adult-style wheelchair. This may increase the tendency of the wheelchair user to flip forward over the front wheels when hitting a threshold (e.g., door threshold, sidewalk crack).

Let us examine the case of an eight-year-old child with spina bifida at thoracic level 12 who uses a manual wheelchair for personal mobility. She is bright, intelligent, and generally a happy child. The child typically wears ankle-foot-orthoses (AFOs), and has been using a wheelchair since age 30–36 months. She uses a hook-and-loop chest strap and hook-and-loop lap belt for postural support. At 18 months, the child used a coaster cart. She has had four different manual wheelchairs. All of these wheelchairs were ultralight models. The child had the ability to perform small wheelies and to negotiate simple common obstacles with her latest wheelchair. She was assessed for a new wheelchair because she was outgrowing her current wheelchair. The child's physician wrote a prescription for it with the assistance from a physical therapist.

Upon receiving the wheelchair, the physical therapist examined it along with a rehabilitation technology supplier. Since the new wheelchair was the child's first adult-sized wheelchair, they should set it up to be as stable as possible for the rearmost position. However, increasing the rearward stability increases the likelihood of tipping forward. As an expert assistive technology provider, the therapist used momentum and energy methods to examine the forward tip stability of the child in her new wheelchair.

The therapist assumed that both front casters would hit a threshold at nearly the same time. When a wheelchair hits a threshold it undergoes an impulse at the point of contact of the front casters and threshold. The wheelchair and user then rotate about the axles of the front casters. Taking moments about the axles of the front caster, the moment of the impulsive force is zero (i.e., because the moment arm is zero) and angular momentum is conserved. The applicable velocity is the component of the wheelchair and user's velocity perpendicular to the threshold (i.e., along the line of progression). The equation for impulsive motion is

$$I\omega = mv_x y \qquad (3.67)$$

where:

     m = total mass of wheelchair and rider;

     I  = moment of inertia of the total mass about the axles of the front casters;

v = forward velocity of the wheelchair/rider when they first strike the threshold;

y = height of center of gravity above the axles of the front wheels;

$\omega$ = angular velocity of the wheelchair and rider.

For the wheelchair and rider to overturn, the center of gravity must be raised above the front axles of the wheelchair (equation 3.68) where x = horizontal location of center of gravity from the axles of the front wheels.

$$\Delta h = \left[\sqrt{x^2 + y^2} - y\right] \tag{3.68}$$

If the wheelchair and rider are to overturn, the kinetic energy remaining after the impact with the door threshold must be sufficient to lift the center of gravity for both through the distance given above ($\Delta h$). This means that the rotational kinetic energy of the wheelchair and rider upon impact with the curb must be greater than the gravitational potential energy obtained when the center of gravity of the wheelchair and rider are above the front casters. This condition is given by equation 3.69, where g = earth's gravitational constant.

$$\text{K.E.}_{\text{impact}} \geq \text{P.E.}_{\text{gravity}}$$

$$\tfrac{1}{2} I \omega^2 \geq mg\Delta h = mg\left[\sqrt{x^2 + y^2} - y\right] \tag{3.69}$$

The critical velocity ($v_x$) for flipping a wheelchair and rider about the front axles when hitting a door threshold or other similar obstacles is determined by combining the equations 3.67–3.69,

$$I\omega = mv_x y \tag{3.70}$$

which if squared becomes

$$I^2 \omega^2 = (I\omega^2) = m^2 v_x^2 y^2 \tag{3.71}$$

This equation can be substituted for the kinetic energy term in equation 3.69,

$$\tfrac{1}{2} I \omega^2 = \frac{m^2 v_x^2 y^2}{2I} \geq mg\Delta h \tag{3.72}$$

Equation 3.72 is now in a form that can be used to solve for $v_x$,

$$v_x^2 \geq \frac{2Ig\Delta h}{my^2} = \frac{2Ig}{my}\left[\sqrt{\left(1 + \frac{x^2}{y^2}\right)} - 1\right] \tag{3.73}$$

A more comprehensive model could be developed to describe this type of overturning, but it is unnecessary for most cases. In order to use this equation for the child in this case, some individual data must be collected from the child and

**TABLE 3.1  Anthropometric data for child**

| | |
|---|---|
| Total body mass | 23.1 kg |
| Lateral malleolus–head metatarsal II | 170 mm |
| Femoral condyles–medial malleolus | 340 mm |
| Greater trochanter–femoral condyles | 270 mm |
| Greater trochanter–glenohumeral joint | 370 mm |
| Head and neck (C7-T1–ear canal) | 170 mm |

her new wheelchair. Published tables and some simple anthropometric and wheelchair measurements can be used to determine the mass (m), inertia (I), and center of gravity position terms (x, y). Earth's gravitational constant is 9.81 m/s². Anthropometric measurements were made with a metric steel tape using standard anatomical landmarks (see Table 3.1). Wheelchair dimensions were also measured using a metric steel tape, a carpenter's square, and a carpenter's level.

Dynamic measurements were made using a stopwatch and two tape markers on a vinyl floor. The tape markers were placed two meters apart. The child was placed in her wheelchair, about 3 meters before the first tape marker. She was asked to push her new wheelchair as fast as she could. The therapist recorded the amount of time required to pass between the two tape markers placed 2 meters apart. The speed was calculated for each of three trials (see Table 3.2).

The therapist used anthropometric and seating measurements to calculate the location of the center of mass of each body segment with respect to the wheelchair's front axles. This will be covered in another chapter. The wheelchair center of mass was assumed to be located at the rear axles, in the sagittal plane. The composite wheelchair and user moment of inertia about the front axles was determined from the moments of inertia of the body segments of the wheelchair user and the moment of inertia for the wheelchair (see Table 3.3).

The moments of inertia for the user's body segments were calculated from each segment's radius of gyration given in standard table, and using the parallel-axis theorem to determine the inertia about the axles of the front casters. From the values in Table 3.3, and equation 3.73, the critical velocity can be calculated for this particular wheelchair and rider. The critical velocity for this subject is

$$v_x^2 \geq \frac{2Ig}{my}\left[\sqrt{\left(1+\frac{x^2}{y^2}\right)}-1\right] = \frac{2(17.1)(9.81)}{(31.2)(.465)}\left[\sqrt{\left(1+\frac{(-.22)^2}{(.465)^2}\right)}-1\right] = 1.57 \text{ m/s}$$

The highest speed that this subject was able to attain was 1.23 m/s. This speed is less than the 1.57 m/s required to flip forward when hitting a threshold. Therefore, the setting for the rear axles would be acceptable if the child were able to

**TABLE 3.2  Linear velocity over approximately 2 meters (N = 3)**

| | |
|---|---|
| $Vx_{mean}$ | 0.74 m/s |
| $Vx_{median}$ | 0.72 m/s |
| $Vx_{min}$ | 0.51 m/s |
| $Vx_{max}$ | 1.23 m/s |

**TABLE 3.3  Wheelchair and rider system characteristics**

| | |
|---|---|
| Moment of inertia front axles | 17.1 kg•m² |
| Earth's gravitational constant | 9.81 m/s² |
| C.O.G. with respect to front axles | x = −.22 m          y = .465 m |
| Mass of wheelchair with rider | 31.2 kg |

demonstrate or learn the ability to safely negotiate obstacles that she would encounter during normal activities of daily living. The center of gravity is often set to minimize the risk of having the person and wheelchair tip backwards. Many wheelchairs are also equipped with rear anti-tip casters. Wheelchairs used by young children should be equipped with forward anti-tip rollers.

## 3.4 Basic Mechanics of Materials

Wheelchairs and their users are subjected to internal forces and moments that relate to performance. Wheelchair standards are defined to simulate loads that the wheelchair would experience during normal and foreseeable use during its expected lifetime. The development of wheelchair standards requires some basic knowledge of materials and material properties. Furthermore, wheelchair users may also experience injuries or secondary disabilities through wheelchair use. Some understanding of material principles is necessary to understand the biomechanics of injury mechanisms.

Stress and strain are commonly used terms that are often confused. *Stress* in terms of the mechanics of materials is the ratio of the applied force divided by the cross-sectional area,

$$\text{stress} = \sigma = \frac{\text{force}}{\text{area}} = \frac{f}{A} \tag{3.74}$$

Stress is a vector quantity with units of Pascals (Pa). Stress is used to estimate when an object will fail. An important characteristic of stress is that it is a property of materials. If we were to take two pieces of steel 7/16 inch and 1/2 inch in diameter to be used as wheelchair axles, and attach one end of each prospective axle to a rigid frame and add weights to the other end, we would find that the force required to break the 1/2-inch axle would be higher than that required to break the 7/16-inch axle, which should not be too surprising. However, the stress at failure would be the same in both prospective axles. The stress at failure is often called the *yield stress*. The yield stress is a characteristic of materials, and can be used to select materials. Engineers when designing a wheelchair measure and calculate forces experienced by the wheelchair during active use and collect this information to select materials. A number of factors must be considered when selecting materials for a wheelchair. Important considerations are how strong does the part need to be, how large can or should it be, and how heavy should it be? By answering these questions the engineer has enough information to select the material based upon its yield stress.

As forces are applied to a material, the material undergoes deformations. The deformation of an object depends upon its dimensions, material properties, the magnitude of the applied force, and the duration of the applied force. Stress is related to the change in cross-sectional area in response to forces. *Strain* is related to the change in length of an object due to an applied load,

$$\text{strain} = \varepsilon = \frac{\text{change in length}}{\text{original length}} = \frac{\Delta l}{l} \tag{3.75}$$

Strain is a unitless vector quantity along the direction of the applied force. Stress and strain are used in studying wheelchair use and in designing wheelchairs. Engineers convert external forces and moments to internal forces and moments, particularly critical forces and moments. Internal forces and moments are used with appropriate formulas to determine stresses and strains, based upon material properties and the geometry of the part.

Elasticity, ductility, stiffness, and brittleness are material properties that are related to stress-strain curves and relations. A tool commonly used by engineers to select materials is the stress-strain curve. If two samples regardless of geometry are tested and their stress-strain curves plotted, then the stiffer of the two materials can be identified (see Figure 3.23). The diagram shows that sample 2 can be deformed more easily than sample 1, which indicates that the stiffness of sample 1 is higher than that of sample 2.

Most important material properties are defined based upon the characteristics of the material's stress-strain curve. We will examine several material properties based upon an example stress-strain curve (see Figure 3.24). There are six distinct points on a stress-strain curve that correspond to properties of the material. We have labeled these o, p, e, y, u, and r. The point o represents the origin, point p represents the *proportionality limit*, point e represents the *elastic limit*, point y represents the *yield point*, point u represents the point of *ultimate stress*, and point r represents the *rupture or failure point*. The line from o to p is the section of the stress-strain curve where stress and strain are linearly proportional. In this range the material behaves much

**FIGURE 3.23** Stress-strain curve for two samples. Sample 1 is stiffer than sample 2.

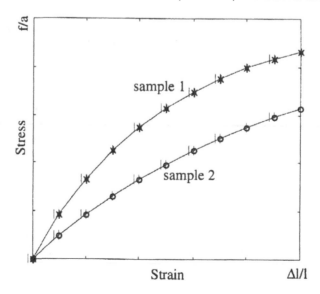

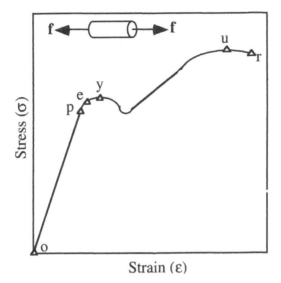

**FIGURE 3.24**  Example stress-strain curve showing critical points related to material properties

like a spring. The elastic limit, point e, represents the maximum stress that can be applied to the material without permanent deformation (i.e., if the force is removed the material will return to its original shape). The *yield strength* of the material is obtained at point y, which corresponds to the yield stress. At the yield stress substantial elongation can occur without increasing force. The ultimate stress of the material is equal to the *ultimate strength* and represents the highest point on the stress-strain curve. Due to a phenomenon called *necking*, the material can continue to elongate past the ultimate strength even after the force has been removed. The final point on a stress-strain curve provides the *rupture strength* of the material.

The slope of the linear portion of the stress-strain curve is called the *elastic* or *Young's modulus* (E). For linearly elastic materials, like most metals, the elastic modulus is a constant. The elastic modulus represents the stiffness of the material. As the elastic modulus increases, the stiffness increases. Elasticity is also defined by stress-strain relationships. *Elasticity* is the ability of a material to return to its original size and shape once the applied force has been removed. Linearly elastic materials act as springs within their elastic region (i.e., the displacement of the material is proportional to the applied force). This elastic property of materials is often exploited to create force sensors in biomechanics, and to add suspension systems to wheelchairs.

In engineering, *plastic deformation* implies that the material has permanently changed shape. Plastic deformations occur when a force is applied above the elastic limit. Plastic deformations are not necessarily undesirable. When making bends to the tubes of a wheelchair frame, the tubes experience plastic deformation. We need to be aware of the effect the bending has on the strength of the material. Once the wheelchair frame is assembled, plastic deformation is to be avoided or the wheelchair may not perform properly. However, elastic deformations may help to dampen some of the small bumps in our path.

More information can be determined from the stress-strain curves. The modulus of elasticity defines the stiffness of the material. The higher the modulus the higher the stiffness, and the greater the resistance to deformation. The *ductility* of a material is defined by the amount of plastic deformation prior to failure (i.e., the distance between points y and u on Figure 3.24). The *brittleness* of a material is the opposite of ductility. A brittle material will experience a rupture without significant plastic deformation (i.e., the distance between points y and r on Figure 3.24 will be small). *Toughness* is also used to describe materials. Toughness is defined as the total area under the stress-strain curve. Toughness is used to define the capacity of a material to sustain permanent plastic deformation.

## 3.5 Properties of Materials

### 3.5.1 Steel for Use in Wheelchairs

Steel is primarily a combination of iron and carbon. Steel also contains varying amounts of other materials. The percent of carbon and other materials mixed with the steel affects the properties and characteristics of the resultant steel. Steel is an important structural material for wheelchair design. The principal raw materials for steel manufacture are iron ore, iron, steel scrap, coal, and limestone. Coal is converted into coke, gas, and chemicals in the coke ovens. Coke is used in the blast furnace as a fuel and reducing agent; the gas is burned in heating units and the chemicals are processed into various organic materials. Limestone is employed as a flux in both the blast furnace and steel-making furnace, where it serves to remove impurities from the melt.

The base material for making steel is pig iron. Pig iron is the product of the blast furnace. Pig iron contains large amounts of carbon, manganese, phosphorus, sulfur, and silicon. In its raw form, pig iron is hard and brittle. Steel-making is the process of removing undesirable elements from pig iron and replacing them with desirable elements in the proper proportions. The final elements may be the same as those originally removed, but in different proportions. Most steel is manufactured using open-hearth, basic oxygen, or electric arc processes. Open-hearth furnaces are used for a wide range of steels that need only nominally restrictive control. It can be used to create high-quality basic steels. Basic oxygen furnaces (BOF) involve the same chemical reactions as open-hearth furnaces, but a BOF introduces nearly pure oxygen into the process at key times. This increases the rate at which steel can be produced. Specialty steels, stainless, tool steel, and high-alloy are made in electric arc furnaces. Electric arc furnaces provide much greater temperature control required for making complex steels.

The percentages of various alloying elements has an effect on the properties of the steel. The steel industry has studied the properties of steel with different alloying elements in varying amounts. The purpose of these studies was to develop some standard steels that engineers could use in their designs. These standards were designed to meet significant metallurgical and engineering needs of steel users. The primary organizations responsible for steel standards are the Society of Automotive Engineers (SAE) and American Iron and Steel Institute (AISI). A number series is used to identify the chemical composition of steel. The most common standard carbon steels used in the design and construction of assistive devices are AISI numbers 1010, 1018, and 1020. These are all readily machinable, formable, and weldable. They have good strength properties and are readily available.

Varying alloying elements and percentages affect different engineering properties. Steel is alloyed with various elements to improve physical properties and to produce special properties. Wheelchairs are commonly constructed using AISI numbers 4130, 4340, and 8620 common alloy steels. AISI 4130 is a chromium-molybdenum alloy that is widely used because of its strength, weldability, and ease in fabrication. It can be treated for higher strength and to resist abrasion. AISI 4340 is chromium-nickel-molybdenum alloy that possesses remarkable ductility and toughness. It has high-fatigue strength and is good for highly stressed parts. AISI 8620 is a chromium-nickel-molybdenum alloy that has excellent machinability and responds well to polishing.

### 3.5.2 Aluminum for Wheelchair Design

Aluminum is the world's most abundant metal. Presently, the only practical source of aluminum is bauxite ore, which is 45%–65% aluminum oxide. Bauxite ore is carefully treated through a series of chemical processes until alumina (aluminum oxide) is produced. The alumina, cryolite, and aluminum fluoride are mixed in an electric smelting furnace where the aluminum is freed and siphoned off to form ingots of usable aluminum. The aluminum industry uses a four-digit index system for the designation of aluminum and its alloys. The first digit indicates the alloy group according to the major alloying elements. The 1xxx series is the basic designation for commercially pure aluminums. In this group the aluminum content is 99% and there are no major alloying elements. The second digit indicates modifications in impurity limits. If the second digit is zero, there are no special controls or impurities. Numbers 1 through 9 are used as the second digit to indicate special control of one or more impurities. The last two digits indicate specific minimum aluminum content. The absolute minimum aluminum content in this group is 99%. The minimum for certain grades may exceed 99%, and these last two digits represent the hundredths of a percent over 99. For example, 1030 would designate 99.30% minimum aluminum content.

If the first number in the designation is any number between 2 and 9, the material is made of an aluminum alloy. In other words, anything but a 1 in the first position of the SAE number designates an alloy. Three aluminum alloys are commonly used in wheelchair engineering: SAE 2024, SAE 6061, and SAE 7075. These are commonly used as structural materials. SAE 2024 is a common high-strength aluminum alloy. It is used for structural parts that require high-fatigue resistance, good strength-to-weight ratio, high machining, but do not require welding. SAE 2024 does not have good corrosion resistance so it is commonly anodized or used with All-Clad (i.e., a fine coating of commercially pure aluminum). SAE 6061 is an inexpensive and versatile structural aluminum alloy. Most aluminum wheelchair frames are made of this alloy. It offers good mechanical properties and corrosion resistance. It can be welded using most common methods. SAE 7075 is one of the highest-strength aluminum alloys. It is ideally suited for high-stress parts. It is not recommended for welded parts.

Aluminum alloy temper designations consist of suffixes to the numeric alloy designations. For example, with 6061 T6, 6061 denotes the alloy and T6 denotes the temper or degree of hardness. The temper designation also indicates the method by which the hardness was obtained. Alloys commonly used for wheelchairs typically use T4 or T6 temper designations. The tempering process that yields the best results is dependent on the type of aluminum alloy. SAE 2024 is commonly specified as 2024 T4, whereas SAE 6061 T6 is used as 6061 T6. Specifying the proper alloy and temper designation can help to make designs successful.

### 3.5.3 Composites for Wheelchair Design

Plastics are the common name for high polymers. High polymers are complex chains of polymers. Polymers are combinations of two or more monomers. Monomers are basic building blocks of chemical elements that have an affinity for linking. The bonding of two monomers is called copolymerization. Under the proper circumstances monomers copolymerize and begin to form chains. These chains can begin to build and form more polymers, leading to the development of plastics. In this sense plastics are composite materials.

Despite having shiny, smooth, and homogeneous appearances, plastics do not exhibit homogeneity down to the molecular level. The properties of plastics are determined largely by how the monomers are arranged. Thermoplastics have linearly linked bonds, whereas thermosetting plastics have cross-linked bonds. High polymers can be made that have very strong bonds. Three-dimensional linkages of carbon atoms can form covalent bonds. Thermosetting plastics are made by creating extensive three-dimensional covalent linkages between molecules. This process is called cross-linking, and often occurs at elevated temperatures. Ultraviolet radiation may break the covalent bonds in the main polymer chains, reducing strength. Manufacturers use additives to reduce this effect. Some common plastics used in wheelchairs are shown in Table 3.4.

Fiber-reinforced composites are deliberate compositions of strong, stiff fibers in a matrix of a softer material. Glass spun to long, consistent, and strong filaments called fiberglass is the most widely used material in composites. Fiberglass has high tensile strength and low cost. Polyester plastic is widely used as a matrix. However, epoxies have become the standard for engineering applications because of their superior properties. A significant advantage of epoxies is that they are addition polymers, i.e., nothing is given off during the curing process. Condensation polymers give off moisture during curing, which must be vented. The principal drawback of fiberglass as a reinforcement material is its low stiffness. Graphite, Kevlar, and boron fibers have high stiffness and nearly the same tensile strength of glass fibers. Other more exotic materials (tungsten and sapphire) have several desirable properties, but their costs are prohibitive for wheelchair use.

Kevlar is an organic fiber that is yellow in color and soft to the touch. It is extremely strong and tough, and forms a very lightweight composite. Kevlar is resistant to impact, but has rather low compression strength. For these reasons, Kevlar is used in bulletproof vests. Graphite fibers are created by extreme stretching and

**TABLE 3.4  Some common plastics used in wheelchairs**

| Thermoplastics | Thermosets |
|---|---|
| ABS | Polyester |
| Nylon | Epoxy |
| Polycarbonate | Epoxy glass |
| Polyethylene | |

heating of rayon fibers, which changes their molecular structure. Graphite fiber has very low density, a high modulus of elasticity, and a high tensile strength.

## 3.6 Fabrication

The quality of a wheelchair is a combination of the design, the materials, the selection of appropriate fabrication processes, and the skill of the workmanship with which the components and total wheelchair are made.

### 3.6.1 Welding

A weld is defined as the local union of materials accomplished by applying heat and pressure with or without fill material (i.e., additional metal) being added. The strength of the weld depends on how the heat and pressure are applied as well as the materials welded and any fill material. Welding permits complex devices to be constructed from readily formable components (e.g., tubes and plates). Welding encompasses three common processes: welding, brazing, and soldering. Brazing refers to the use of brass as a filler material when bonding two metals. Soldering refers to the process of bonding two metals at low temperatures ($< 425°$ C), and is commonly used for the assembly of electric circuits. Welding implies that the melting point of the filler material is near that of the materials being bonded. Welding includes a number of high-temperature bonding processes.

Torch welding is a process whereby the adjoining edges of the materials to be bonded are heated until they reach a molten state. The materials flow together and form a local bond. The flame, usually oxygen-acetylene, is adjusted to a narrow point, at which the temperature is nearly 6000° F. A high level of skill is required to get full penetration through the materials being welded and proper flow of the fill material. The greatest advantage of torch welding is that the equipment is inexpensive and portable and requires no external power. Torch welding works well for most common standard carbon steels. Torch welding does not work well with many steel alloys or with other metals (e.g., aluminum or titanium).

Electric arc welding uses either direct current or alternating electricity to create localized heating at the points to be joined. Electric arc welding does not require oxygen to create heat and can thus be used for a greater variety of metals. Shielded metal arc welding (also known as stick welding) is the most common form of electric arc welding. Stick welding uses a consumable electrode (i.e., the electrode is the device through which the current flows from the machine through the parts being welded). As the weld progresses the electrode melts into the weld to provide filler material. The electrode can be covered with flux to help remove impurities and oxidants from the weld, in which case the electrodes are short "sticks," or the flux can be in the center of the electrode, which permits using a spool of cored wire. Most common steels can be stick welded with the proper electrode.

Gas metal arc welding, metal inert gas (MIG), or $CO_2$ welding uses a continuous bare metal wire electrode. The welding zone is shielded by an inert gas, such as $CO_2$ or argon. This method requires less skill by the user and is suitable for most common aluminums and steels. It is only recommended for pieces less than or equal to 0.25 inch thick. Gas tungsten arc welding, or tungsten inert gas (TIG), uses a nonconsumable electrode shielded by an inert gas, helium or argon, and a separate filler rod. TIG can be used with most weldable metals (e.g., steel, aluminum, or titanium). It requires a substantial degree of skill to achieve good welds. TIG welding is the process used to assemble most ultralight and lightweight wheelchairs.

Thermal plastics can also be welded by heating with electrical filaments. Typically, thermal plastics are welded by applying a heated metal surface to the materials to be bonded and then applying moderate pressure.

### 3.6.2 Fasteners

Joints assembled with screws, bolts, and studs can be readily disassembled and reassembled. Threaded fasteners have been standardized in such a way that the selection of the proper fastener is resolved by determining critical dimensions. There are a wide variety of screw types: flat, round, oval, pan, binding, truss, fillister, and hexagon. The selection of the proper screw type depends on the amount of space available, the probability that someone will come in contact with it, and the amount of force the screw must support. The heads may be slotted or recessed (Phillips, frearson, or torque). Machine screw points are not finished, i.e., they are flat. They are used in threaded holes or with nuts. Machine screws are commonly used on thin metal sections like those found on electrical equipment. Slotted cap screws come with round, flat, and fillister head styles. Capscrews are available in fluted socket, for a typical wrench, and recessed socket, the Allen cap screw. Capscrews have fine tolerances and finishes. They are typically used on tapped holes or with nuts. They are used in applications where high reliability and strength are required. Setscrews are used to set the position of collars or pulleys on soft shafts. They are available with a variety of recessed heads. Setscrews come with flat, cone, oval, cup, dog, and half-dog points. Machine bolts are available with square, hex, rounded, or flat countersunk heads. They make snug, full-fit connections and are usually held in place with a nut. They are used for general fastening. Tap bolts are regular hexhead bolts with fully threaded shanks. They are used in threaded holes wherever a machine bolt or capscrew would be impractical.

### 3.6.4 Working with Adhesives

Epoxy systems differ greatly in their working properties. Useful epoxies require the proper combination of workability and strength. Good epoxies must have very low toxicity. Other desirable characteristics are low water absorption, good material wetting properties without drainage, and low density for a lighter laminate. Composite materials are bonded by wetting the cloth to be used with epoxy. Just enough epoxy to wet all of the fibers should be used. Excess epoxy will make the end product heavier. Once the cloth has been wetted it is laid-up on the mold. For small quantities a Styrofoam mold covered in plastic wrap works well. The wetted cloth should be laid in criss-crossing layers until the desired number of layers is achieved. All materials have to be free from oil, grease, and dirt or a strong bond will not be achieved.

## 3.7 Summary

Some readers may wish to browse through the mathematical sections of this chapter. However, the interested reader should find much of the information necessary to understand the mechanical aspects of wheelchairs and wheelchair propulsion. As the research and development of wheelchairs and their usage advances, rehabilitation professionals will need to be more familiar with the concepts introduced in this chapter. The advances made into the understanding of the biomechanics of wheelchair propulsion depend heavily on kinematic and kinetic analysis. The application and understanding of wheelchair standards also rely on many of the concepts presented in this chapter. Most students of rehabilitation medicine, physical therapy, rehabilitation science, and rehabilitation engineering will have had sufficient background coursework and training to become quite conversant in the topics presented here. A thorough understanding of the mechanical engineering material should prepare readers for that aspect of assistive technology practitioner certification.

## References and Further Reading

Beer F. P., Johnston E. R. Jr. (1977) *Vector Mechanics for Engineers: Statics and Dynamics*, 3d ed. New York, NY, McGraw-Hill.

Cook A. M., Hussey S .M. (1995) *Assistive Technologies: Principles and Practice*. St. Louis, MO, Mosby-Year Book.

Cook A. M., Webster J. G. (1982) *Therapeutic Medical Devices: Application and Design*. Englewood Cliffs, NJ, Prentice-Hall.

Cooper R. A. (1995) *Rehabilitation Engineering Applied to Mobility and Manipulation*. London, UK, Institute of Physics Publishers.

Edwards K. S., McKee R. B. (1991) *Fundamentals of Mechanical Component Design*. New York, NY, McGraw Hill.

Jacobs K., Bettencourt C. M. (1995) *Ergonomics for Therapists*. Boston, MA, Butterworth-Heinemann.

Johnson A. T. (1991) *Biomechanics and Exercise Physiology*. New York, NY, John Wiley & Sons.

Jones I. S. (1976) *The Effect of Vehicle Characteristics on Road Accidents*. Elmsford, NY, Pergamon Press.

Kapit W., Elson L. M. (1977) *The Anatomy Coloring Book*. New York, NY, Harper & Row.

Kroemer K. H. E., Kroemer H. J., Kroemer-Elbert K. E. (1990) *Engineering Physiology: Basis of Human Factors/Ergonomics*, 2d ed. New York, NY, Van Nostrand Reinhold.

Nahum A. M., Melvin J. W. (1993) *Accidental Injury: Biomechanics and Prevention*. New York, NY, Springer-Verlag.

Özkaya N., Nordin M. (1991) *Fundamentals of Biomechanics: Equilibrium, Motion, and Deformation*. New York, NY, Van Nostrand Reinhold.

Pietrocola F. (1991) Plastics: Will their success story continue? *Medical Design and Material*, April, 42-49.

Sherrill C. (1984) *Sport and Disabled Athletes*, Champaign, IL, Human Kinetics.

Trefler E., Hobson D. A., Taylor S. J., Monahan L.C., Shaw C. G. (1993) *Seating and Mobility for Persons with Physical Disabilities*. Tucson, AZ, Therapy Skill Builders.

Van Vlack L. H. (1980) *Elements of Materials Science and Engineering*. Menlo Park, CA, Addison-Wesley.

Webster J. G. (1991) *Prevention of Pressure Sores.* Philadelphia, PA, Adam Hilger.

Whitman J. D. (1991) *An Automated Process to Aid in Wheelchair Selection.* California State University at Sacramento, unpublished thesis.

Wilson A. B. (1992) *Wheelchairs: A Prescription Guide.* New York, NY, Demos.

Winter D. A. (1990) *Biomechanics and Motor Control of Human Movement.* New York, NY, John Wiley & Sons.

| CHAPTER | Biomechanics |
|---------|--------------|
| **4** | and Ergonomics of Wheelchairs |

*Chapter Goals*

☑ To understand basic human physiology
☑ To understand elements of kinesiology and biomechanics
☑ To know principles of human factors/ergonomics
☑ To know the types of measurements of physical conditions and performance

## 4.1 Wheelchair User Disability Etiology

Disability involves limitations in actions and activities because of mental and physical impairments. About 14% of the U.S. population is limited in selected activities, with some of these limitations making wheelchair use necessary. Each year the National Center for Health Statistics conducts a National Health Interview Survey on Assistive Devices. This survey has shown that there were 1,411,000 wheelchair users in the United States in 1992 (NCHS 1992). Arthritis is one of the leading causes of activity limitation in the United States and is second in prevalence to orthopedic impairments (LaPlante 1991). The incidence and epidemiology of wheelchair user etiology has changed over the past 40 years. Between 1980 and 1990 alone, the use of wheelchairs increased 96.1% (McNeil 1993). Advances in the medical arena have led to numerous methods of prolonging life, thus increasing the demand for wheelchairs. There are numerous grounds for a person to use a wheelchair for mobility. These causes fall into two major categories: traumatic injury and chronic/degenerative disease. Table 4.1 presents data obtained in a survey conducted by the British Ministry of Health, which gave the diagnosis per hundred persons who obtained wheelchairs.

It is estimated that 5% of people over 70 years use wheelchairs (Sonn and Grimby 1994). This age-specific prevalence of disability is therefore higher for elderly persons, which places them in a large subcategory of wheelchair users (MMWR 1994). For the elderly, the more common causes for wheelchair requirement are arthritis/rheumatism, hypertension, diabetes, cardiac and respiratory disease (Pickles and Topping 1994). The prevailing reasons these people gave for requesting a wheelchair were arthritis and unsteadiness (18.2%), with strokes and

**TABLE 4.1    Etiology of wheelchair users**

| | |
|---|---|
| Arthritis | 28% |
| Organic nervous disease | 14% |
| Cerebral vascular disease | 13% |
| Other bone injuries and deformities | 11% |
| Lower limb amputations | 9% |
| Cerebral palsy | 8% |
| Traumatic paraplegia/quadriplegia | 7% |
| Respiratory and cardiac disease | 3% |

frequent falls ranked second and third, respectively. Most of these people (54.5%) use their wheelchairs all of the time (Brooks 1994).

## 4.2 Anthropometry Related to Wheelchairs and Seating

Anthropometry can be simply defined as the physical measurement of the human body. There are two basic types of anthropometric measures commonly made. *Static measurement* is the characterization of fixed properties of the body (e.g., mass, density, limb lengths). *Functional measurements* are those taken with people assuming common movement positions or performing movement tasks that help to determine the properties of the body (e.g., range of motion, reach).

Often when making a biomechanical analysis the body is considered a system of mechanical links. The physical size and form of the body segments are some of the most common anthropometric measures. Segment lengths are determined using anatomical landmarks, commonly readily identifiable joints. Scientists have carefully dissected cadavers and estimated joint centers of rotation and have determined model sets of data lengths as a function of total body length. Measurements based on palpable bony landmarks are highly correlated with measurements from cadaver study. Each body segment has a unique composition of bone, muscle, fat, and other tissue. Gravity influences the motion of segments, as well as other external and internal forces. Control and support mechanisms for people with severe mobility impairments must consider the effect of gravity. One need only hold the arms elevated in front for any length of time to experience the effect of gravity. Cadaver studies have been used to determine estimates of segment densities. Segment densities are related to their mass and volumes.

$$density = \frac{mass}{volume} \tag{4.1}$$

Body segment volumes can be derived from living subjects; hence, segment mass on living people can be estimated using their actual segment volume and a segment density estimate. Segment densities are typically closely related to total body density. Segment center of mass is also an important anthropometric measure. The mass of a segment can be represented by the sum of the mass of small portions of the limb,

$$m_{segment} = \sum_{i=1}^{n} m_i = \sum_{i=1}^{n} \delta_i V_i \approx \delta \sum_{i=1}^{n} V_i \tag{4.2}$$

where $m_i$ is the mass, $\delta_i$ is the density, and $V_i$ is the volume of the $i$th portion of the segment, respectively. The center of mass must create the same moment due to gravity with respect to any point along the segment as the original mass distribution. The center of mass can be defined as the distance $q$ from the proximal end of the segment.

$$mq = \sum_{i=n}^{n} m_i q_i \Rightarrow q = \frac{1}{m}\sum_{i=1}^{n} m_i q_i \tag{4.3}$$

When performing many biomechanical analyses the center of mass of multiple segments is required. When a person is moving one or more segments the body center of mass location is changing, so the center of mass must be calculated as a time series (see Figure 4.1).

$$x_o(t) = \frac{m_1 x_1(t) + m_2 x_2(t) + m_3 x_3(t) + \cdots m_n x_n(t)}{m}$$
$$y_o(t) = \frac{m_1 y_1(t) + m_2 y_2(t) + m_3 y_3(t) + \cdots m_n y_n(t)}{m} \tag{4.4}$$

The center of mass location is most useful for helping to provide support for posture and stability. If rotational accelerations are involved in movements then inertial resistance must be factored into analyses. Inertia is a measure of the ability of the segment to resist changes in angular velocity. The magnitude of inertia depends on the axis about which rotation takes place, and is minimum about the center of mass. The moment of inertia is a constant, and can be calculated with respect to the segment's distal end given the mass of each small portion.

$$I = \sum_{i=1}^{n} m_i q_i^2 \quad \text{or} \quad \int q^2 dm \tag{4.5}$$

**FIGURE 4.1**   Illustration of dividing a limb segment into sections

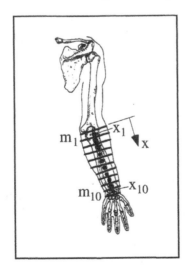

For most analyses the moments of inertia are considered to act around either a joint or segment mass center. The moment of inertia multiplied by the segment angular acceleration provides an estimate of the instantaneous joint moments and forces. This information can be combined with static measurements for functional postures to produce useful kinetic analysis. In cadaver studies or with paralyzed limbs, segments can be swung as a pendulum around the appropriate joint axes. The period of oscillation of the pendulum can be used to estimate moment of inertia,

$$I = \frac{WL}{4\pi^2 f^2}$$                                                            (4.6)

where $W$ is the weight of the segment, $L$ is distance from pivot to segment center of mass, and $f$ is the frequency of oscillation. Several other effective techniques have been developed to determine moments of inertia on living people. Many tables of anthropometric values use the radius of gyration ($\rho$) as a means of presenting moment of inertia data:

$$I_o = m\rho_o^2$$                                                                     (4.7)

Often it is convenient to calculate the moment of inertia about some axis parallel to the center of mass, but located at some other point in the plane. This is extremely useful in biomechanical and postural analyses. The *parallel axis theorem* permits translating the moment of inertia about the center of mass to another axis in the plane.

$$I = \frac{m}{2}(x - \rho_o)^2 + \frac{m}{2}(x + \rho_o)^2 = m\rho_o^2 + mx^2 = I_o + mx^2$$        (4.8)

The distance $x$ can be any direction from the center of mass as long as the axis of rotation is parallel to the axis of the moment of inertia about the center of mass.

Anthropometric measures are useful in evaluating simple measurements of an individual's ability to perform some tasks. Strength, reach, and dexterity tests are required to assess a person's ability to operate devices or perform job functions. Well-motivated or trained individuals can voluntarily improve their performance on functional tests. It is important to make multiple measurements to assure reliable data.

### 4.2.1 Seated Anthropometry

Several specialized measurements are used to define sitting. Functional relations are based upon anthropometry of seating. These measurements can be used to define wheelchairs, seating systems, and workspace requirements. Sitting height is the vertical distance from the floor to the horizontal midsection of the back portion of the thigh while in contact with the seat, with a knee flexion angle of 90 degrees and the feet resting flatly on the footrests. Elbow height is the vertical distance from the floor to the posterior tip of the olecranon when the arm is flexed at 90 degrees at the elbow and the shoulder in its neutral position. Thigh height is the vertical distance from the floor to the highest part of the thigh while in the seated position. Patellar height is the vertical distance from the floor to the superior tip of the patella while seated. Orbital height is the vertical distance from the floor to the orbit when sitting with the spine erect. Shoulder height is the vertical distance from the floor to the superior aspect of the acromion while seated. Hand-grip height is the vertical distance from the floor to the midpoint of the hanging fist while seated. Internal seating depth is the sagittal distance from the posterior aspect of the popliteal fold to the posterior aspect of the buttock. External seating depth is the sagittal distance from the anterior aspect of the knee to the posterior part of the buttock. Abdominal depth is the sagittal distance from the anterior abdominal wall to the posterior part of the buttock. Buttocks width is the maximum transverse distance across the buttocks. Shoulder width is the maximum transverse distance across the shoulders. External elbow width is the maximum transverse distance between the tips of the olecrani when the arms are abducted to 90 degrees.

Wheelchair seating measurements vary somewhat from those used for seated anthropometry. Some simplification is employed because of tasks specific to wheelchair prescription and design (Figure 4.2). These measurements are used to determine seating and wheelchair dimensions. Wheelchair measurements should be made with the chair loaded. This helps to simulate the dimensions of the chair when occupied. ANSI/RESNA and ISO standards specify using a seating dummy

**FIGURE 4.2**  Common seat anthropometry measurements

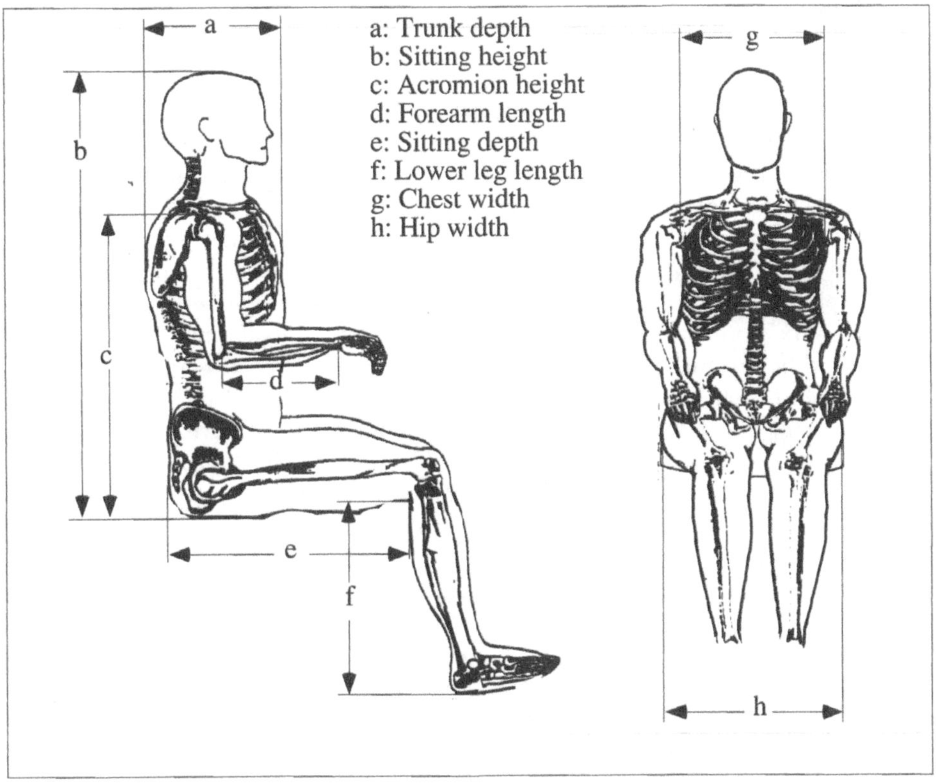

a: Trunk depth
b: Sitting height
c: Acromion height
d: Forearm length
e: Sitting depth
f: Lower leg length
g: Chest width
h: Hip width

The most commonly cited extrinsic factor is impingement of the rotator cuff by surrounding structures. Changes in the undersurface of the structures forming the coracoacromial arch may be related to impingement. Most rotator cuff tears can be attributed to impingement, with the arm abducted and forward flexed. Specific shapes of the acromion are correlated with an increased risk for tears of the rotator cuff. Wylie et al. reported that 18% of active wheelchair users had joint space narrowing in the shoulder. It is likely that both the shape of the coracoacromial arch and the vascularity of the rotator cuff tendons contribute to pathology. Any activity that forces the humeral head further into the glenohumeral joint can cause impingement under the acromioclavicular arch and thus inflammation. The humeral head is placed in close proximity to the acromioclavicular arch during overhead activities. In manual wheelchair users the vast majority of activity is not overhead, but there are forces that tend to drive the humeral head up into the glenohumeral joint. These forces occur during transfer activities and during wheelchair propulsion.

Another extrinsic factor leading to impingement and rotator cuff tear is instability of the glenohumeral joint. The instability is thought to relate to a combination of attenuation of supporting structures of the glenohumeral joint, such as the glenoid labrum, and to muscle imbalance. Muscle imbalance, caused by overuse, is thought to lead to abnormal biomechanics and thus injury. The most common disparity in strength associated with rotator cuff tear is an imbalance between the internal and external rotators of the shoulder. Burnham et al. were able to demonstrate muscle imbalance in a group of wheelchair athletes and correlated this imbalance with shoulder pain.

Rotator cuff tear can be diagnosed with a thorough history and physical examination. Typically, the patient will complain of pain with shoulder movement, commonly in the overhead position. Physical examination findings consist of pain with resisted internal or external rotation and pain at end range of motion. The impingement test described by Neer involves forward flexion and internal rotation, which if it causes pain is considered positive. Other findings on physical examination include pain on palpation of the subdeltoid bursa and biceps tendon. The most sensitive noninvasive test for rotator cuff tear is magnetic resonance imaging (MRI). MRI has been found to be nearly 100% sensitive and about 95% specific for complete tears, approximately 93% specific and about 87% sensitive for tendinitis. MRI is the noninvasive gold standard for rotator cuff examination.

Although the shoulder is the most common site of musculoskeletal injury in manual wheelchair users, elbow, wrist, and hand pain are also commonly reported. Significant pain is defined as that requiring analgesia, occurring with two or more activities of daily living, or requiring cessation of activity. Using this definition the prevalence of forearm, wrist, and hand pain is between 8% and 55%. Arm pain is related to overuse of the arm during transfers or wheelchair propulsion.

The most common neurologic cause of upper extremity pain in wheelchair users is carpal tunnel syndrome, with a prevalence between 49% and 73%. The incidence of carpal tunnel syndrome has been found to increase with increased duration of wheelchair use. To add objective criteria to the diagnosis of carpal tunnel syndrome, a number of investigators have performed nerve conduction tests. Electrodiagnostic evidence of carpal tunnel syndrome appears in about 50% of wheelchair users. Forty-four percent of patients with electrical abnormalities are asymptomatic. Duration of disability has been found to correlate with electrodiagnostic tests.

Ulnar nerve damage is quite common among wheelchair users. Slowing of the ulnar nerve has been seen in both the above-elbow-to-below-elbow segment and the below-elbow-to-wrist segment. The prevalence of ulnar nerve injury varies between 15% and 40%. It is apparent that carpal tunnel syndrome and ulnar nerve injuries are common problems among wheelchair users. Most of the studies found a greater prevalence of abnormalities on nerve conduction studies than actual clinical symptoms. This may signify that subclinical nerve damage exists in a number of wheelchair users. Whether this subclinical damage goes on to become clinically important has yet to be determined. Carpal tunnel syndrome is generally thought to be caused by compression of the median nerve within the carpal tunnel. Extremes of wrist flexion and extension have been shown to greatly increase the pressure within the carpal tunnel. Thickening of the flexor tendon sheaths secondary to repetitive motion and contraction of the tendons within the carpal tunnel have been implicated as a cause for compression of the median nerve. The majority of scientists who have investigated carpal tunnel syndrome in wheelchair users have implicated transfer and the repetitive activity of propelling the chair as a causative factor.

The symptoms of carpal tunnel syndrome include numbness and paresthesias in a median distribution in the hand. The pain is often described as stinging, burning, or aching. Symptoms typically worsen at night and are commonly worse with activities that involve pinching or grasping objects. Two clinical tests for carpal tunnel syndrome are the Phalen's and Tinel's signs. Unfortunately, the sensitivity and specificity of these two tests are relatively poor. More sensitive tests for carpal tunnel syndrome are nerve conduction studies. A number of studies have looked at the most appropriate nerve conduction tests for carpal tunnel syndrome. Two of the most sensitive nerve conduction studies are median and ulnar mixed mid-palmars, and radial and median sensory to the thumb. Mid-palmar studies have been found to be 97% specific and between 70% and 85% sensitive in symptomatic hands. Radial and median sensory studies to the thumb have been found to be 99% specific and 60% to 70% sensitive in symptomatic hands. Each of these tests has an established protocol and an established upper limit of normal.

### 4.3.2 Accidental Injuries

Falling and tipping-related accidents are the primary accidents accompanied with wheelchair use. In a study involving 651 records collected by the Medical Device Reporting System of the U.S. Food and Drug Administration between 1975 and 1993, type of wheelchair injury and engineering factors leading to injury were examined (Kirby 1995). Table 4.2 gives the breakdown of recorded wheelchair injuries, and Table 4.3 lists the recorded engineering factors involved in injury.

Axle position, camber, the position of the user, and the location of any added masses directly affect the tipping angles of the wheelchair. Making the proper adjustments to the wheelchair can help prevent falling and tipping-related accidents. Many wheelchairs offer rear wheel adjustability. This feature allows the user to position the rear axle to personal preference. Moving the rear wheels rearward increases uphill stability and decreases the chance of a rear tipping accident. Camber is the degree of angling of the rear wheels outward at the bottom of the chair and inward where the user's hands contact the handrim. Greater camber increases the sideways wheelchair stability, and is important for users' negotiating

TABLE 4.2   Distribution of recorded wheelchair injuries

|  | Number of Incidences | Percentage of Incidences |
|---|---|---|
| Fracture | 143 | 45.5 |
| Laceration | 70 | 22.3 |
| Contusions/abrasions | 63 | 20.1 |
| Concussions/subdurals | 9 | 2.8 |
| Dislocation | 5 | 1.6 |
| Dental injury | 4 | 1.3 |
| Puncture | 4 | 1.3 |
| Strain/sprain | 4 | 1.3 |
| Burns, thermal | 4 | 1.3 |
| Other | 8 | 2.6 |

cross slopes. The user can change the wheelchair's stability depending on upper body strength and mobility. Rearward stability can be increased by the user leaning forward, and forward stability can be increased by the user leaning backwards. A user with good upper body strength might opt for a less stable and more maneuverable wheelchair adjustment, relying on trunk mobility to avoid tipping. If the user has asymmetric body weight distribution or poor trunk control, the wheelchair can be modified by adding weights where needed. By calculating the center of gravity of the wheelchair and user, weights can be placed at appropriate points on the wheelchair to make it safer.

Some wheelchair accidents occur as a result of poor design. Wheelchair stability, frame and component material strength, environmental interaction, and braking ability are important factors in designing a safe wheelchair. American National Standards Institute (ANSI)/RESNA and International Standards Organization (ISO) have developed standardized tests for wheelchairs for disclosure to the public. These standards allow the user to select a wheelchair based upon performance, safety, and dimensions. The standards serve as a guide to avoid design-related accidents that may occur, based on the disclosed information.

## 4.4 Physical Activity and Wheelchair Propulsion

### 4.4.1 Coronary Heart Disease Among Wheelchair Users

Coronary heart disease and stroke have many causes. Modifiable risk factors include smoking, high blood pressure, blood lipid levels, obesity, diabetes, and physical activity. Lifestyle improvements can control these risk factors and this has

TABLE 4.3   Wheelchair factors leading to accidents

|  | Number of Failures | Percentage of Failures |
|---|---|---|
| Mechanical/frame | 305 | 77.3 |
| Electrical/electronic | 48 | 12.2 |
| Brakes | 24 | 6.1 |
| Motor | 18 | 4.6 |

played a major role in the decline of heart disease and stroke. Medically, physical activity is defined as bodily movement produced by skeletal muscles that requires energy expenditure. Exercise is a type of physical activity. Exercise is defined as planned structured and repetitive bodily movements done to improve or maintain one or more components of physical fitness. Physical inactivity denotes a level of activity less than that needed to maintain good health. Physical activity has been demonstrated to protect against the development of cardiovascular disease and to modify several of its risk factors. Physical inactivity is widespread among wheelchair users. The least active wheelchair users are not well educated and are socially or economically disadvantaged. Physical inactivity is associated with osteoporosis, diabetes, and some cancers.

Traditionally, it has been assumed that rigorous activity and the use of large muscle groups were required to benefit from exercise. Many people believed that wheelchair users could not benefit from exercise. Recently, it has been learned that structured or vigorous activities are not required to reduce risk factors for cardiovascular disease. The National Institutes of Health recommend a cumulative total of 30 minutes of activity each day with individual bouts of activity lasting at least 10 minutes. Longer duration or greater intensity activity need only be done three times per week to achieve cardiovascular benefits. Resistance and flexibility training can assist in performing activities of daily living.

Behavioral and attitudinal factors that influence motivation for and ability to sustain physical activity are strongly determined by social experiences, cultural background, physical disability, and health status. Table 4.4 shows the factors that influence whether a person will sustain exercise. Health care providers have substantial influence in reducing risk behaviors and with making people feel competent in their ability to participate in physical activity. There is evidence that a significant percentage of the wheelchair user population may be at greater risk of acquiring cardiovascular disease. In studies of exercise performance of middle-aged or elderly wheelchair users, it has been reported that nearly 50% of the people had to be excluded from the study for cardiovascular disease. Several attempts have been made to modify the Astrand-Ryhming submaximal cycle test to predict an individual's peak oxygen uptake during arm cranking. Chambers et al. derived three equations to predict oxygen uptake during arm-crank exercise in six-minute stages at 25, 50, and 75 Watts. A few attempts have been made to develop submaximal stress tests during wheelchair exercise. However, current wheelchair tests may not be suitable clinically for patients with lower limb disabilities. This is because the tests are based on unimpaired people pushing wheelchairs or by wheelchair athletes. This has led most clinics to develop protocols specific to their local population. Arm-cranking exercise has been demonstrated to be effective in eliciting angina and ischemic ST segment responses suitable for diagnosing coronary heart disease. Arm-crank exercise is not as sensitive as tread-

**TABLE 4.4  Factors that influence sustaining physical activity**

Perception of benefit
Feeling of competency and safety
Easy access and fits within schedule
No additional financial or social cost associated with activity
Balance between labor-saving devices and physical activity

mill exercise for people who are capable of walking on a treadmill. For individuals who cannot perform a treadmill test, because of either peripheral vascular disease or lower limb disability, an arm-crank stress test can induce significant electrocardiogram (ECG) changes to diagnose coronary artery disease. Currently, there is no consensus on the value of arm-exercise stress testing to detect coronary artery disease. However, several methods appear promising and present lower risk than invasive techniques.

Some work has been done to develop fitness norms for wheelchair users. Normative values are useful for assisting healthcare professionals and wheelchair users in assessing an individual's health status against people with a similar impairment. Based on an individual's results, an exercise program can be developed to improve fitness and reduce risk for coronary artery disease. Langbein and Cooper have worked to develop normative values for fitness among apparently healthy manual wheelchair users (see Tables 4.5 and 4.6). The normative values are based on peak exercise stress tests during arm-crank and wheelchair ergometry.

## 4.4.2 Pulmonary Function Among Wheelchair Users

As a result of improved medical treatment of infectious diseases, formerly leading causes of mortality in the United States have been supplanted in rank by such chronic events as coronary artery disease, respiratory disease, and cancers. It has been reported that 21% of the mortality rate among people with spinal cord injury is related to respiratory incidents, not far behind cardiovascular incidents (25%), the leading cause of mortality. The level of physical impairment affects the functions of the various aspects of the respiratory apparatus such as the intercostal muscles and diaphragm. Lower pulmonary functions have been documented among wheelchair users in several studies. More specifically, individuals with higher levels of impairment have poorer pulmonary functions than people with lower levels of impairment. Cooper et al. collected pulmonary function data from a diverse group of 109 wheelchair users. Their subjects came from culturally and ethnically diverse backgrounds, and ranged in age from 17 to 69 years. Their study combined the results of smokers and nonsmokers. The pulmonary functions of the men are presented in Table 4.7. Insufficient data have been collected to produce percentile values for women wheelchair users. Prediction equations for male and female wheelchair users are presented in

**TABLE 4.5   Normative values for cardiorespiratory fitness among men wheelchair users**

|  | Upper Level Impairment | Middle Level Impairment | Low Level Impairment |
|---|---|---|---|
| Fitness | ml•kg$^{-1}$•min$^{-1}$ | ml•kg$^{-1}$•min$^{-1}$ | ml•kg$^{-1}$•min$^{-1}$ |
| Poor | < 4.03 | < 8.36 | < 6.55 |
| Moderate | 4.03–11.27 | 8.36–17.08 | 6.55–19.86 |
| Average | 11.28–18.52 | 17.09–25.83 | 19.87–33.19 |
| Good | 18.53–25.77 | 25.84–34.26 | 33.20–46.51 |
| Excellent | > 25.77 | > 34.56 | > 46.51 |

Upper level = C5–T2; Middle level = T3–T10; Lower level = T11–L5.

**TABLE 4.6**  Normative values for cardiorespiratory fitness among women wheelchair users

|  | Upper Level Impairment | Middle & Low Level Impairment |
|---|---|---|
| Fitness | ml•kg⁻¹•min⁻¹ | ml•kg⁻¹•min⁻¹ |
| Poor | < 5.81 | < 8.32 |
| Moderate | 5.81–13.63 | 8.32–18.22 |
| Average | 13.64–21.48 | 18.23–28.15 |
| Good | 21.49–29.31 | 28.16–38.06 |
| Excellent | > 29.31 | > 38.06 |

Upper level = C5–T2; Middle & Low = T3–L5.

**TABLE 4.7**  Male wheelchair user pulmonary function percentiles

|  | 10th | 25th | 50th | 75th | 90th |
|---|---|---|---|---|---|
| **Upper Level Injury** |  |  |  |  |  |
| FEVC (L) | 2.78 | 3.23 | 4.10 | 4.63 | 5.48 |
| FEV1 (L) | 2.27 | 2.55 | 3.18 | 3.89 | 4.59 |
| FEVC 25–75% (L) | 1.43 | 2.70 | 3.60 | 4.93 | 5.17 |
| PEF (L/min) | 3.20 | 4.82 | 6.41 | 7.69 | 8.26 |
| FIVC (L) | 3.18 | 3.65 | 4.07 | 4.49 | 5.77 |
| PIF (L/min) | 2.65 | 2.87 | 3.60 | 5.85 | 7.09 |
| RV (L) | 1.14 | 1.47 | 2.25 | 2.53 | 3.03 |
| MVV (L/min) | 77.4 | 97.2 | 122.7 | 157.3 | 176.0 |
| SVC (L) | 2.88 | 3.30 | 3.90 | 4.47 | 4.84 |
| TV (L) | 0.48 | 0.60 | 0.90 | 0.98 | 1.48 |
| FEV1/FVC | 0.65 | 0.75 | 0.84 | 0.87 | 0.91 |
| **Middle Level Injury** |  |  |  |  |  |
| FEVC (L) | 3.23 | 3.72 | 4.34 | 4.98 | 5.48 |
| FEV1 (L) | 2.61 | 3.05 | 3.70 | 4.12 | 4.44 |
| FEVC 25–75% (L) | 3.21 | 3.75 | 4.24 | 5.66 | 6.81 |
| PEF (L/min) | 4.15 | 4.96 | 7.71 | 9.40 | 9.82 |
| FIVC (L) | 3.50 | 4.21 | 4.79 | 5.32 | 5.79 |
| PIF (L/min) | 2.85 | 3.55 | 5.22 | 7.39 | 8.74 |
| RV (L) | 1.55 | 1.95 | 2.37 | 2.58 | 2.90 |
| MVV (L/min) | 98.9 | 117.6 | 149.4 | 174.6 | 201.5 |
| SVC (L) | 3.30 | 3.68 | 3.93 | 4.48 | 5.15 |
| TV (L) | 0.52 | 0.82 | 1.10 | 1.40 | 1.67 |
| FEV1/FVC | 0.67 | 0.78 | 0.84 | 0.90 | 0.94 |
| **Lower Level Injury** |  |  |  |  |  |
| FEVC (L) | 3.36 | 3.96 | 4.52 | 5.36 | 5.49 |
| FEV1 (L) | 2.81 | 3.31 | 3.86 | 4.28 | 4.63 |
| FEVC 25–75% (L) | 3.93 | 4.11 | 4.91 | 5.30 | 5.91 |
| PEF (L/min) | 5.79 | 7.26 | 8.22 | 10.27 | 11.76 |
| FIVC (L) | 3.52 | 4.12 | 5.13 | 5.29 | 6.04 |
| PIF (L/min) | 3.36 | 3.52 | 5.50 | 7.15 | 9.45 |
| RV (L) | 1.24 | 1.47 | 1.80 | 2.27 | 2.80 |
| MVV (L/min) | 112.4 | 134.8 | 169.6 | 190.8 | 208.4 |
| SVC (L) | 3.75 | 4.14 | 4.88 | 5.15 | 5.67 |
| TV (L) | 0.78 | 0.94 | 1.11 | 1.28 | 1.66 |
| FEV1/FVC | 0.74 | 0.77 | 0.85 | 0.89 | 0.93 |

**TABLE 4.8   Pulmonary function prediction equations for people with spinal cord injuries based on age, height, weight, injury level, and years of injury ($p < .05$)**

*MEN*

FEVC (L) = −0.041 Years Injured + 0.085 Injury Level + 3.978
FEV1 (L) = −.038 Years Injured + 0.075 Injury Level + 3.318
PEF (L/min) = −0.137 Years Injured + 0.325 Injury Level + 5.658
FIVC (L) = −0.097 Years Injured + 0.172 Injury Level + 0.097 age + .801
PIF (L/min) = 0.236 Injury Level + 3.589
RV (L) = 0.036 Height − 0.019 Weight − 2.762
MVV (L/min) = −1.989 Height + 506.66
SVC (L) = 0.065 Injury Level + 3.234

*WOMEN*

FEVC (L) = 0.037 Injury Level + 0.075 Height − 0.027 Weight −7.941
FEV1 (L) = 0.046 Height − 5.013
PEF (L/min) = 0.092 Age + 1.632
FIVC (L) = −0.036 Age + 0.054 Height − 4.229
PIF (L/min) = 0.035 Weight + 1.922
RV (L) = −0.03 Years Injured + 1.823
MVV (L) = −3.644 Years Injured + 146.863

Prediction equations for male and female wheelchair users are presented in Table 4.8.

The basis for determining health status is provided by the work of Cooper et al. in developing pulmonary function prediction equations based on measured performances of apparently healthy wheelchair users establishing pulmonary function normative values, including forced expired vital capacity (FEVC), forced expired volume after one second (FEV1), forced expired vital capacity from 25% to 75% (FEVC 25%–75%), peak expiratory flow (PEF), forced inspired vital capacity (FIVC), peak inspiratory flow (PIF), residual volume (RV), maximal voluntary ventilation (MVV), slow vital capacity (SVC), tidal volume (TV), and the ratio of FEV1/FVC.

## 4.5 Biomechanics of Wheelchair Propulsion

It has been reported that wheelchair propulsion is inefficient. The low efficiency and high strains seen in manual wheelchair propulsion have been associated with four conditions:

1) a discontinuous motion, with an idle recovery phase;
2) a complex hand-arm movement during the propulsion phase, requiring additional coordinative muscular action;
3) a complex coupling of the hand to the pushrim, leading to braking forces at the start of the propulsion phase and a negative torque; and
4) the shoulder complex requires (static) muscular actions to stabilize and adjust the shoulder complex with respect to the trunk during the push phase.

These factors, among others, may subject the upper extremity joint structures to forces and movement patterns which cause them to fail over time. An understanding of the kinematics and kinetics of wheelchair propulsion will allow the clinician and rehabilitation engineer to effect changes in wheelchair design, the user-wheelchair interface, and stroke technique in order to reduce the potential for injury. Efficiency has been shown to be approximately 10% for depot-type wheelchairs and as high as 38% for racing wheelchairs. The high efficiency of racing wheelchairs accounts for the faster road-racing times of wheelchair athletes, and demonstrates that proper design and fitting can have a dramatic impact on efficiency. Properly fitting ultralight wheelchairs designed for activities of daily living have efficiencies of about 20%, which makes their efficiency equivalent to walking.

### 4.5.1 Kinematics of Wheelchair Propulsion

The phases of the wheelchair propulsion stroke have been described by a number of researchers. Flexion and extension of the joints of the upper limb are described as the main motions produced each stroke or cycle time (CT). The stroke has generally been divided into propulsion or drive and recovery phase, which are referred to as propulsion time (PT) and recovery time (RT), respectively. The propulsive phase usually begins with the hands contacting the pushrim close to top dead center and ending when the hand is in a forward, downward position. During the recovery phase the arms are brought back into position to allow for the beginning of the next propulsive phase (see Figure 4.4).

The amount of time subjects spend in propulsion during the cycle has been reported close to 25% for both adult and pediatric groups pushing an everyday wheelchair, between 30% and 45% for subjects pushing a wheelchair on a treadmill, and between 33% and 37% for athletes pushing racing wheelchairs. The stroke has been divided into 5 phases based on racing wheelchair propulsion. These include (1) hand drive forward and downward, (2) pushrim impact, (3)

**FIGURE 4.4**   Example manual wheelchair pushrim propulsion moment curve. Time (1) indicates initial contact. The period (1)–(2) is accommodation time required to establish hand-pushrim coupling. Time (3) peaks at the impact spike. Time (4) peaks the moment curve. Period (5)–(6) is retardation due to release of complex coupling between hand and pushrim. Phase (1)–(6) is the propulsion phase. Phase (6)–(7) is the recovery phase. Phase (1)–(7) is a stroke.

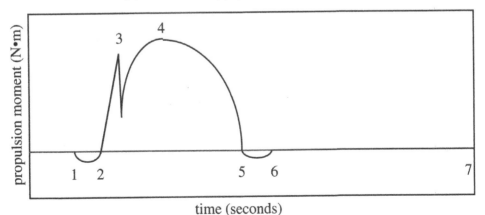

hand on the pushrim, (4) hand off pushrim, and (5) elbow drive to the top. It is suggested that these phases might also be used for analyzing the propulsion stroke for individuals pushing an everyday wheelchair.

The range of motion and movement patterns of joint segments have been studied in relationship to various conditions of propulsion. Veeger et al. found that maximum elbow extension occurred at the end of the push phase with a greater extension angle as resistance increased, while trunk flexion stayed the same. Vanlandewijck et al. characterized the elbow movement while subjects pushed on a treadmill as a push-pull action, which involves a flexion at the elbow joint followed by extension. They noted that at lower speeds, half of the push time was equally divided over a pull-and-push phase, while at higher speeds (2.21 m/s) only one-third of propulsion time was spent on elbow flexion. At hand contact with the pushrim the shoulder joint was in maximum abduction, shoulder flexion occurred during the entire push phase, and increasing speed of propulsion increased shoulder flexion range of motion in the first 50% of the stroke. During recovery they noted that the motion pattern was extremely variable. Increasing seat height for subjects pushing on a treadmill resulted in decreased extension and adduction-abduction of the arm at the shoulder. There is evidence that the stroking pattern is not symmetrical between left and right sides. Within a subject, variations are small, but between subjects variations are large. Skilled wheelchair users use a circular pattern rather than a pumping action and inexperienced subjects have larger angles for the left elbow and shoulder than the right. In studies comparing non–wheelchair users versus wheelchair users, the non–wheelchair users leaned farther forward, started and ended the push with the arms farther back, and had greater arm extension during the stroke. Studies have also shown that different wheelchairs produced differences in stroke patterns for the same subject with paraplegia.

Changes in the phases of the stroke have been described for different conditions of propulsion. Researchers have measured the effects on the stroke during protocols on a treadmill or a wheelchair ergometer and with changes in speed, seat height, resistance, and power. Increasing seat height was shown to decrease push range (the amount of rotation the wheel undergoes during propulsion) and propulsion time. Fatigue has been shown to minimally affect propulsion time and recovery time. Studies have shown that increasing cycle frequency and the amount of work per cycle, while decreasing cycle time, caused an increase in mean power output.

Different modes of propulsion have been investigated in terms of their influence on kinematics. Comparison of treadmill to ergometer modes of wheelchair propulsion demonstrated that there were only small differences in kinematics and both propulsion time and cycle time decreased with increases in propulsion velocity. Lever versus pushrim propulsion resulted in differences kinematically in upper extremity motion with pushrim propulsion requiring less elbow motion, greater shoulder extension, less shoulder rotation, and less arm abduction. Seat position has a greater effect on joint range of motion for pushrim propulsion than for lever propulsion, with a forward position increasing shoulder abduction/adduction, a backward position increasing shoulder flexion/extension, and a lower position increasing overall upper extremity motion.

Analysis of the electrical activity of the upper extremity musculature during wheelchair propulsion revealed that the anterior deltoid and pectoralis major were highly active during the propulsion phase. The biceps brachii was active during the initial part of the propulsion phase (pull motion) and during the latter part of the recovery phase. The triceps brachii was active during the end of the push phase. Seat position was shown to affect the activation pattern to the greatest extent in the triceps brachii, pectoralis major, and posterior deltoid, with the backward-low position having the lowest overall activity.

### 4.5.2 Kinetics of Wheelchair Propulsion

The complexity of developing a system for measuring pushrim forces is evidenced by the paucity of data in the literature on the kinetics of wheelchair propulsion. A number of researchers have attempted to develop a force sensing system with varying degrees of success. The wheelchair kinetic data reported in the literature can be divided into three categories: (1) static force measurements, (2) external devices for measuring forces and torques, and (3) measurement of force components at the pushrim—indirectly or directly.

Brauer and Hertig used a system of springs to restrain a pushrim. Static torque was measured for wheelchair and non–wheelchair users at six different positions ranging from 10 to 40 degrees relative to the vertical. Males were found to generate more torque than females. Ranges of torque values were from 27.9 to 46.6 N•m for males (wheelchair and non–wheelchair users) and 17.1 to 32.1 N•m for females. The authors concluded that the amount of torque produced by the user at the pushrim varies with frictional characteristics of the pushrim, grip location, handedness, grip strength, and/or how well the wheelchair fit the anthropometric measurements of each subject. Brubaker et al. measured static pushing and pulling force for four grip positions using strain-gaged beams mounted to the pushrims. A moveable set allowed various seat positions. The range of forces between 500 and 750 N varied considerably by rim and seat position.

Tupling et al. used a force plate to measure the force generated during the initiation of wheelchair propulsion for the grab-and-start techniques. They found that the grab start was more effective in initiating the movement and that the individual's strength determines the ability to generate an impulse. Samuelsson et al. described a wheelchair ergometer that was a wheelchair with a gear attached to the hub connected by a chain and gear to an isokinetic dynamometer. This device allowed torque and power output to be calculated. Results of a pilot study showed that subjects could produce peak torque values in the range of 70 N•m at 120 deg/s. Ruggles et al. tested three different wheelchairs through a roller system connected to a Cybex Isokinetic Machine. Peak torque, angular displacement, work, and angular impulse were compared. Differences among wheelchairs were found and the authors suggest that wheelchair design and dimensions relative to the anthropometry of the user have a great influence on the mechanical characteristics of propulsion.

These studies and the static studies have provided useful information; however, they can only estimate the actual forces at the pushrim during propulsion and they do not allow for calculation of joint moments. Niesling et al. described a stationary ergometer capable of measuring pushrim forces using a three-dimensional force transducer mounted on the support brackets. This device has been used in a number of studies of wheelchair propulsion biomechanics. Roeleveld et al. tested nine wheelchair athletes during a 30-second sprint test on the same system. Results showed that the fraction of effective force was low for these subjects and only

slightly higher than what was found for less experienced subjects. This was attributed to the total force not being tangentially directed and to the geometry of the
wheelchair. Utilizing a similar protocol on the device, Dallmeijer et al. in addition
to physiological measurements compared forces applied to the pushrim by a group
of spinal cord injured (SCI) subjects during a 30-second sprint test. FEF was also
found to be low in this study and although a number of differences were found in
performance between the high-lesion group (C4–C8) and the other lower-lesion
groups, FEF was not different. This and other studies by Veeger and Van der
Woude's group concluded that the FEF was adversely affected by nonoptimal wheelchair dimensions, ineffective propulsive technique, and the need for friction
between the hand and pushrim.

Cooper and Cheda described a force-sensing pushrim to dynamically measure
racing wheelchair pushrim forces and torques. A slotted disk was used to mount different size pushrims, which mounted to the hub with three beams instrumented
with strain gages. A later version of this force-measuring wheel (Smart[Wheel]) allows
measurement of three-dimensional pushrim forces and moments. The unique
quality of this device is that it can be mounted to the user's own everyday wheelchair. Measurement of pushrim forces with this device has shown that a large radial
and vertical component of force is apparent in the stroke of most individuals, an
impact spike is seen early in the propulsion phase, and the magnitude of these
forces is dependent on experience using a wheelchair.

### 4.5.3 Net Joint Forces and Moments

Joint forces have been studied by few authors. Larger joint moments have been
noted with increases in external power output, with the highest moments occurring
at the shoulder during flexion and adduction with the anterior deltoids and pectoralis major acting as primary movers. Fatigue was shown not to affect the magnitude of joint moment or joint reaction forces, and joint moments and joint power
measures were highest during shoulder joint flexion. Shoulder joint moments were
found to be much higher than at the wrist or the elbow when subjects pushed a
wheelchair on a treadmill. Higher speed and greater slope resulted in greater loads
on the three joints, with the effect of slope being more significant than that of
speed. It has also been shown that there is a larger moment at the shoulder than
either the wrist or elbow, a large component of vertical reaction force at the
shoulder, and differences between wheelchair users and non–wheelchair users in
terms of peak values and when these values occurred during the propulsion stroke.

### 4.5.4 The Wrist During Manual Wheelchair Propulsion

Using the marker system shown in Figure 4.5, we were able to place forces,
moments, and movements in terms of actual wrist anatomy. The mathematics used
to calculate the parameters in a local coordinate system are based on vector mathematics as presented in an earlier chapter. This is necessary because forces and
moments are typically measured with respect to horizontal and vertical, and injury
is based on the orientation and position of the limb. We will define the hand coordinate system as $O_H$ ($i_H$, $j_H$, $k_H$), illustrated in Figure 4.6. Based on the positions of
the markers given by the video system and applying the right-hand rule, we can
define the axes of the hand coordinate system,

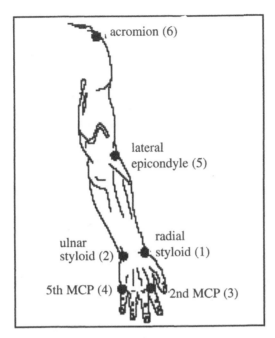

**FIGURE 4.5**   Marker location and number: Location of the six markers used to collect kinematic data (MCP = metacarpal phalangeal joint)

**FIGURE 4.6**   Axis of local coordinate system: Axis indicates the location of the forces and moments as well as the positive direction specified in the mathematical model.

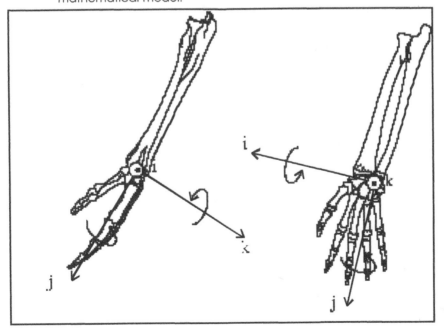

$$i_H = \frac{V_{1-2}}{\|V_{1-2}\|} \qquad j_H = \frac{V_{1-3}}{\|V_{1-3}\|} - \left[\frac{V_{1-2}}{\|V_{1-3}\|} \bullet i_H\right] i_H \qquad k_H = i_H \times j_H \qquad (4.9)$$

The first part defines a unit vector from markers 1 to 2 (see Figure 4.5 for marker numbers and locations). By defining $i_H$, an axis of the local coordinate system is established. The second axis $j_H$ is the unit vector from markers 1 to 3, minus the portion of the vector that lies along the vector $i_H$. These vectors by definition are perpendicular. $k_H$ is perpendicular to the plane defined by $i_H$ and $j_H$, the cross product of the two unit vectors. The basis vector local coordinate system is then used to define a rotation matrix between the world and hand coordinate systems.

$$\mathbf{R}_{WH} = \begin{bmatrix} i_{Hx} & i_{Hy} & i_{Hz} \\ j_{Hx} & j_{Hy} & j_{Hz} \\ k_{Hx} & k_{Hy} & k_{Hz} \end{bmatrix} \quad \mathbf{R}_{HW} = \mathbf{R}_{WH}^{T}$$

$$(4.10)$$

Using the rotation matrix in equation 4.10, the vector between markers 2 and 5 can be placed in the hand coordinate system:

$$\begin{bmatrix} {}^H V_{2-5,x} \\ {}^H V_{2-5,y} \\ {}^H V_{2-5,z} \end{bmatrix} = \mathbf{R}_{WH} \left( \begin{bmatrix} {}^H V_{0-5,x} \\ {}^H V_{0-5,y} \\ {}^H V_{0-5,z} \end{bmatrix} - \begin{bmatrix} {}^H V_{0-2,x} \\ {}^H V_{0-2,y} \\ {}^H V_{0-2,z} \end{bmatrix} \right) \qquad (4.11)$$

This can be reduced to $\mathbf{R}_{WH}$ times $V_{2-5}$. The normalized vector between markers 2 and 5 in the hand coordinate reference frame is converted to a unit vector:

$$\frac{{}^H V_{2-5}}{\|{}^H V_{2-5}\|} \equiv \begin{bmatrix} a & b & c \end{bmatrix} \qquad (4.12)$$

Each term on the right side of the equation is a component of the unit vector on the left side of the equation. Since each term is known, we are able to determine specific angles.

In Figure 4.7, we are looking along the i axis, which travels from the radial styloid to the ulnar styloid. The unit vector **k** travels straight out from the palm, and

**FIGURE 4.7**  Illustration of how wrist angles can be determined

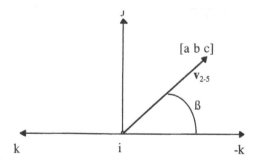

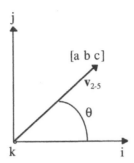

**FIGURE 4.8** Graphical representation of radial and ulnar deviation

$V_{2-5}$ is the unit vector from markers 2 to 5 along the ulna. Therefore ß is the flexion-extension angle and when ß = 0° the wrist is flexed at 90°.

$$\beta = atan2(b,-c) \tag{4.13}$$

Defining flexion and extension at the wrist as being 0° when the wrist is in an anatomically neutral position, we must add 90° to ß. To determine radial and ulnar deviation, we look down the **k** axis (see Figure 4.8):

$$\theta = atan2(b,a) \tag{4.14}$$

When θ = 0° the vector is along a line from the radial to the ulnar styloid. In order to define anatomically neutral as 0° we must subtract 90°. Supination-pronation angle (δ) can be found using similar methods. We define a unit vector that is perpendicular to the plane formed by markers 2, 5, and 6 ($v_{sp256}$) as:

$$v_{sp\,256} = \frac{V_{5-2} \times V_{5-6}}{\|V_{5-2} \times V_{5-6}\|} \tag{4.15}$$

This unit vector is then rotated into the hand coordinate system. To determine δ we look down the **j** axis (see Figure 4.9):

$$\delta = atan2(-a,c) \tag{4.16}$$

When δ = 0° the hand is halfway between supination and pronation with $v_{sp256}$ pointing along **i**. When δ = 90° the hand is fully pronated. Wrist forces can be

**FIGURE 4.9** Graphical representation of supination-pronation model

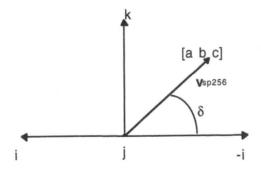

computed by placing the forces as measured at the hub, in the local coordinate system:

$$\begin{bmatrix} F_{w,x} \\ F_{w,y} \\ F_{w,z} \end{bmatrix} = R_{WH} \begin{bmatrix} F_x \\ F_y \\ F_z \end{bmatrix} \qquad (4.17)$$

Wrist moments can be determined by adding the moments that occur at the hub ($M_o$) to the moments caused by the forces at the hub ($F_o$) multiplied by the lever arm or distance between the origin of the local coordinate system and the hub ($V_{0-2}$). The hub is the designated origin of the global coordinate system.

$$M_{w,2} = M_o + F_o \times v_{0-2} \qquad (4.18)$$

$$F_o = \begin{bmatrix} F_x & F_y & F_z \end{bmatrix}^T \quad M_o = \begin{bmatrix} M_x & M_y & M_z \end{bmatrix}^T \qquad (4.19)$$

The moments are then placed in the local system:

$$^H M_{w,2} = R_{WH} \left( M_{w,2} \right)^T \qquad (4.20)$$

The hand markers (see Figure 4.5) can be used to define the axes of the local coordinate system. The first axis, **i**, is defined as a line between the radial and ulnar styloid (see Figure 4.6). Movement about the **i** axis represents flexion and extension. A moment about **i** represents the flexion/extension moment, and forces acting along **i** represent a shear force at the wrist. The second axis, **j**, is defined as being perpendicular to **i** and running in the direction of a line from the radial styloid to the second metacarpal head. Movement and the moment about the **j** axis represent supination or pronation and the moment acting to cause this movement. The **k** axis is defined as being perpendicular to the plane formed by **i** and **j** and comes out of the back of the hand. Movement and a moment about **k** represent ulnar and radial deviation and the moment acting to cause this movement.

In calculating wrist forces and moments, we assumed inertial components caused by the hand are negligible. This assumption is based on the small mass of the hand compared to the relatively large forces and moments occurring at the wrist. For the motion data presented, an angle of 0° represents the anatomically neutral position of the wrist and forearm.

Figures 4.10 through 4.13 present force, motion, and moment data for four propulsive strokes at the same speed. A different subject was used for each plot to demonstrate the stability of the curves in different subjects. In each of these figures, the plot begins at the onset of the stroke as defined above. Differences exist in the length of the stroke in an individual and thus individual curves are of different length. Although variation existed between subjects, general patterns of force, moment, and angle curves were seen.

As subjects impacted the pushrim, the beginning of propulsion, their hands tended to be slightly extended, radially deviated and supinated (Figure 4.10). During the propulsive or drive phase all subjects went from flexion to extension. The majority of subjects showed an initial increase in extension when the hand impacted the pushrim. Radial deviation increased slightly at the beginning of the drive phase in the majority of subjects. All subjects moved from a position of radial deviation to

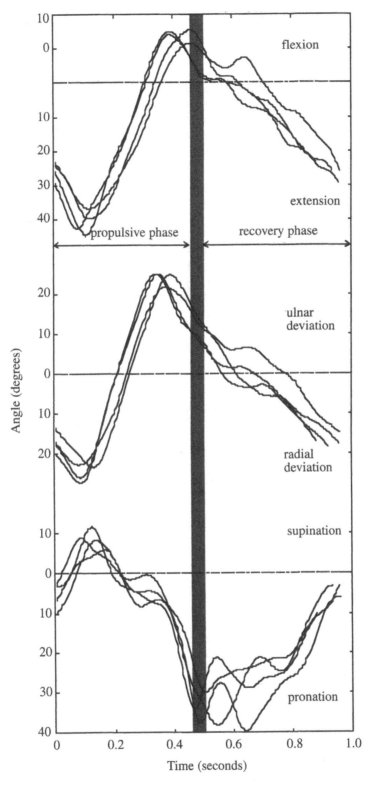

**FIGURE 4.10** Movement of the wrist during propulsion: The beginning of the stroke is at zero seconds. The gray area indicates the time during which the subject went from the propulsive to the recovery phase.

ulnar deviation during the remainder of the propulsive phase. More variability was seen in the supination-pronation motion although the majority of subjects started slightly supinated and then pronated during the drive phase of the stroke.

Using the local coordinate system (Figure 4.6), forces at the wrist were broken down into three components. Two shear forces occur at the wrist, one acting along a line joining the radial and ulnar styloids (i axis) and one acting perpendicular to the plane of the hand (k axis). A third force acts along the long axis of the hand (j axis) and causes either a compressive or distractive force. Figure 4.12 shows four force curves along each axis for a single subject at 3 mph. During the majority of the propulsive phase there is a shear force acting from the radial to the ulnar styloid and a shear force acting from the palm to the dorsum of the hand. The force acting along the j axis is compressive throughout the stroke and is also the largest force acting at the wrist. At the very beginning and very ending of the stroke all of the forces tend to act in the reverse direction. This is likely caused by the hand transiently slowing the pushrim at the beginning and ending of the propulsive phase.

The three moments acting at the wrist are also displayed in Figure 4.13. All of the moments seen at the wrist can cause motion and/or act to maintain stability about the axis described. The moment about the i axis, formed by a line from the radial to the ulnar styloid, can act to flex or extend the wrist. During the majority of the propulsive phase there is an extension moment acting at the wrist. Another

**FIGURE 4.11**   The movement acting to extend the wrist is plotted against the extension/flexion angle. A single stroke at each of two speeds is shown. The beginning of the stroke is in the upper left corner of the curves when the moment first deviates from zero. Larger moments and less motion are seen at the faster speed. Note that larger moments occur at the extremes of flexion and extension.

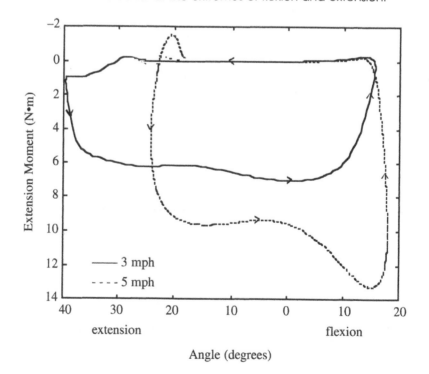

moment acts about the **k** axis, perpendicular to the plane of the hand, and can cause radial or ulnar deviation. A radial deviation moment is seen during the majority of the propulsive phase and this is the largest moment acting at the wrist. Finally the moment acting about **j**, the long axis of the hand, can cause either supination or pronation. During the majority of the propulsive phase a pronation moment is seen.

With increasing speed a number of parameters were found to change. With increasing speed the only motion parameter found to change significantly was radial deviation. As subjects increased their speed the mean radial deviation decreased by approximately four degrees. Thus, with increasing speed, less radial deviation was seen at the wrist. Other stable measures found to change with speed were the peak mean extension moment and peak mean flexion moment. With increasing speeds both of the moments were seen to increase. The mean flexion moment increased by approximately 2 N•m while the mean extension moment increased by approximately 3 N•m. Finally, as speed increased the mean compression force acting along the long axis of the hand increased by approximately 15 N while the mean shear acting from ulnar to the radial styloid increased by approximately 6 N.

Figure 4.11 illustrates the changes in moments and angles with speed. The moment-angle plot is representative of the movement as well as the moment acting about the **i** axis. Both the movement and the moment are in flexion and extension. In this figure, when the moment is zero the hand is off the pushrim. It can be seen that with increased speed both the peak flexion and extension moments increased, while the amount of extension at the wrist decreased. This figure also demonstrates how the peak moments tended to occur at the extremes of range. This was seen in all subjects at all speeds and in all planes of motion.

The force-angle plot (Figure 4.12) is representative of the movement as well as axial force acting along the **j** axis for two different speeds. It should be noted that this force acts along the long axis of the hand, not the forearm. The wrist is usually extended and radially or ulnarly deviated as this force is applied. Thus, although this force acts to compress the wrist a shear component is also present. This force was found to increase significantly with speed and is also the largest force seen. As with the moments, peak forces occurred at extremes of range.

The ultimate goal of much of the effort toward investigating propulsion biomechanics is to reduce injury. Studies have shown that the biomechanics of wheelchair propulsion are affected by changes in wheelchair setup. If modifiable parameters can be found which cause wrist injuries, it may be possible to prevent their occurrence. A first step in the goal of reducing wheelchair propulsion-related injuries is to provide a robust methodology that enables characterization of the forces, moments, and motion at the wrist during wheelchair propulsion. In addition, reliable biomechanical parameters that describe the forces, moments, and motion, and are capable of differentiating between two conditions, are needed.

It is helpful to look at the pathophysiology and ergonomics of the most common wrist injury in manual wheelchair users. Carpal tunnel syndrome is generally thought to be caused by compression of the median nerve within the carpal tunnel. Extremes of wrist flexion and extension have been shown to greatly increase the pressure within the carpal tunnel, more so in patients with carpal tunnel syndrome. Gellman studied patients with spinal cord injuries and found that pressures in the carpal tunnel were higher in wrist flexion in this group than in a group of controls. In all of these studies, extremes of passive wrist flexion and extension were studied. Interestingly, our study found that the largest moments

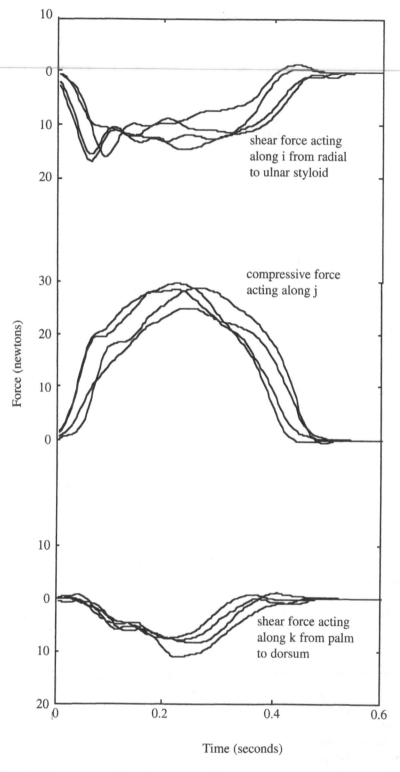

**FIGURE 4.12** Force versus time curve. Forces acting in each axis of the local coordinate system are shown. When the force is zero the subject's hand is off the pushrim; the remainder of the time is the propulsive phase.

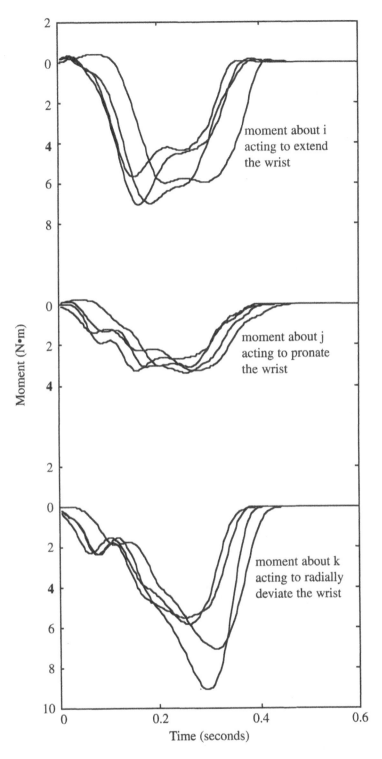

**FIGURE 4.13** Moment versus time curve. Four consecutive strokes for a single subject are presented. Moments acting in each axis of the local coordinate system are shown. When the moment is zero the subject's hand is off the pushrim; the remainder of the time is the propulsive phase.

occur in the direction of ulnar deviation, not extension. In addition, the amount of movement in radial and ulnar deviation was equal to that in flexion and extension. Although ulnar deviation has not been studied as extensively as flexion and extension, it too has been linked to the development of carpal tunnel syndrome.

There is a large body of epidemiologic and ergonomic literature relating carpal tunnel syndrome to worksite risk factors. A number of studies have shown that high force–high repetition jobs are associated with a high incidence of carpal tunnel syndrome. Silverstein et al. performed biomechanical investigation of a number of jobs and stratified these to determine the risk of carpal tunnel syndrome. Silverstein found that high force and high repetition jobs were associated with carpal tunnel syndrome. Their definition of high repetition was a cycle time of less than 30 seconds. Clearly the cycle time of the propulsive stroke (approximately 1 sec) fits this category. High force was defined as average hand force of more than 39 N while low force was defined as below 9.8 N. In our study, the mean compressive force at the wrist over the propulsive cycle was usually somewhere between these two forces. Loslever et al. studied factors associated with the early development of CTS in high-risk jobs. The time spent exerting forces over 20 N was found to correlate with the early development of CTS. Data for wheelchair propulsion show the compressive force to be over 20 N during a large percentage of the propulsive phase.

## 4.6 Biomechanics of Seating

When seated, the body is positioned such that its weight is supported mainly by the ischial tuberosities of the pelvis and the surrounding soft tissues. Depending on the wheelchair and posture, some proportion of the total body weight will be transferred to the seat, backrest, legrests, and armrests of the wheelchair. Proper seating posture can provide stability to perform precise visual and motor control tasks. Proper seating can reduce the strain on muscles, tendons, and joints. Proper seating posture can reduce hydrostatic pressure and improve venous return in lower extremities.

The spine is particularly important to seating posture, as are the upper and lower extremities. Many people with disabilities develop or have developed spinal deformities. Curvature of the spine requires special consideration when designing seating support structures. For the purpose of designing seating and postural support devices, the spine can be divided into three regions: the flexible cervical and lumbar spine, and the rigid thoracic spine. The thoracic spine is sandwiched between the cervical and lumbar spine. The cervical spine is attached to the head, which is assumed rigid, whereas the lumber spine is connected to the sacrum, which is rigidly affixed to the pelvis.

Sitting can be divided into three postures: anterior, median, and posterior. The distinction is based on the location of the person's center of mass, which affects the distribution of body mass over the seat, backrest, and legrests. The shape of the spine is also affected by posture. When in a relaxed median position the center of mass is directly above the ischial tuberosities, and the lumbar spine is either straight or in slight kyphosis. Forward rotation results from forward rotation of the pelvis with a straight spine or by little rotation of the pelvis and large kyphosis. Contoured seating structures offer reduced pressure and shape deformation around the ischial tuberosities in a relaxed median position. This cushion design may reduce the risk of decubitus ulcers; however, the pelvis must remain free to rotate to prevent extreme kyphosis when the person moves to an anterior posture. In a posterior posture the person's center of mass is behind the ischial tuberosities, and corresponds to rearward rotation of the pelvis and kyphosis of the spine. The design of the backrest has substantial effect on posterior seating posture.

The postures of the cervical spine, shoulders, and upper extremities are often dependent on the assistive devices used and the work layout. Hence, seating posture and task performance are interrelated. The posture of people with disabilities is dependent on their anthropometry, disability etiology, level of impairment, and sitting habits. The height, inclination, and depth of the seat affect seating posture. The position, shape, height, and angle of the backrest influence seating posture. The length, angle, and shape of the legrests influence seating posture. Other structures of the wheelchair or seating system (e.g., armrests) influence seating as well. Therefore when designing/selecting a seating system and wheelchair the tasks to be performed in the system must be considered as well as the physical attributes of the person. Also it is important that alterations in posture be permitted.

Radiographic studies have shown pelvis rotation and flattening of the lumbar spine lordosis while seated. A properly designed lower back support can mitigate flattening of lumbar lordosis. The shape of the lumbar spine during sitting depends on the rotation of the pelvis. When seated the sacral endplate become nearly horizontal and normal lumbar lordosis becomes flattened. Providing some sacral horizontal angle can help to provide a more neutral lumbar lordosis. Several suggestions have been made with respect to preventing flattening of the lumbar spine: a forward tilted seat, pelvis fixation, increased seat height, increased backrest height. Lumbar or total back support (provided scapula movement is unrestricted) are most successful in providing healthy seating posture.

Certain postures place greater pressure on the discs of the lumbar spine. There is an increase in trunk load moment upon the lumbar discs when the pelvis is rotated backwards and the lumbar spine and torso are rotated forwards. There is deformation of the discs themselves with lumbar lordosis flattening. Inclination of the backrest angle can result in decreased disc pressure. An optimal of about 110 degrees has been published. Studies have also shown a decrease in disc pressure when lumbar support was added at the level of the fourth and fifth lumbar vertebrae. The use of armrests has also been shown to reduce disc pressure.

Head and neck position is usually determined by visual requirements. Head and neck flexion are often related to visual tasks. For some people the head and neck provide an important control input. By altering the position of devices and monitors, the amount of head and neck flexion can be controlled. This is a common problem among users of augmentative communication devices who have certain demands on their arms for control of the device, and other demands on their head and neck for observing the display. There is little variation in the values of the muscle moment arms with changes in posture, therefore the spine muscle forces are approximately proportional to the load moments. A flexed neck posture should be avoided when possible.

Bending and reaching have been shown to increase disc pressure due to large external moments imparted on the spine. This factor should be considered when integrating multiple assistive technologies with the wheelchair. For people who use wheelchairs for many hours during the day a zero-shear reclining system should be used to permit changes in posture. The layout of other assistive devices should be such that lifting and moving is minimized. Operation of such devices should be performed with the person's joints and limbs in their near-neutral position.

It is not uncommon for therapists, rehabilitation engineers, and users to integrate assistive devices with the wheelchair. Even simple devices (e.g., lap trays) may alter the working seating position. The placement of the work surface and devices relative to the person is important not only because they influence the spine, but because they influence the posture of and loads on the upper extremity as well. When performing work on a lap tray or countertop, a shoulder abduction angle of less than 20 degrees and a flexion angle of less than 25 degrees should be attempted.

The ball-in-socket arrangement of the glenohumeral joint provides the arm with a large amount of mobility. This mobility is enhanced by six additional joints that comprise the trunk-arm complex or shoulder girdle. This extreme mobility is at the sacrifice of intrinsic stability. Stability is provided by the ligaments, joint capsules, and musculature of the upper extremity. The head of the humerus is held in the glenoid socket by the scapula through the combined actions of the rotator cuff muscles and the pectoral muscles. Many muscle and skeletal structures are involved in movement of the shoulder. During many movements demand on one set of muscles is compromised at the expense of another set of muscles.

When integrating technologies or designing a workspace for the wheelchair user, a particular concern should be to minimize the length and number of times the hands must be lifted above shoulder height. This type of activity may aggravate the stress induced on the shoulder by manual wheelchair propulsion, and may lead to degenerative tendinitis in the biceps and supraspinatus muscles. In extended reach positions the shoulder joint is flexed and the elbow is extended. Load moments at the elbow and shoulder can become large relative to the flexor strength moments required at both joints. Use of an adjustable elbow support can reduce the moments on the shoulder and elbow.

Arm and forearm postures are not only dictated by the location of the hand, but also by hand orientation around the long axis of the forearm. If the hand is supinated, then the arm will normally be adducted and close to the torso. If operation of a device requires the hand to be prone, then the arm will normally be abducted and elevated. The relation between hand posture and arm orientation is important when designing or selecting devices to integrate with a wheelchair workstation.

Legrests provide critical support not only while mobile, but while stationary as well. Proper leg support can help the reduce the load on the buttocks and thighs. Legrests should be adjusted so that the feet sit squarely and firmly on the footrests. The weight of the lower legs and feet should be supported solely by the legrests, and not by the front of the thighs. Pressure to the thighs behind the knee can increase edema in the legs and place pressure on the sciatic nerve. Range of motion exercises and changes in seating posture can reduce edema in the legs. The seat base pan should be about 3 to 5 centimeters below the knee when loaded. The edge of the cushion or seat should be contoured to relieve pressure. About 5 to 10 centimeters of clearance should be provided between the edge of the seat pan and the center of the knees.

A seat angle of about five degrees is typical. Some wheelchair users prefer a larger seat angle because of the greater stability it provides. However, seat angles in excess of 15 degrees are not recommended. Excessive seat angle can result in small knee flexion angle, which may transfer the weight of the trunk over a small area at the ischial tuberosities. The spine may also become flexed as the pelvis rotates backward. In addition, the abdominal organs are compressed in this posture when one leans forward.

## 4.7 Access System Biomechanics

Many power wheelchair users require multiple assistive devices (e.g., wheelchair, environmental control unit, communication device, computer access device). Integrated controls allow the user to control more than one assistive device through a single input device. Typically, this is the device chosen to control the power wheelchair. If the power wheelchair is optimized to the driver as described previously, then the appropriate hardware and software protocol can be used to interconnect various devices. This would provide the user effective control of a variety of electronic assistive devices. Integrated controls is the term used to describe plug-and-play for assistive devices. Ideally, all electronic assistive devices would use compatible communication protocols and interconnected hardware. The need for integrated controls is illustrated by the walking/talking problem. Many power wheelchair users who use augmentative communication devices cannot operate both systems simultaneously (i.e., the walking and talking problem). Neither of these systems requires constant vigilance, but they are limited by their input structure and inability to communicate over a common communications bus. If both the power wheelchair and augmentative communication system could be controlled with the same input device and communicate over a common data bus, then shared control would permit the user to toggle between driving and talking states. The two subsystems maintain speech and safe driving while the other subsystem is being controlled by the user. This case and others like it have prompted work on a worldwide assistive device electronic communication standard.

The RESNA Serial Interface Standards Committee and Trace Center have made significant advances toward developing a worldwide serial interface communications standard between power wheelchairs and other devices. This work and the work of European groups has formed the basis for a draft ISO standard (TC 173/SC-1/WG-7). The Multiple Master Multiple Slave (M3S) initiative is a European Economic Community (EEC) effort to develop a standard interface between various electronic assistive technologies. M3S is based upon the CAN (controller area network) protocol used in many modern automobiles.

Many assistive devices include at least one input device (e.g., joystick, head-operated switch, extremity-operated switch, or voice recognition system) and at least one actuator (e.g., wheelchair, environmental control unit, robot, voice synthesizer). The M3S bus is suitable for general purpose applications with the proper systems and subsystems (see Figure 4.14). The M3S standard is essentially the CAN bus with additional lines used to increase margins of safety and reliability. The advantage of M3S over current technology is the ability to simply interface multiple assistive devices and other technical products within the user's environment. The M3S bus permits control of multiple actuators with a single input device. This allows the input device to be optimized to the user's abilities, and subsequently used to control a number of actuators.

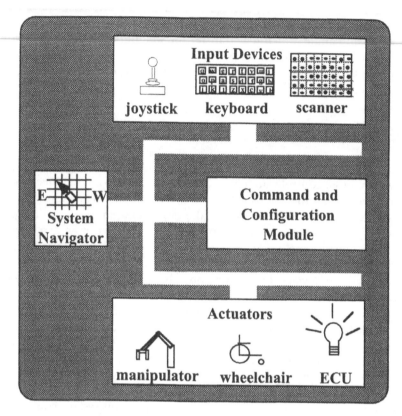

**FIGURE 4.14**  Illustration of multiple master multiple slave (M3S) architecture. Multiple input devices and multiple actuators can be on the M3S bus simultaneously. A system navigator works with the command and configuration module (CCM) to set priorities, perform handshaking, and for device identification. The CCM monitors and controls communication between various components of the system.

The M3S standard would specify a basic hardware architecture, a bus communication system, and a configuration method. A basic M3S bus consists of 7 wires: 2 power lines, 2 CAN lines, 2 safety lines, 1 shield, and 1 special support line (harness number). The M3S bus is intelligent in that it is easily configured to meet each user's individual needs. The intelligence in the system exists in the controllers of the individual input devices, actuators, and control and configuration module (CCM). The CCM deals with the processing necessary to configure the system and the ongoing need to monitor the safety of the system. The CCM is linked to a simple display that allows the user to select and operate each actuator. The CCM processor itself contains the master menu used to select individual actuators. The M3S system possesses the capability to access a wide range of devices via wireless link (infrared or radio) to a home bus.

Joysticks and switches can be used effectively to control a powered wheelchair or power base (see Figure 4.15). The joystick is the most common control interface between the user and the wheelchair. Joysticks produce voltage signals proportional to displacement, force, or switch closures. Displacement joysticks are most popular. Displacement joysticks may use either potentiometers, variable inductors (coils), or

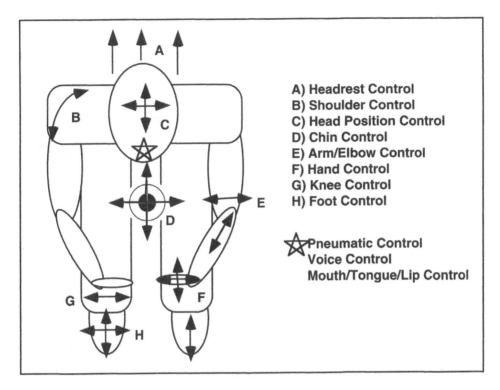

A) Headrest Control
B) Shoulder Control
C) Head Position Control
D) Chin Control
E) Arm/Elbow Control
F) Hand Control
G) Knee Control
H) Foot Control

Pneumatic Control
Voice Control
Mouth/Tongue/Lip Control

**FIGURE 4.15** Potential interface sites for use in controlling a powered wheelchair

optical sensors to convert displacement to voltage. Inductive joysticks are most common because they wear well, the stick is not physically in contact with the windings, and they can be made quite sensitive. Joysticks can be modified to be used for chin, foot, elbow, tongue, or shoulder control. Typically, short-throw joysticks are used for these applications. Force-sensing joysticks use three basic transducers: simple springs and dampers on a displacement joystick, cantilever beams with strain gages, and fluid with pressure sensors. Force-sensing joysticks that rely on passive dampers or fluid pressure generally require the user to have range of motion within normal values for displacement joystick users. Beam-based force-sensing joysticks require negligible motion, and hence may be used for people with limited motion abilities.

People who exhibit intention tremor require special control considerations. Signal processing techniques are often required to grant the user greater control over the wheelchair. Typically, signal averaging or a low-pass filter with a cutoff frequency of below 5 Hertz is used. The signal processing is typically incorporated into the controller. Some people lack the fine motor control to use a joystick effectively. An alternative for these people is to use switch control or head-position control. Switch control simply uses either a set of switches or a single switch and a coded input, i.e., Morse code or some other simple switch code. The input of the user is latched by the controller and the wheelchair performs the task commanded by the user. The user may latch the chair to repeatedly perform a task a specified number of times, e.g., continue straight until commanded to do otherwise. Switch control is quite functional, but it is generally slower than joystick control. Switch inputs can be generated in many ways. Typically, low-pressure switches are used. The input can come from a sip-&-puff mechanism that works off a pressure transducer. A switch contact is detected when the pressure exceeds or drops below a threshold. The pressure sensor may be configured to react to pressure generated by the user blowing into or sipping from an input or by the user simply interrupting the flow in or out of a tube. Sip-&-puff may also be used as a combination of proportional and switch control. For example, the user can put the control in the "read speed" mode and then the proportional voltage output from the pressure transducer will be latched as the user-desired speed.

Simple switches of various sizes can be used to control the chair with many parts of the body. Switches may be mounted on the armrests or a lap tray for hand or arm activation, on the footrest(s) for foot activation, or on a headrest for head activation. The motion of the head can also be used for proportional control by using ultrasonic sensors. Ultrasonic sensors can be mounted in an array about the headrest. The signal produced by the ultrasonic sensors is related to the position of the head. Hence, motion of the head can be used to create a proportional control signal. Ultrasonic head control and switch control can be combined to give some users greater mastery over their power wheelchair. Switches can be used to select the controller mode, whereas the ultrasonic sensors give a proportional input signal.

A critical consideration when selecting or designing a user interface is that the ability of the user to accurately control the interface is heavily dependent on the stability of the user within the wheelchair. Often custom seating and postural support systems are required for a user interface to be truly effective. The placement of the user interface is also critical to its efficacy as a functional control device.

## References and Further Reading

Aljure J., Eltorai I., Bradley W. E., Lin J. E., Johnson B. (1985) Carpal tunnel syndrome in paraplegic patients. *Paraplegia* 23; 182–186.

Armstrong T. J., Foulke J. A., Joseph B. S., Goldstein S. A. (1982) Investigation of cumulative trauma disorders in a poultry processing plant. *American Industrial Hygiene Association Journal* 43:103–116.

Aronson R. M., Carley D. W., Onal E., Wilborn J., Lopata M. (1991) Upper airway muscle activity and the thoracic volume dependence of upper airway resistance. *Journal of Applied Physiology* 70(1):430–438.

Axelson P., Minkel J., Chesney D. (1994) A guide to wheelchair selection: How to use the ANSI/RESNA wheelchair standards to buy a wheelchair. Washington DC, Paralyzed Veterans of America.

Bartolucci M. (1992) Making a chair able by design. *Metropolis* 12(4):29–33.

Bayley J. C., Cochran T. P., Sledge C. B. (1987). The weight-bearing shoulder. The impingement syndrome in paraplegics. *Journal of Bone and Joint Surgery–American Volume* 69:676–678.

Bergenudd H., Lindgarde F., Nilsson B., Petersson C. J. (1988). Shoulder pain in middle age. A study of prevalence and relation to occupational work load and psychosocial factors. *Clinical Orthopaedics and Related Research:* 234–238.

Bigliani L. U., Morrison D. S., April E. W. (1986). The morphology of the acromion and its relationship to rotator cuff tears. *Orthopaedic Transactions* 10:216.

Briskorn C. N. (1994). Composing the composite. *Team Rehab Report* 5(2):35–39.

Brooks L. (1994) Use of devices for mobility by the elderly. *Wisconsin Medical Journal,* January.

Brubaker C. E. (1986) Wheelchair prescription: An analysis of factors that affect mobility and performance. *Journal of Rehabilitation Research and Development* 23(4):19–26.

Burnham R. S., May L., Nelson E., Steadward R., Reid D. C. (1993) Shoulder pain in wheelchair athletes. The role of muscle imbalance. *American Journal of Sports Medicine* 21:238–242.

Burnham R. S., Steadward R. D. (1994) Upper extremity peripheral nerve entrapments among wheelchair athletes: Prevalence, location, and risk factors. *Archives of Physical Medicine and Rehabilitation* 75:519–524.

Cherniack R. M. (1977) *Pulmonary Function Testing.* Philadelphia, PA, W.B. Saunders Co.

Church G., Glennen S. (1992) *The Handbook of Assistive Technology.* San Diego, CA, Singular Publishing Group.

Cole T. M., Edgerton V. R. (1990) Report of the task force on medical rehabilitation research. Hunt Valley, Maryland National Institutes of Health.

Cooper R. A. (1990) A comparison of pulmonary functions of wheelchair racers in their racing and standard wheelchairs. *Proceedings RESNA 14th Annual Conference,* Kansas City, MO, 245–247.

Cooper R. A. (1995) *Rehabilitation Engineering Applied to Mobility and Manipulation.* London, U.K., Institute of Physics Publishers.

Cooper R. A., Baldini F. D., Robertson R. N., Jones D., Monical S., Vosse A. (1992) Pulmonary function of elite wheelchair athletes. *Palaestra* 8(4):10.

Crapo R. O., Morris A. H. (1981) Standardized single breath normal values for carbon monoxide diffusing capacity. *American Review Respiratory Disease* 123:185–189.

Crapo R. O., Morris A. H., Clayton P. D., Nixon C. R. (1982) Lung volumes in healthy non-smoking adults. *Bulletin European Physiopathology Respiratory* 18:419–425.

Crapo R. O., Morris A. H., Gardner R. M. (1981) Reference spirometric values using techniques and equipment that meet ATS recommendations. *American Review Respiratory Disease* 123:659–664.

Davidoff G., Werner R., Waring W. (1991) Compressive mononeuropathies of the upper extremity in chronic paraplegia. *Paraplegia* 29:17–24.

Delgrosso I., Boillat M. A. (1991) Carpal tunnel syndrome: Role of occupation. *International Archives of Occupational and Environmental Health* 63:267–270.

Ferrara M. S., Buckley W. E., McCann B. C., Limbird T. J., Powell J. W., Robl R. (1992) The injury experience of the competitive athlete with a disability: Prevention implications. *Medicine and Science in Sports and Exercise* 24(2):184–188.

Frieman B. G., Albert T. J., Fenlin J. M., Jr. (1994) Rotator cuff disease: A review of diagnosis, pathophysiology, and current trends in treatment [Review]. *Archives of Physical Medicine and Rehabilitation* 75:604–609.

Fu F. H., Harner C. D., Klein A. H. (1991) Shoulder impingement syndrome. A critical review [Review]. *Clinical Orthopaedics and Related Research,*162–173.

Gelberman R. H., Hergenroeder P. T., Hargens A. R., Lundborg G. N., Akeson W. H. (1981) The carpal tunnel syndrome. A study of carpal canal pressures. *Journal of Bone and Joint Surgery–American Volume* 63:380–383.

Gellman H., Chandler D. R., Petrasek J., Sie I., Adkins R., Waters R. L. (1988a) Carpal tunnel syndrome in paraplegic patients. *Journal of Bone and Joint Surgery* 70:517–519.

Gellman H., Sie I., Waters R. L. (1988b) Late complications of the weight-bearing upper extremity in the paraplegic patient. *Clinical Orthopaedics and Related Research:*132-135.

Gross D., Ladd H. W., Riley E. J., Macklem P. T., Grassino A. (1980) The effect of training on strength and endurance of the diaphragm in quadriplegia. *American Journal of Medicine* 68:27–35.

Hagberg M., Morgenstern H., Kelsh M. (1992) Impact of occupations and job tasks on the prevalence of carpal tunnel syndrome [Review]. *Scandinavian Journal of Work, Environment and Health* 18:337–345.

Hardy D. C., Vogler J. B., White R. H. (1986) The shoulder impingement syndrome: Prevalence of radiographic findings. *American Journal of Roentgenology* 147:557–561.

Herberts P., Kadefors R., Andersson G., Petersen I. (1981) Shoulder pain in industry: An epidemiological study on welders. *Acta Orthopaedica Scandinavica* 52:299–306.

Herberts P., Kadefors R., Hogfors C., Sigholm G. (1984) Shoulder pain and heavy manual labor. *Clinical Orthopaedics and Related Research*:166–178.

Hinton R. Y. (1988) Isokinetic evaluation of shoulder rotational strength in high school baseball pitchers. *American Journal of Sports Medicine* 16:274–279.

Hullemann K. D., List M., Matthes D. (1975) Spiroergometric and telemetric investigations during the XXI International Stoke Mandeville games 1972 in Heidelberg. *Paraplegia* 13:109–123.

Iannotti S. P., Swiontkowski M. F., Esterhai J. L. (1989) Intraoperative assessment of rotator cuff vascularity using laser Doppler flowmetry. New York, NY, 4th International Conference on Surgery of the Shoulder.

Jobe F. W., Kvitne R. S., Giangarra C. E. (1989) Shoulder pain in the overhand or throwing athlete. The relationship of anterior instability and rotator cuff impingement. *Orthopaedic Review* 18:963–975.

Kamenetz H. (1969) *The Wheelchair Book: Mobility for the Disabled.* Springfield, IL, C.C. Thomas.

Kirby R., Ackroyd-Stolarz S. (1995) Wheelchair Safety—Adverse Reports to the United States Food and Drug Administration. *American Journal of Physical Medicine and Rehabilitation* 74(4).

Kokkola K., Moller K., Lehtonen T. (1975) Pulmonary function in tetraplegic and paraplegic. *Annals of Clinical Research* 7:76–79.

Laplante M. (1991) The demographics of disability. *Milbank Quarterly* 69(1–2):55–77.

Leaf D. A., Adkins R. H., Greenwood J., Bahl R. A. (1990) Maximal aerobic capacity and theoretical implications for longevity revisited in spinal cord injury patients. *Annals of Sports Medicine* 5:133–137.

Leith D. E., Bradley M. (1976) Ventilatory muscle strength and endurance training. *Journal of Applied Physiology* 41(4):508–516.

Loslever P., Ranaivosoa A. (1993) Biomechanical and epidemiological investigation of carpal tunnel syndrome at workplaces with high risk factors. *Ergonomics* 36:537–555.

Lundborg G., Gelberman R. H., Minteer-Convery M., Lee Y. F., Hargens A. R. (1982) Median nerve compression in the carpal tunnel—functional response to experimentally induced controlled pressure. *Journal of Hand Surgery* 7:252–259.

McMaster W. C., Long S. C., Caiozzo V. J. (1991) Isokinetic torque imbalances in the rotator cuff of the elite water polo player. *American Journal of Sports Medicine* 19:72–75.

McNeil J. M. (1991–92) *Americans with Disabilities.* Data From the Survey of Income and Program Participation, P70, 33.

Miles D. S., Sawka M. N., Wilde S. W., Durbin R. J., Gotshall R. W., Glaser R. M. (1982) Pulmonary function changes in wheelchair athletes subsequent to exercise training. *Ergonomics* 25(3):239–246.

Moore J. S. (1992) Carpal tunnel syndrome [Review]. *Occupational Medicine: State of the Art Reviews* 7:741–763.

*Morbidity and Mortality Weekly Report* (1994) Prevalence of Disabilities and Associated Health conditions—United States, 1991–1992. *MMWR* 43(40) (The On-line Journal of Current Clinical Trials).

*National Center for Health Statistics* (1992) National Health Interview Survey of Assistive Devices, 1990, NCHS (Hyattsville, Maryland).

Neer C. S., II. (1972) Anterior acromioplasty for the chronic impingement syndrome in the shoulder: A preliminary report. *Journal of Bone and Joint Surgery* 54:41–50.

Neer C. S., II. (1983) Impingement lesions. *Clinical Orthopaedics and Related Research* 173:70–77.

Nichols P. J., Norman P. A., Ennis J. R.(1979) Wheelchair user's shoulder? Shoulder pain in patients with spinal cord lesions. *Scandinavian Journal of Rehabilitation Medicine* 11:29–32.

Ohry A., Molho M., Rozin R. (1975) Alterations of pulmonary function in spinal cord injured patients. *Paraplegia* 13:101–108.

Ozaki J., Fujimoto S., Nakagawa Y., Masuhara K., Tamai S. (1988) Tears of the rotator cuff of the shoulder associated with pathological changes in the acromion. A study in cadavera. *Journal of Bone and Joint Surgery* 70:1224–1230.

Pickles B., Topping A. (1994) Community care for Canadian seniors: An exercise in educational planning. *Disability and Rehabilitation* 16(3):181–189.

Pentland W. E., Twomey L. T. (1991) The weight-bearing upper extremity in women with long term paraplegia. *Paraplegia* 29:521–530.

Powers S. K., Lawler J., Criswell D., Lileu F., Martin D. (1992) Aging and respiratory muscle metabolic plasticity: Effects of endurance training. *Journal of Applied Physiology* 72(3):1068–1073.

Rathbun J. B., Macnab I. (1970) The microvascular pattern of the rotator cuff. *Journal of Bone and Joint Surgery* 52:540–553.

Shephard R. (1988) Sports medicine and the wheelchair athlete. *Sports Medicine* 4:226–247.

Sie I. H., Waters R. L., Adkins R. H., Gellman H. (1992) Upper extremity pain in the post-rehabilitation spinal cord injured patient. *Archives of Physical Medicine and Rehabilitation* 73:44–48.

Silverstein B. A., Fine L. J., Armstrong T. J. (1987) Occupational factors and carpal tunnel syndrome. *American Journal of Industrial Medicine* 11:343–358.

Sonn U., Grimby G. (1994) Assistive devices in an elderly population studied at 70–76 years of age. *Disability and Rehabilitation* 16(2):85–93.

Stefaniwsky L., Bilowit D. S., Prasad S. S. (1980) Reduced motor conduction velocity of the ulnar nerve in spinal cord injured patients. *Paraplegia* 18:21–24.

Stenlund B., Goldie I., Hagberg M., Hogstedt C., Marions O. (1992) Radiographic osteoarthrosis in the acromioclavicular joint resulting from manual work or exposure to vibration. *British Journal of Industrial Medicine* 49:588–593.

Stenlund B., Goldie I., Hagberg M., Hogstedt C. (1993) Shoulder tendinitis and its relation to heavy manual work and exposure to vibration. *Scandinavian Journal of Work, Environment and Health* 19:43–49.

Stone D., Keltz H. (1964) The effect of respiratory muscle dysfunction on pulmonary function. *Journal of Applied Physiology* 43:621–629.

Trefler E., Hobson D. A., Johnson Taylor S., Monahan L. C., Shaw G. C. (1993) *Seating and Mobility for Persons with Physical Disabilities*. Tucson, AZ, Therapy Skill Builders.

Tun C. G., Upton J. (1988) The paraplegic hand: Electrodiagnostic studies and clinical findings. *Journal of Hand Surgery* 13:716–719.

Van Loan M. D., McCluer M. D., Loftin J. M., Boileau R. A. (1987) Comparison of physiological responses to maximal arm exercise among able-bodied paraplegics and quadriplegics. *Paraplegia* 25:397–405.

Wells C. L., Hooker S. P. (1990) The spinal injured athlete. *Adapted Physical Activity Quarterly* 7:265–285.

Werner C. O., Elmqvist D., Ohlin P. (1983) Pressure and nerve lesion in the carpal tunnel. *Acta Orthopaedica Scandinavica* 54:312–316.

Wilson A. B. (1992) *Wheelchairs: A Prescription Guide.* New York, NY, Demos.

Winter D. A. (1990) *Biomechanics and Motor Control of Human Movement,* 2nd ed. New York, NY, John Wiley & Sons.

Wylie E. J., Chakera T. M. (1988) Degenerative joint abnormalities in patients with paraplegia of duration greater than 20 years. *Paraplegia* 26:101–106.

Zwiren L. D., Bar-Or O. (1974) Responses to exercise of paraplegics who differ in conditioning level. *Medicine and Science in Sport* 7(2):94–98.

# CHAPTER 5

# Wheelchair Electronics Fundamentals

*Chapter Goals*

☑ To understand electrical and electronic principles
☑ To appreciate basic computer literacy related to power wheelchairs, record keeping, and information access
☑ To understand the relationship between technology and its environment
☑ To know how to problem-solve and integrate technical and functional information
☑ To understand the roles, constraints, and perspectives of designers and fabricators

## 5.1 Introduction

Many assistive devices have been made possible through developments in electronics. Electric-powered wheelchairs make extensive use of electronics and electrical principles. Electricity and magnetism have a long history, and have had a profound impact on our quality of life. Electricity results when two charged particles are placed in the vicinity of each other. Magnetism results from the motion of charged particles. *Electrical engineering* focuses on the study and application of electricity and magnetism. *Electronics* is a branch of electrical engineering that focuses on signal processing and electrical systems. Electronics is commonly associated with semiconductor devices.

Electricity occurs in nature, and has been a source of fear and wonderment for centuries. Lightning is a form of electricity that most people have witnessed. Other forms of natural electricity exist. The natural attraction of the mineral magnetite to soft iron was first discovered by Thales of Miletus. Electricity and magnetism can also be generated. In 1551, Jerome Cardan began to distinguish materials by rubbing them together to see if they were electric or magnetic. Jerome Cardan also developed the first theory of electricity founded on fluid concepts. In 1747, Benjamin Franklin developed the first single fluid theory of electricity and introduced the concept of positive and negative electrification. Franklin defined excess fluid as positive electrification, and fluid deficiency as negative electrification. Current theories no longer consider electricity to be a fluid, but the concept of positive and negative charge persists. Charge is an important concept in electricity. The force between two particles is related to their charge. This relationship is called *Coulomb's Law*, in honor of C. A. Coulomb's discovery in 1785. Coulomb's Law provides a foundation for many electrical devices. Electricity was not a useful source of energy until A. Volta developed the *voltaic cell* in 1800. The voltaic cell is more commonly called a battery cell and is used as the basis of batteries. Batteries are an important source of electrical energy, which powers all current electric wheelchairs. Because of this significant discovery, Volta is remembered by having the unit of electrical potential, the volt, named in his honor. The relationship between electricity and magnetism was exploited in 1827 by Joseph Henry to develop the electromagnet. An electromagnet is a coil of wire that acts like a magnet when current flows through the wire. In 1840, Samuel F. B. Morse was granted a patent for the electromagnet telegraph. Electromagnets are key components to electric motors; Michael Faraday, in 1831, showed that changing magnetic fields induces electrical currents. Michael Faraday's discoveries eventually led to the development of the first electric power plant in New York City in 1882. These developments were all based on *direct current* (d.c.). As the name implies, direct current flows in only one direction; later, alternating current was developed. *Alternating current* flows in one direction part of the time and in the opposite direction the remainder of the time. Alternating current is the most commonly used form of electrical energy. However, most electric-powered wheelchairs use batteries and direct current motors.

The 1900s saw many more developments in electrical engineering. Television and radio were developed, as well as a host of other consumer electronics. With the development of electrical motors and batteries simple electric-powered wheelchairs could be developed, but many new discoveries were required to arrive at the microprocessor-controlled electric-powered wheelchair. Batteries and electric motors led to constant speed electric-powered wheelchairs that were controlled by direction switches (i.e., one switch for forward, one for reverse, one for left, and another for right). This provided limited control over the power wheelchair, and was unsuitable for many people. The invention of the *transistor* revolutionized the design of electric-powered wheelchairs, and made them useful for many people with physical impairments. The transistor is a semiconductor device that was invented at Bell Telephone Laboratories by J. Bardeen, W. Brattain, and W. Shockley in 1947. *Semiconductor* devices are made of materials whose abilities to control the flow of current can be regulated. The transistor is able to efficiently amplify signals, and forms the basis for modern electronics. The transistor is the basic component of an integrated circuit. An *integrated circuit* (IC) is a complete circuit performing a specific electrical function which is made on a single chip of semiconductor material, usually silicon. Hence the name *chip* is used to describe many common electronic components. Manufacturing processes and electrical engineering design have progressed to the point where entire computers, called *microprocessors*, can be made from a single chip of silicon. The advantage of this process is that it increases reliability, lowers cost, and reduces size. With the increasing demand for ICs, there is continuous improvement in manufacturing and design processes, which partially explains why computers become exceedingly more powerful while becoming less expensive, and why people can buy musical greeting cards with ICs. Power wheelchairs have numerous ICs and transistors, which control the motors and provide many possible access devices for consumers.

Electric-powered wheelchairs incorporate many aspects of electrical engineering. Some electrical concepts will be addressed in this chapter. A basic understanding of electrical concepts is necessary to fully appreciate the operation and manufacture of wheelchairs and to be able to critically evaluate new products as they are introduced.

## 5.2 Basic Electrical Parameters

In 1885, C. A. Coulomb applied Newton's "Inverse Square Law" to electricity to develop what is known today as "Coulomb's Law." Coulomb's Law states that the force of attraction or repulsion between two charged bodies is proportional to the product of their charges, and inversely proportional to the square of the distance between them. Charge is customarily represented by $q$, and the distance between the two bodies will be represented by $l$. Therefore, the force acting on the bodies ($F$) is

$$F \propto \frac{q_1 q_2}{l^2} \qquad (5.1)$$

From the relationship described by equation (5.1), A. M. Ampere developed the fundamental law of electrodynamics known as Ampere's Law. *Ampere's Law* is important because it recognizes electric current as the rate of flow of electric charge due to a driving force. *Current* is the term used to describe the motion of charged bodies. Because of this important contribution, the unit for current is named ampere after him. Ampere's Law states that current $I$ in amperes is proportional to the change in charge $\Delta q$ in coulombs, divided by the change in time $\Delta t$ in seconds,

$$I = \frac{\Delta q}{\Delta t} \qquad (5.2)$$

The movement of charges requires a driving force, or a difference in electrical potential. *Voltage* is the property used to describe the driving force acting on charged particles to create a current. Voltage, $V$, is equal to the amount of work performed, $W$, divided by the change in charge, $\Delta q$, to perform the work,

$$V = \frac{W}{\Delta q} \qquad (5.3)$$

Current and voltage are related in different ways, depending on the layout of the circuit and the components involved. One of the most fundamental components is the resistor. In 1833, G. S. Ohm presented *Ohm's Law* defining the relationship between current, voltage, and resistance. Subsequently, the units of resistance, ohms, were named in his honor. Ohm's Law states the voltage across a resistor, $V$, is equal to the resistance, $R$, times the current through the resistor, $I$,

$$V = IR \qquad (5.4)$$

Electrical resistance is much like resistance to flow of a fluid. Electrical resistance ($R$) is related to the length of the resistive material ($l$), the cross-sectional area of the resistive material ($A$), and the *resistivity* of the material ($\rho$):

$$R = \rho \frac{l}{A} \qquad (5.5)$$

In equation (5.5) the units of the resistivity are ohm•meter ($\Omega$•m), the length is measured in meters, and the area in meters squared. Materials with low resistivity are identified as good *conductors*, whereas materials with high resistivity are good *insulators*. Materials that are between conductors and insulators are called *semiconductors*. Copper is a good conductor and for this reason it is often used to make wire. Plastic is a good insulator, and is commonly used as a covering for wire.

Voltage is the work done per unit charge. Work is the expenditure of energy. It is important to remember that work can be done by both mechanical and electrical systems, and that work can be exchanged through energy between mechanical and electrical systems. This fundamental concept is the basis for electric-powered wheelchairs. Energy is a fundamental property which exists in nature. Energy cannot be created or destroyed; it can only be transformed from one form to another. This is known as the law of conservation of energy. For example, an electric-powered wheelchair uses energy stored as chemical energy within the batteries; the batteries transform the chemical energy into electrical energy, which is used to drive an electric motor, which transforms electrical energy into mechanical energy. Mechanical energy propels the wheelchair and driver.

Power is the amount of work done per unit time (see equation (3.63)). Power is a very important quantity and has the same definition for electrical, mechanical, and chemical systems. Power may be transformed from one form to another.

$$P = \frac{dW}{dt} \approx \frac{\Delta W}{\Delta t} = \frac{W_f - W_s}{t_f - t_s} \tag{3.63}$$

Another important property of power is that the total amount of power expended by a system can be determined by the sum of the power consumed by each of the components whether electrical, mechanical, or chemical. For example, the power consumed by the motors, controller, access system, friction, and moving the wheelchair and rider may be summed. The total power consumed must not exceed the total amount of power produced by the batteries.

The power in a d.c. electrical circuit is simply the product of the voltage across the circuit and the current through the circuit,

$$P = VI \tag{5.6}$$

The power absorbed by a resistor can be found using equation (5.6) and applying Ohm's Law,

$$P = VI = (IR)I = I^2 R \tag{5.7}$$

Equation (5.6) can be used to find the power for many practical devices and systems. In order to gain a better understanding of electrical power, some new concepts must be introduced. Previously the concepts of direct current and alternating current were introduced. The batteries produce direct current, whereas electrical power plants produce alternating current. Both types of current are used widely for different applications. Integrated circuits used in power wheelchair controllers and computers use direct current. In the case of computers, alternating current is converted to direct current through a device called a direct current power supply. Direct current flows in one direction and is always either positive or negative. Alternating current changes the direction of flow at regular intervals. Direct current can be described by an amplitude and direction, whereas alternating current must be described by an amplitude, direction, and frequency (see Figure 5.1).

Alternating current can be represented as a sinusoid with amplitude $I$, and period $T$,

$$I(t) = I \sin\left(\frac{2\pi}{T}t\right) = I \sin\left(2\pi f t\right) \qquad (5.8)$$

The frequency $(f)$ of the alternating current is equal to the reciprocal of the period for one complete oscillation,

$$f = \frac{1}{T} \qquad (5.9)$$

The concept of phase must be introduced before power for an alternating current circuit can be introduced. Some electrical components, including some motors, may shift the timing of the current and voltage. This has an effect on power calculations. Phase can be viewed as a time or frequency shift between voltage and current (see Figure 5.2).

The difference between the zero-crossing times can be used in equation (5.10) to determine the phase shift between the voltage and current,

$$\varphi = \pi\left(1 + \frac{2\tau}{T}\right) \qquad (5.10)$$

**FIGURE 5.1**  Plot of alternating current over time. The amplitude of the current is given by I, and the period of the current is T.

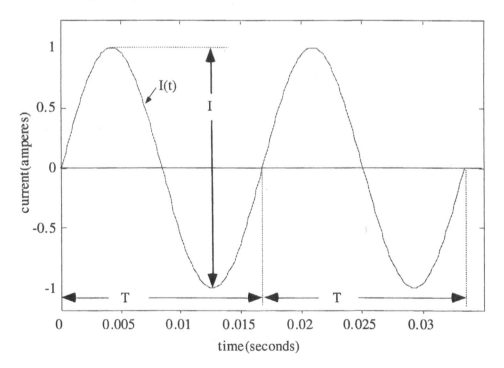

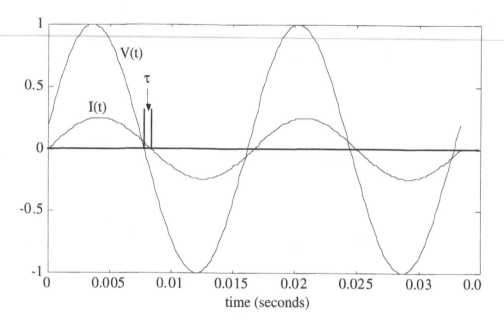

**FIGURE 5.2** Graph of alternating current and alternating voltage with a phase shift between them. The phase shift is demonstrated by the difference in the zero crossing point.

The units of phase are radians. Voltage is usually assumed to be zero phase; however, there may be a phase shift in the current induced by the circuit or device through which it flows. Alternating current voltage with zero phase is represented by

$$V(t) = V \sin (2\pi f t) \tag{5.11}$$

The current with a phase shift is similar to equation (5.8), but a term ($\varphi$) is added to the argument of the sine function,

$$I(t) = I \sin (2\pi f t + \varphi) \tag{5.12}$$

The power for the voltage and current described by equations (5.11) and (5.12) is given by their magnitudes and the phase angle,

$$P = VI \cos \varphi \tag{5.13}$$

The current and voltage plotted in Figure 5.2 can be described by equation (5.14),

$$I(t) = 0.25 \sin (2\pi 60t + 0.10) \qquad V(t) = \sin (2\pi 60t) \tag{5.14}$$

The power for the current and voltage in equation (5.14) is described by $I$, $V$, and the phase 0.10 radians,

$$P = (1)(0.25) \cos (0.10) = 0.249 \quad \text{Watts} \tag{5.15}$$

The principles introduced in this section provide a foundation for understanding aspects of electric-powered assistive devices. This is important to understanding the operation of electric-powered wheelchairs, wheelchair battery chargers, and other electrical devices.

## 5.3 Basic Electronic Components

### 5.3.1 Resistors

The resistor is one of the oldest and most commonly used electrical components. Resistors are considered passive elements because they do require an external energy source in order to function. Resistors obey Ohm's Law as described in section 5.2. Practical resistors are only available in distinct value, or as adjustable resistors known as potentiometers. Potentiometers are used on some wheelchairs to adjust their driving behavior for a specific individual. Fixed value resistors are marked by colored bands; see Figure 5.3.

Resistors are also rated for accuracy, expressed as the percent variation from the nominal value. Most resistors used in assistive devices have a 5% accuracy. Resistors are also rated for the amount of power that they can dissipate. Typical power

**FIGURE 5.3** Illustration of how resistor values are calculated

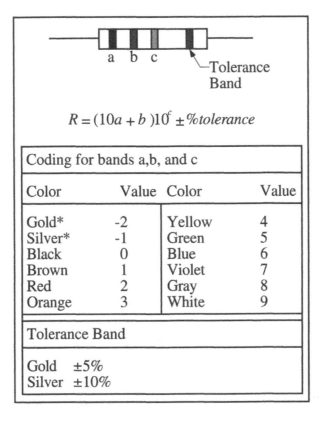

$$R = (10a + b )10^c \pm \%tolerance$$

| Coding for bands a,b, and c | | | |
|---|---|---|---|
| Color | Value | Color | Value |
| Gold* | -2 | Yellow | 4 |
| Silver* | -1 | Green | 5 |
| Black | 0 | Blue | 6 |
| Brown | 1 | Violet | 7 |
| Red | 2 | Gray | 8 |
| Orange | 3 | White | 9 |

| Tolerance Band | |
|---|---|
| Gold | ±5% |
| Silver | ±10% |

values are 1/4, 1/2, 1, and 10 Watts. Resistors with 1/4 Watts power rating are suit-able for electronic circuits; however, engineers typically calculate or estimate the power to be dissipated by the resistor before selecting a power rating. Engineers use symbols to represent resistors and potentiometers; these symbols are illustrated in Figure 5.4.

Potentiometers can be used as position sensors, because their resistance may be varied by moving a wiper attached to the potentiometer and the device whose position is to be measured. Position has been measured using potentiometers for a variety of published experiments. Potentiometers are also commonly used to make electric goniometers by using a rotary potentiometer, which changes its resistance in response to changes in angle. An example application of a potentiometer is pre-sented in Figure 5.5.

The goniometer presented in Figure 5.5 provides a convenient means of recording elbow angle with a computer. With a few simple components and the appropriate computer interface hardware and software, elbow angle can be dynam-ically recorded directly by a computer. This can make measurements more conve-nient and accurate.

### 5.3.2 Capacitors

Capacitors are passive elements that are commonly used in electric circuits, and are used as sensors. Capacitors can store energy that is provided from an external source. Capacitors are used in some wall-mounted flashlights that do not require batteries. The flashlight is connected to a wall outlet which provides energy to charge the capacitor. When the flashlight is used the energy stored in the capacitor is used to power a lightbulb. Capacitors are also used in some calculators to provide energy to the memory of the calculator for a few minutes so that batteries can be changed without losing the information stored in the calculator's memory. There are two symbols commonly used to describe capacitors in electric circuits, shown in Figure 5.6.

Some capacitors are directional, polarized, so that the voltage applied across them is supposed to be in a specific direction. Other capacitors may be placed in any orientation. A capacitor is a two-terminal element that can be modeled by two conducting plates separated by a dielectric material. Electric charge can be stored

**FIGURE 5.4**  Symbols for fixed and variable resistors used in electric circuits

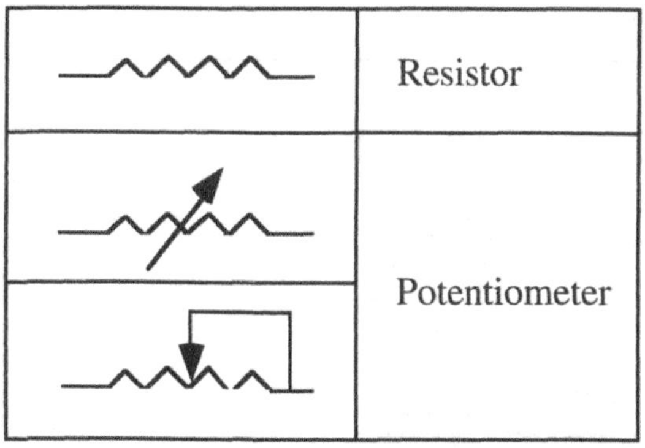

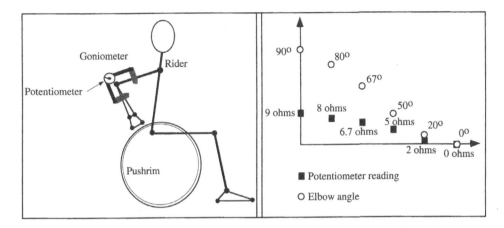

**FIGURE 5.5** Example use of a potentiometer to measure elbow angle as a change in resistance.

on the plates. The capacitance is proportional to the dielectric constant ($\varepsilon$), which determines the energy stored per unit volume per unit voltage difference across a capacitor (equation (5.16)).

$$C = \frac{\varepsilon A}{d} = \frac{q}{v} \qquad (5.16)$$

The area of the plates is given by $A$, and $d$ describes the space between the plates. The units of capacitance are farads. The current through a capacitor can be found by differentiating equation (5.17). Hence, if the voltage applied across a capacitor is constant, then the current will be zero. The capacitor type is determined by its dielectric material. As a practical matter capacitors are given a voltage rating which is the maximum voltage that can safely be applied to the capacitor. Common types of capacitors include ceramic (barium titanate), Mylar, Teflon, polystyrene, and tantalum. These types of capacitors range in value from 100 pF to 1 mF having tolerances 3%, 10%, and 20%. Larger capacitance values require use of electrolytic capacitors. Electrolytic capacitors are constructed of polarized layers of aluminum oxide or tantalum oxide and can yield values of 1 to 100,000 mF. Electrolytic capacitors are polarized and must be connected to the circuit with the proper voltage polarity.

$$q = Cv \Rightarrow \frac{dq}{dt} = i = C\frac{dv}{dt} \qquad (5.17)$$

**FIGURE 5.6** Electrical symbols used to represent capacitors

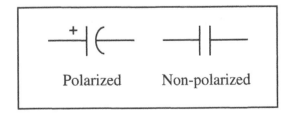

Capacitors have been used as seating pressure sensors, by exploiting the relationships in equations (5.16) and (5.17). If we examine equation (5.16), the capacitance will vary by changing the dielectric material, increasing or decreasing the distance between the two parallel plates, or by changing the area of overlap between the plates (see Figure 5.7).

If the changes made in the capacitance are in response to a pressure or force, then the possibility exists to use it as a sensor. Two methods have been used to make capacitance sensors for wheelchairs or seating. Pressure has been measured by using a dielectric material that is compressible like a spring. For example, rubber or foam has been used as a dielectric material sandwiched between two pieces of copper foil. One side of the copper foil is placed on the seating surface and the person sits on the other piece of copper foil. The rubber or foam between the copper foil compresses due to the person's weight, and the distance, $d$, decreases causing an increase in the capacitance. Hence, a capacitive sensor can be used to measure seating or backrest pressure. Multiple sensors can be used to create a pressure-sensing mat. Another approach is to change the overlapping area of the two parallel plates. The torque applied to the wheels of an electric-powered wheelchair can be measured by using two concentric parallel plates that are connected by a torsional spring, a spring that resists twisting (see Figure 5.8). As

**FIGURE 5.7**    Examples of how capacitance can be changed to be used as a sensor

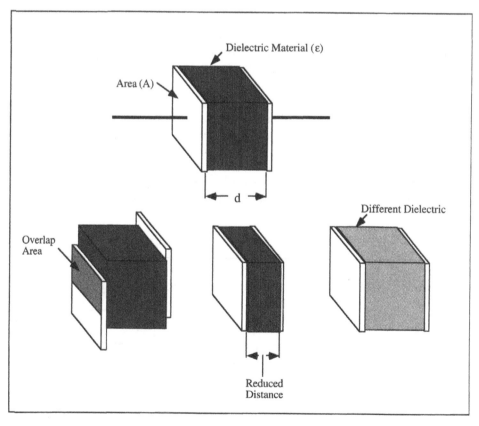

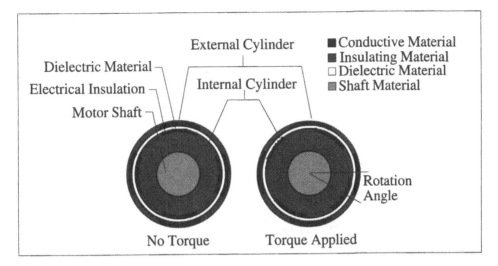

Dielectric Material
Electrical Insulation
Motor Shaft

External Cylinder
Internal Cylinder

■ Conductive Material
■ Insulating Material
□ Dielectric Material
■ Shaft Material

Rotation Angle

No Torque          Torque Applied

**FIGURE 5.8**  Schematic for a motor torque sensor using a capacitive sensor. The sensor operates by attaching the internal cylinder to the motor shaft via an insulator material, and attaching an external cylinder to a flexible shaft coupling. As torque is applied by the motor to the wheels through the flexible shaft coupling, the internal cylinder rotates with respect to the external cylinder. This causes a change in the overlapping area of the conductive material on the two concentric cylinders, which causes a change in the capacitance between the two concentric cylinders.

torque is applied, the overlapping area of the two concentric parallel plates changes, and the capacitance changes. Hence, torque can be measured as a change in capacitance.

There are meters that exploit equation (5.17) to measure capacitance. Many higher-quality hand-held multimeters can measure capacitance. However, close examination of equation (5.17) reveals how a change in capacitance can be observed. If the voltage $v$ across the capacitor is held constant, then the current through the capacitor will be

$$q = Cv \Rightarrow i = \frac{dq}{dt} = \frac{dCv}{dt} = v\frac{dC}{dt} + C\frac{dv}{dt} \tag{5.18}$$

Since $v$ is held constant, equation (5.18) simplifies to

$$i = v\frac{dC}{dt} \tag{5.19}$$

By measuring the current with a known voltage, the capacitance can be found at each instant by integration. Other more complex methods can also be used, but this method provides a simple alternative. Equation (5.18) shows that if the voltage is not held constant, then the current will have a component due to the change in the voltage. Engineers have worked to develop stable voltage sources to minimize the change in $v$, and computer algorithms to compensate for it. It is important to remember the basic principles of how capacitance can be used to measure variables like force, torque, and pressure. Capacitors are important components for electric-powered wheelchairs, and one should be aware of their existence and principle of operation.

### 5.3.3 Inductors

A conductor, wire, may be shaped into a multiturn coil. The voltage across the coil is proportional to the rate of change of the current (equation (5.20)). The inductance ($L$) is the constant of proportionality, which is measured in henrys.

$$v = L\frac{di}{dt} \tag{5.20}$$

Inductors are commonly available with values ranging from 1 mH to 100 H. Large inductors are obtained by using many turns and an iron core; the combination of these two characteristics often increases the power dissipation. Inductors are commonly used in joysticks to control wheelchairs. Inductors can be characterized by the number of turns ($N$), the permeability of the core material ($\mu$), the area of the core ($A$), and the average length of the core ($l$),

$$L = \frac{N^2\mu A}{l} \tag{5.21}$$

Joysticks use variable inductors. Variable inductors exploit the change in inductance due to change in the permeability of the core material. Permeability describes how well a material promotes and shapes magnetic fields. Iron has a much higher permeability than does air. By using a sleeve with a moveable iron core, the inductance varies with the position of the moveable core within the sleeve. As the iron core moves, the permeability increases and decreases as the core material varies from being mostly iron to being mostly air. Variable inductors are quite durable, and make good sensors for wheelchair joysticks.

### 5.3.4 Common Transducers

The principles that describe resistors, capacitors, and inductors are used to make a variety of transducers. A transducer is a device that converts a mechanical, chemical, optical, or electrical property into an electrical signal. Voltage is the most common electrical form of signal used to represent a property being measured. This is because several devices are available to record and interface voltage signals to a computer. A sensor is a device that incorporates a transducer or transducers to measure a desired quantity.

Potentiometers, variable capacitors, and variable inductors were introduced in previous sections. Other transducers are used with wheelchairs and seating. The strength and durability of a wheelchair can be studied using strain gages. Strain gages are simply specialized resistors that can be bonded to metals or plastics. Strain gages are made of flexible material that moves with the surface of the material to which it is bonded. Therefore, as the material stretches or shrinks due to applied forces, the strain gage will also stretch or shrink. As a strain gage stretches its resistance increases; as the strain gage shrinks its resistance decreases. Metal pieces can be shaped to act like springs, which bend, stretch, or compress due to an applied force. By applying strain gages to such metal pieces, the applied forces can be measured. This is the basis for force sensors used in biomechanics (i.e., for force platforms), and for measuring forces with wheelchairs. Strain gage–based force sensors have also been used to develop input devices for electric-powered wheelchairs that respond to the force applied by a hand, foot, or chin.

Strain gages are also used to measure seating pressure. This can be done by placing strain gages onto a thin metal diaphragm. Either air pressure or water pressure is applied to the diaphragm, which flexes causing a change in the resistance of the strain gages. Seating pressure can be measured by using a small sack of water connected through a thin inelastic tube to a strain gage pressure transducer. When pressure is applied to the sack of water, it will compress sending water through the tube, which in turn places pressure on the transducer. This method is used in some pressure-sensing systems. Another method used in several pressure-sensing mats relies on the use of a resistive material applied to a flexible substrate that is separated from another substrate covered with a conductive material (see Figure 5.9). Conductive polymer ink is often used as the resistive material. Gold- or silver-based metals are used to form the conductors. As force or pressure is applied to one or both of the substrates, the gap between them narrows and the surfaces begin to touch. As force/pressure increases, the contact area increases, which, as shown in equation (5.5), decreases the resistance. The change, decrease, in resistance is related to force. Force-sensing mats use a series of this type of sensor to create a seating pressure profile.

**FIGURE 5.9**  Illustration of the construction of a conductive polymer force-sensing resistor. As force is applied to the flexible substrate material, the interlaced conductive material and the conductive polymer ink begin to make contact. This reduces the electrical resistance between the external connectors. As force increases, the contact area between the conductive polymer ink and interlaced conductive material increases, which decreases the resistance across the external connectors.

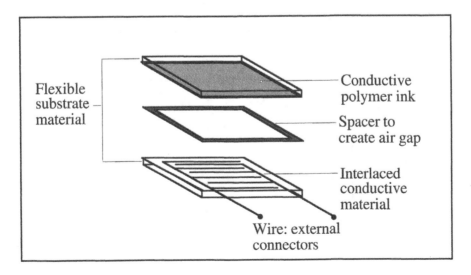

### 5.3.5 Basic Circuit Concepts

Resistors, capacitors, inductors, and transducers all must be connected to an electric or electronic circuit. A circuit is the interconnection of multiple electrical or electronic devices. Engineers use two basic concepts to define and analyze electric circuits. A node is a point of connection of two or more electrical or electronic components. A loop is a closed path through which current can flow to perform a desired function. Engineers use two fundamental laws to analyze electric circuits. Gustav-Robert Kirchhoff formulated these voltage and current laws. These laws are now called Kirchhoff's Voltage Law (KVL) and Kirchhoff's Current Law (KCL). KCL states that the sum of the currents entering a node equals the sum of the current leaving that node (Figure 5.10). KVL states that within a closed loop, the sum of the voltage rises equals the sum of the voltage drops (Figure 5.11).

A few other fundamental concepts are required to understand basic circuits. An open circuit is a loop with a disconnected or interrupted path. Opening a switch causes an open circuit, which stops current flows. A short circuit is a path of zero or no resistance. A series circuit is composed of two or more components connected end to end. A parallel circuit is composed of one or more components connected between the same two nodes. Open and short circuits effect the behavior of a device or system. Many electric-powered wheelchairs and scooters include protection against short circuits. Open circuits are often necessary to control electric power. The on/off switch on an electric-powered wheelchair causes an open circuit between the batteries and the controller. An undesired open circuit can result in the wheelchair stopping or behaving undesirably.

### 5.3.6 Amplifiers and Filters

Amplifiers convert small signals into larger signals (see Figure 5.12). A simple amplifier can be represented as a constant multiplier. In other words, if a signal

**FIGURE 5.10**   The node is defined by the interconnection of the three components (resistors). Nodal analysis uses the fact that the sum of the current entering and leaving a node must be zero. In this illustration, $I_3 = I_1 + I_2$.

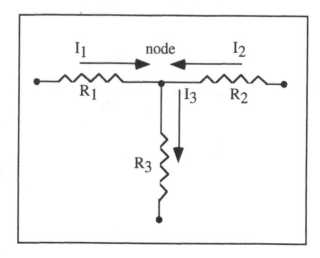

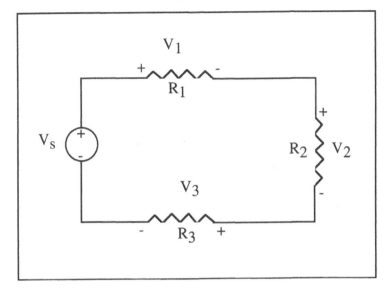

**FIGURE 5.11**  Loop analysis applies the fact the sum of the voltages around a loop are zero. In this illustration, the source (battery) voltage is equal to the sum of the voltage drops across each of the resistors in the loop: $V_s = V_1 + V_2 + V_3$.

that is one tenth of a volt is input into an amplifier with a gain of ten, then the output from the amplifier will be one volt. Amplifiers are used with most common transducers. This is because transducer signals are often small and require amplification to be properly interfaced to a computer or other instrument. Amplifiers can be used to perform mathematical functions. As described previously, an amplifier can be used to multiply a signal by a constant. Amplifiers can also be used to add two signals together. Amplifiers also have dynamic properties that are affected by the gain, the size of the multiplier, and the frequency of the signal.

**FIGURE 5.12**  Illustration of the effect of amplification on a signal. The original signal is five times larger after it has been passed through an amplifier with gain of five. Amplifiers help to make small signals large enough to record.

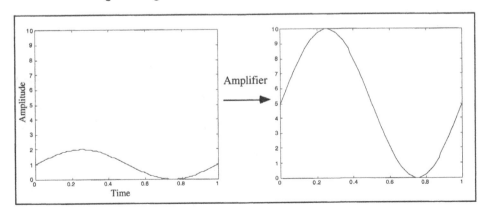

Amplifiers are rated by a gain-bandwidth product, which is a constant. Engineers estimate the frequency and gain required to perform the desired function and then select or design an amplifier that is appropriate. There are several types of amplifiers that are used in electric and electronic circuits. The two most common type of amplifiers used with wheelchairs and accessories are inverting amplifiers and instrumentation amplifiers. Both of these types of amplifiers can be purchased in predesigned packages that require only a few external resistors to tune them for a particular application. Figure 5.13 provides descriptions of a few common amplifier configurations.

A filter is a circuit that alters the frequency and phase of a signal. This is in contrast to an amplifier, which changes the amplitude of a signal. Filters are used to remove tremor sensed by joysticks, which may not be related to intended motion. Filters also remove noise present in the atmosphere due to lights and other electric-powered devices. There are four basic types of filters: low-pass, high-pass, band-pass, and notch. Low-pass filters remove frequency components above the cut-off frequency. High-pass filters remove frequency components below the cut-off frequency. Band-pass filters remove the components of a signal outside of two cut-off frequencies. A notch filter removes the components of a signal between two cut-off frequencies. A filter can be thought of as multiplication in the frequency domain. The French mathematician Baron Jean Baptiste Fourier showed in 1826 that arbitrary periodic functions can be represented as an infinite series of sinusoids. The sinusoidal series is called the *Fourier series*. A Fourier series consists of sinusoids whose frequencies are multiples of the lowest or *fundamental* frequency. The higher frequencies in the Fourier series are integer multiples of the fundamental frequency and are called harmonics. The Fourier series for an arbitrary periodic function can be described by an equation of the form

$$f(t) = a_0 + a_1 \cos \omega_0 t + a_2 \cos 2\omega_0 t + a_3 \cos 3\omega_0 t + \cdots$$
$$+ b_1 \sin \omega_0 t + b_2 \sin 2\omega_0 t + b_3 \sin 3\omega_0 t + \cdots \tag{5.22}$$

Equation (5.22) is often written in compact form,

$$f(t) = a_0 + \sum_{n=1}^{\infty} (a_n \cos n\omega_0 t + b_n \sin n\omega_0 t) \tag{5.23}$$

The Fourier series of f(t) = 3 + sin2t is simply the function itself, and it would be graphed in the frequency domain with two points: one at zero radians (d.c.) and the other at 2 radians ($1/\pi$ Hertz). More complex signals result in a higher number of terms in the Fourier series. As stated earlier a filter can be viewed as multiplication in the frequency domain, and an amplifier can be viewed as multiplication in the time domain. The time domain is a quaint way of saying that the signal is viewed as changing with time (i.e., the signal can be plotted with time along the dependent axis and f(t) along the independent axis). The frequency domain is used to analyze and shape signals with a periodic component. If the signal has a periodic component, then it can be represented by a Fourier series. A frequency domain plot uses the frequency, in radians or Hertz, along the independent axis and the vector sum of the $a_n$'s and $b_n$'s along the dependent axis. The vector sum of the $a_n$'s and $b_n$'s is given by

$$c_n = \sqrt{a_n^2 + b_n^2} \tag{5.24}$$

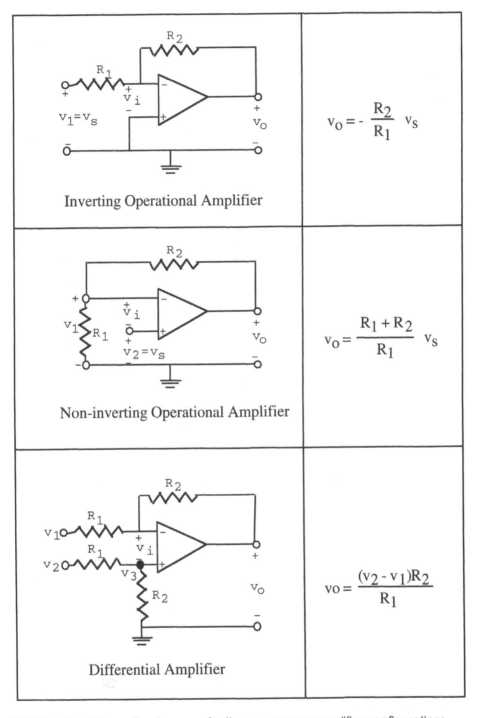

**FIGURE 5.13** Schematic diagrams for three common amplifier configurations. Engineers use the "triangle" symbol to represent amplifier in their circuit diagrams. The input voltage for the amplifier is represented by $v_i$, whereas the output voltage of the amplifier is represented by $v_o$. The R's represent external resistors, which the engineer adds to the commercial chip to obtain the desired gain.

A filter has the effect of suppressing or eliminating some components of the Fourier series. For example a low-pass filter eliminates all of the harmonics above the cut-off frequency. Figure 5.14 shows the idealized frequency domain representations of the most common filter types.

Most electric-powered wheelchairs use several filters and amplifiers. In fact the motors themselves are used as filters to smooth the speed control signals. Access devices use filters as well. Many people experience some tremor while driving an electric-powered wheelchair, whether related to the impairment or due to normal vibrations experienced while driving. This tremor is higher in frequency than the normal signal provided to the joystick to drive the wheelchair in forward or reverse, and while turning. Hence, a low-pass filter can be used to minimize the unwanted effects of tremor on driving. In some cases, wheelchair or access device manufacturers allow the cut-off frequency to be adjusted for a particular user.

### 5.3.7 Transformers and Chargers

Some devices receive their power from a wall outlet and require the voltage converted to be compatible with the device. The most common examples are devices that convert the alternating current of the wall outlet into direct current for some devices. Devices that convert alternating current to direct current are called direct current power supplies. Battery chargers for electric-powered wheelchairs are essentially direct current power supplies that sense the change in voltage and current at the battery terminals. A *transformer* is a device that transfers energy from one circuit to another by stepping the voltage up or down. Wheelchair applications use step-down transformers. Transformers can also be used to isolate one circuit from another. This property is used in many medical instruments and devices that receive their power from a wall outlet and are connected to a person.

A transformer is made of two magnetically coupled coils. The two coils are electrically isolated, but are magnetically coupled through the iron core, which serves as the frame of the transformer. One coil is called the primary coil, usually the one connected to the a.c. wall outlet, and the other coil is called the secondary coil, which is often connected to the device. Faraday's Law states that the voltage induced in a coil is proportional to the number of turns of the coil, and the rate of change of the magnetic flux linking the coil. The change in the magnetic flux is equal to the frequency of the source, 60 Hz in North America or 50 Hz in Europe. An ideal transformer transfers energy from the primary coil to the secondary coil without loss of energy within the coil. Most practical coils are better than 90% efficient; therefore, the idealized coil model is useful. In an idealized coil, the voltages across the primary $(V_p)$ and secondary $(V_s)$ coils are proportional to the ratio between the turns of the coils:

$$\frac{V_p}{V_s} = \frac{N_p}{N_s} = c \qquad (5.25)$$

The power available from the primary and secondary coils is equal. This results in a useful relationship between the voltages and current in the primary and secondary coils:

$$\frac{V_p}{V_s} = \frac{I_s}{I_p} = c \qquad (5.26)$$

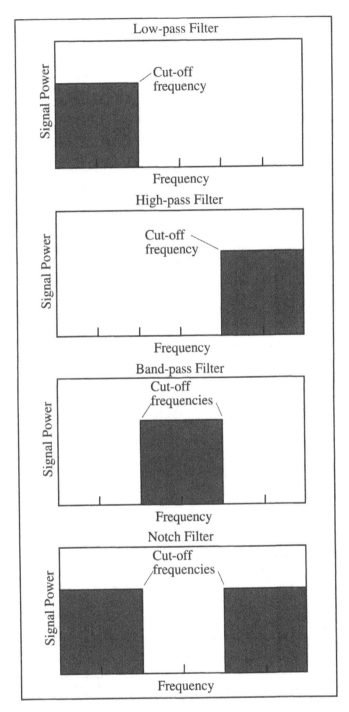

**FIGURE 5.14** Depictions of the frequencies that remain unaffected by common types of ideal filters. There are many ways to implement the filters presented. The filters are differentiated by the frequencies of the input signal, which remain unaltered (shown in gray). Engineers select the type of filter and its cut-off frequency to remove noise and other unwanted signals.

When using a transformer, there is always a trade-off between current and voltage. A simple battery charger or power supply can be constructed using the circuit depicted in Figure 5.15.

In Figure 5.15, a standard wall outlet is used to supply power. Most residential wall outlets in North America supply 115 to 125 volts of alternating current at a frequency of 60 Hertz, with a circuit breaker used to set the current limit to 15 amperes. The voltages after each critical stage are illustrated in Figure 5.16.

The transformer is used to step the voltage down from 125 V a.c. to 38 V a.c., which is the value required by the batteries. The full-bridge rectifier is used to convert the alternating current to direct current. A full-bridge rectifier accomplishes this by flipping the negative portion of the sine wave. The output of the full-bridge rectifier is a rough direct current voltage and current that looks like the lobes of a sine wave. The low-pass filter smoothes the voltages and current values to reduce the ripple. The current choke is used to limit the amount of current that can be supplied to the batteries. For commercial battery chargers more sophisticated controls are used for the output current of the battery charger. The end-stage capacitor is used to reduce ripple in the output voltage and current. Ripple is used to define the small variations in the direct current output voltage. The goal of this section is not to teach the design of battery chargers or power supplies, but to gain an appreciation for their function and principles of operation.

### 5.3.8 Power Transistors

There are many types of transistors. In fact, semiconductor chips may contain millions of them in as small as 10 mm by 10 mm. The transistors within semiconductor chips behave much like the discrete transistors that will be introduced in this section. Power wheelchairs rely mostly on metal oxide semiconductor field effect tran-

**FIGURE 5.15**   Schematic diagram for a 24-volt direct current wheelchair battery charger. Commercial wheelchair battery chargers contain several safety features to protect the user and battery from possible harm. This circuit is to illustrate the concepts behind battery chargers and transformers.

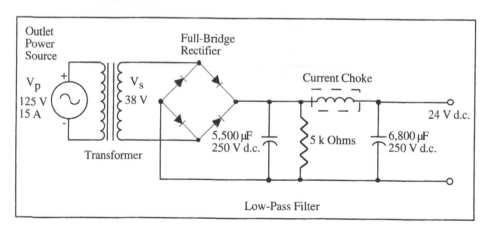

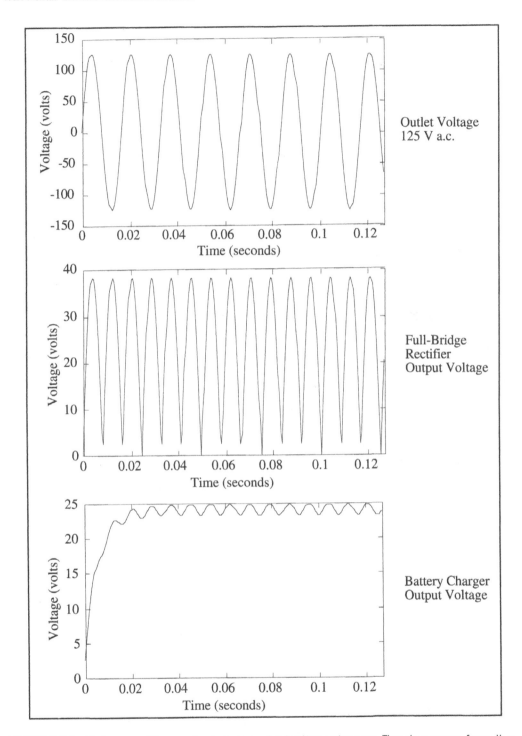

**FIGURE 5.16**    Voltages of the various stages of a battery charger. The sine wave from the wall outlet is stepped down and then full-wave rectified. The rectified voltage provides direct current, but the voltage variation, ripple, is quite large. The low-pass filter reduces the ripple, but at the cost of lowering the voltage.

sistors or MOS-FETs. Power MOS-FETs are key components to the power train of electric-powered wheelchairs. They are the key components in the power stage of modern power wheelchair controllers. The power MOS-FETs are used as switches to control the application of the battery voltage to the motors.

MOS-FETs can be used in many configurations, but the most commonly used mode within power wheelchair controllers and related devices is as a switch. Simply, the MOS-FET can be used to act as a switch, which can be controlled by a microcontroller. A MOS-FET can be described by three states: off-state, linear-state, and on-state. An advantage of a MOS-FET is that it has little resistance when turned on. When being used as a switch a MOS-FET is driven from the off-state where it has high resistance to the on-state where it has low resistance. In the off-state MOS-FETs can have resistances in the millions of ohms, whereas in the on-state they can have resistances in the hundreds of milliohms. This means that when they are off little current is drawn from the batteries, and when in the on-state little power is dissipated by the MOS-FETs. MOS-FETs are driven from the off-state through the linear-state to the on-state by applying a voltage between gait and source. MOS-FETs have three external electrical connections: drain, gait, and source. The circuit symbol for a MOS-FET is depicted in Figure 5.17.

MOS-FETs used in most power wheelchairs and their powered accessories have an on threshold voltage of between 0.8 and 1.5 volts. Power MOS-FETs are switched on and off to control the speed of the motors. The faster the switching frequency the less noise that is generated, and the more efficiently the motors operate. Typically, power wheelchair controllers use a switching frequency of 20 kilohertz. Power MOS-FETs are given a voltage and a current rating. Since power wheelchairs are capable of drawing up to 60 amps for short periods of time (i.e., during acceleration) power MOS-FETs are often rated for 100 amps. Most power wheelchairs rely on two 12-volt batteries in parallel to create a 24-volt system. Hence the power MOS-FETs must be rated greater than 24 volts. Power MOS-FETs rated between 60 and 100 volts are common. MOS-FETs can be used in parallel to accommodate higher currents with lower current ratings required per MOS-FET. This also provides some redundancy to the controller's power stage. A brief description of how MOS-FETs can be used to control motors is provided in the section on electromechanical components.

**FIGURE 5.17**   Circuit symbol for a MOS-FET

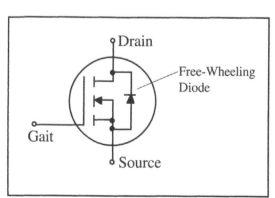

## *5.3.9 Receivers and Transmitters*

The concept of a transmitter and receiver is very old. Early versions of transmitting and receiving include smoke signals, alp horns, semaphore flags, and lights. Communication requires a transmitter and receiver pair. Both the transmitter and receiver must understand the code in order to transmit information. By definition, information can only be transmitted when the receiver does not know in advance exactly what message the transmitter is going to send. The transmitter and receiver must speak a common language, but the message is unknown until it is sent and received. All communication schemes have two basic components: a common language, and a means of transmitting the information.

Electronic devices use a variety of means of communicating. The simplest and most common means of transmitting a signal is through the use of wires. Two devices are connected via wires. One sends a signal and the other receives the signal and interprets it. Communication can be one way, which is sometimes called blind communication or no-handshaking, or it can be two way, which commonly requires handshaking. Handshaking means that the transmitter sends a message along with the protocol for communication, the receiver interprets the signal and responds to having received the communication protocol. A common means of direct wire communication is the telephone system, which uses a series of wires and digital switches to connect telephones together.

Other mediums can also be used to transmit signals. Cellular telephones transmit electromagnetic signals through space. The cellular telephone produces high-frequency electromagnetic waves, which are received by a local antenna commonly called a cell. The cell amplifies the signal from the phone and transmits the signal to another nearby cell on the same network or to a satellite. Cellular phones use a digital code to recognize individual telephones. The telephone sends a brief message with each transmission identifying itself. When the satellite or cell transmits, the first thing it does is send a code that identifies to which telephone the message is directed. This helps to keep conversation private as each telephone has a unique address. Garage door openers work along the same lines, but with lower frequency and much simpler coding schemes. A garage door opener only recognizes a unique transmission frequency. If that frequency is detected with enough power, then the garage door opens or closes depending upon what its last action was. Although the communication scheme is very simple, it is very effective for the purpose.

Light can also be used to transmit and receive information. Most television remote controls use infrared light to communicate. Television remote controls use simple one-way communication. The remote control transmits a burst, a short transmission, of infrared light which contains a code. The burst is received by a sensor on the television which interprets the meaning of the signal and performs the desired function. In many cases, communication back to the user is accomplished by having the television screen display the command that it received. Televisions and similar appliances use a standardized serial data scheme to code signals from a remote control. Each burst from the remote control is of the same length. However, the burst consists of a rapid series of turning an infrared light on and off. First the infrared light is turned on for a period, then it starts turning on and off. When the light is on, the appliance interprets a one and, conversely, when the light is off the appliance interprets a zero. Each function on the remote is coded with a unique pattern of ones and zeros. The rate of communication depends on the speed that the remote can send and that the appliance can receive signals reliably. To have more functions, more ones and zeros are required. If the only function were to turn the television on and off, then only one bit of information is required. A bit represents a single one or zero. In this example, to turn the television on, a one could be sent by the remote to the television. To turn the television off, a zero would be sent. This type of code is called bi-state, in that there is either a one (on) or zero (off). With a bi-state code, the number of unique codes that can be generated is equal to two to the power of the number of bits (n),

$$\text{number of unique codes} = 2^n \qquad (5.27)$$

In the case of the television n = 1, two codes are available. If n were equal to three, than eight unique codes would be available. Engineers and computer specialists have given codes with eight bits a special name called a "byte." Many computers and printers are available with wireless communication or infrared links. These systems use the same type of communication as a television remote control. However, some computers and peripherals use two-way infrared communication. Infrared communication only requires that the devices be placed pointing to one another and in close proximity.

Electric-powered wheelchairs and accessories can use a variety of means to communicate. Communication for the access device (e.g., joystick) to the controller can be analog or digital through wires. Communication between the wheelchair controller and a computer or environmental control unit is normally done with infrared. Control of a garage door or a communication via a cellular modem/phone to a wheelchair repair station can be accomplished with radio frequency communication.

## 5.4 Basic Electrical Safety

Electrical safety is often overlooked when learning about electric-powered wheelchairs and associated electrical devices. Injuries related to electrical shock among wheelchair users are uncommon. Most injuries are attributable to improper use due to inadequate training or lack of experience. Wheelchair users rarely read owners' manuals until a problem has occurred. Furthermore, all electric-powered wheelchairs eventually fail, and engineers must design them with fail-safe mechanisms. This section focuses on basic electrical safety, and does not address the multitude of other safety concerns that must be addressed when designing or manufacturing a wheelchair.

### 5.4.1 Electricity and the Human Body

For a person to be affected by electricity the body must be part of an electric circuit. Current must enter the body at some point and exit the body at another point. Engineers examine the risk of injury based upon the impedances of the body tissues, and of the impedances of the entry and exit points. Skin often has the highest impedance of body tissues. When a person becomes part of an electric circuit three reactions are possible: tissue may become excited (e.g., nerve, muscle); tissue may experience resistive heating; and electrochemical burns may occur.

When using electric-powered wheelchairs two cases need to be considered: contact with the battery power bus or an auxiliary battery-powered circuit; and contact with an alternating current power source connected to the wheelchair (e.g., a battery charger plugged into a wall outlet). The level of current influences the reaction of the body. If a person has moist hands and grasps copper wires connected to a power source then the lowest threshold current perceptible is about 0.5 milliamps at 60 Hz alternating current, or between 2 and 10 milliamps for direct current. A person with intact sensation will feel slight warming or tingling. However, many wheelchair users may not be able to sense small current. Therefore, the individual's sensation cannot be relied on to provide notice of an impending problem.

As current increases, it may stimulate muscles and nerves. This can cause severe pain sensations among intact tissue. It can also cause involuntary muscle contractions that may lead to secondary accidents. Involuntary contractions can lead to losing control over the wheelchair or severe contractions can lead to falling out of the wheelchair. Engineers define the threshold of muscle stimulation as the *let-go current*. As current rises higher, more severe reactions may follow. Higher currents can cause involuntary contractions of respiratory muscles leading to asphyxiation. Dalziel et al. showed that currents of 18 to 22 milliamps are sufficient to cause contraction of respiratory muscles.

When current passes through the chest, the risk of potential injury is considerably increased. As current passes through the chest, some current passes through the heart. This current can stimulate the heart and raise heart rate to 300 beats per minute. At this rate, the pumping action of the heart ceases and the person dies within a few minutes. This process is called *ventricular fibrillation*, and occurs at currents between 75 and 400 milliamps. Ventricular fibrillation is most commonly related to cord-connected appliances such as battery chargers. Animals studies indicate that currents of 1 to 6 amps cause the entire heart muscle to contract. These currents can be applied for very short periods without permanent damage. Currents above 10 amperes are known to shut down activity within the central nervous system, and to produce muscle contractions severe enough to separate muscles from their attachments to bone.

### 5.4.2 Macroshock

Large currents applied directly to the surface of the body are called *macroshocks*. The magnitude of the current to cause damage or ventricular fibrillation is much higher than would be necessary if the current were applied directly to the heart. The location of the entry and exit points plays an important role in the potential for harm. If the current passes primarily through an extremity, then the risk of fibrillation or organ damage is reduced. Current passing through the heart poses the greatest risk because of the heart's susceptibility to electric current. Substantial current may pass through the heart if current passes from one arm to another (see Figure 5.18).

Skin and body resistance and the distribution of current across the surface of the body reduce the danger of injury. However, electric-powered wheelchairs and associated devices must be designed to minimize the possibility of people coming in contact with dangerous voltages. The resistance of the skin limits the amount of current that can flow through the body. Skin resistance varies from 15 kilo-ohms to 1 mega-ohm depending on moisture and sweat concentration. When the skin is

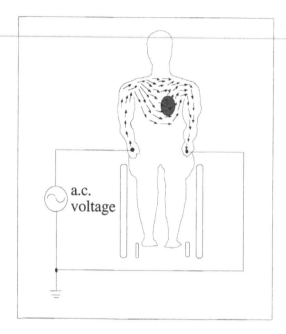

**FIGURE 5.18**   Current path through the heart due to macroshock

broken the resistance drops to about 1% of its normal value. The internal resistance of the body is about 500 ohms. Wheelchairs must be designed to minimize the risk of macroshock, and electrical connections should not be permitted to puncture the skin.

### 5.4.3 Microshock

People are particularly vulnerable to electric shock when devices are placed in direct contact with the heart. Some devices provide the possibility of current flowing directly to the heart (e.g., external pacemakers, cardiac catheters). Very small currents called *microshocks* can cause fibrillation of the heart if applied directly to cardiac muscle. The acceptable safety limit for microshock is 10 microamps. People should use extra caution when using electric-powered wheelchairs in hospital environments.

### 5.4.4 Common Hazards

Devices connected to wall outlets pose potential hazards. Wall outlets use two conductors supplying a 120-volt device. The neutral wire (white) on a 120-volt circuit is connected to ground. Therefore, any connection between the hot connector (black) and any grounded object poses a shock hazard. The National Electrical Code requires that the potential between any two exposed conductive surfaces within hospitals be less than 500 millivolts. Even a good grounding system cannot prevent hazardous voltages that can result from *groundfaults*. A groundfault is a short circuit between the hot conductor and ground that ejects large currents into the grounding system. This type of fault is rare, but occurs often enough that most residential bathroom circuits are equipped with groundfault detectors. A ground-fault detector on circuits used to charge electric-powered wheelchair batteries can help prevent injury.

Electric-powered wheelchairs and associated electrically powered devices are designed to minimize exposure of people to hazardous voltages and currents. However, electric-powered wheelchairs and other devices have metal chassis that occupants or other people may touch. Devices that are connected to a wall outlet must be grounded to prevent a shock should the insulation wear or a wire break, causing a macroshock hazard. Electric-powered wheelchairs cannot be grounded since they are battery operated, and must travel independently over a wide variety of surfaces. International Standards Organization (ISO) guidelines specify that the minimum allowable resistance between the power circuit and the chassis of the wheelchair is 10 kilo-ohms.

Failures in electrical systems which may result in shock hazards can be caused by worn insulation, shorted components, or mechanical failures that cause short circuits. Fluids such as blood, urine, intravenous solutions, and food can conduct enough electricity to cause temporary short circuits when they spill on what might otherwise be a safe device. The mechanical design of the wheelchair or other device should protect people from this type of hazard. Most accidents result from carelessness and failure to correct known deficiencies in power connections or the devices themselves.

## 5.5 Electromechanical Components

### 5.5.1 Controllers

If one thinks of a MOS-FET as a simple switch that can be controlled by a microprocessor, than this concept can be built on to form the framework for a motor controller. Most electric-powered wheelchairs and their powered accessories use simple permanent magnet direct current motors. This means that if a voltage is applied to the motor it will turn, and the direction of the current flow determines the direction that the motor will turn. Figure 5.19 illustrates how a motor can be controlled by a MOS-FET.

When the MOS-FET is turned on current flows through the loop. This current causes the motor to rotate. If the MOS-FET is turned off no current flows and the motor stops rotating. In this case, the speed of the motor is controlled by the amount of mechanical resistance that the motor experiences. This circuit can be modified to control speed and current for more precise control over the motor. The amount of current delivered to the motor can be controlled by varying the amount of time that the MOS-FET is turned on.

Figure 5.20 shows a motor controller circuit that allows driving the motor in forward and reverse. This is, obviously, necessary for driving an electric-powered wheelchair. The circuit used for controlling forward and reverse motor speed is called an H-bridge. This is because the circuit resembles an H, with the motor in the cross-bar and the MOS-FETs making up the uprights. Again, the MOS-FETs are used as switches. However, they are turned on in pairs in order to control the path of the current and, hence, control the direction of rotation of the motor. Current will flow in the direction indicated by arrow A when MOS-FETs 1 and 4 are turned on, and MOS-

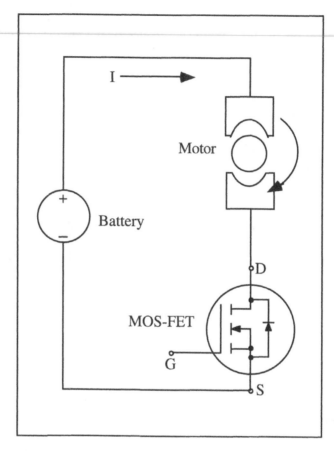

**FIGURE 5.19**  Unidirectional motor control circuit using a battery and a single MOS-FET

FETs 2 and 3 are turned off. The motor will turn in a clockwise fashion. To drive the motor in a counterclockwise direction, MOS-FETs 2 and 3 are turned on, while MOS-FETs 1 and 4 are turned off. The current will flow in the direction indicated by arrow B. We have seen that one MOS-FET is required to control a motor in one direction, but four are required to control a motor in two directions. Typically, MOS-FETs 2 and 4 are simply turned either on or off to select the direction of current flow (i.e., motor rotation). In such cases, MOS-FETs 1 and 3 are pulsed in order to control speed.

Some precautions must be taken when designing a bi-directional motor controller. If MOS-FETs 1 and 2 or 3 and 4 are turned on simultaneously, then the battery will be shorted, possibly causing it damage. This phenomena is called *vertical conduction*. Vertical conduction is eliminated during normal operation by using a small *deadzone* in the command signal response. When the command signal changes from forward to reverse, it transitions through zero speed, which could lead to vertical conduction. This is eliminated by not having the MOS-FETs command signals active until the person's intentions are clearly for forward or reverse. Small movements of the access device (e.g., joystick) are interpreted to mean that the person intends to remain stopped. The deadzone is typically quite small (i.e., a few millivolts) and goes unnoticed by the driver.

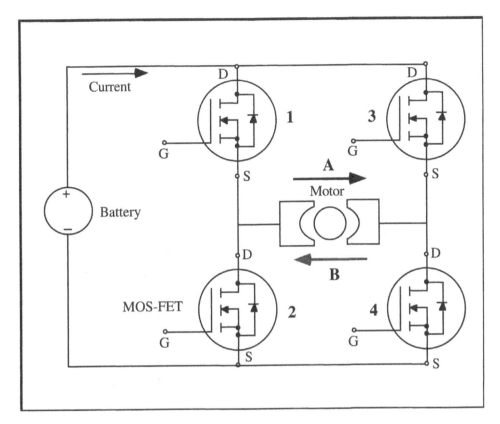

**FIGURE 5.20**  Bidirectional motor control circuit for a permanent magnet d.c.
motor using an H-bridge and four MOS-FET transistors

## 5.5.2 Motors

Electric-powered wheelchairs and their electric-powered accessories typically use
permanent magnet direct current motors. In many cases one motor is used to
drive each wheel. A permanent magnet d.c. motor is illustrated in Figure 5.21. The
motor faceplate is mounted to the wheelchair frame. Permanent magnets are
inserted into the motor housing at even spacings. The permanent magnets are
placed with alternating poles (i.e., north–south–north–south). Motors are often
characterized by the number of permanent magnet poles that they have (e.g., a
four-pole motor has four permanent magnets). The armature is the part of the
motor that rotates. Armatures are made by winding wire around an iron core to
form an electromagnet. The armature also has several poles when current is
applied to the wires of which it is made. Current is applied to the windings of the
armature through the commutator and brushes. Current from the controller is
applied directly to the brushes of the motor. The brushes are made of carbon or
copper and carbon. This makes them soft, and allows them to conform to the commutator. The commutator is made up of a series of copper bars placed around a
cylinder. An insulating material (e.g., phenolic) is placed between the copper bars.
Each copper bar makes an electrical connection to one of the armature windings.
The alignment of the commutator is such that when current is applied the elec-

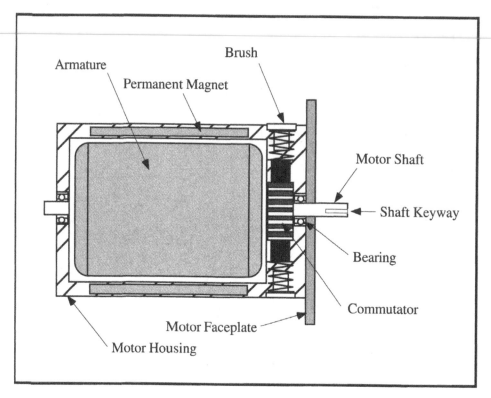

**FIGURE 5.21**   Cut-away view of a permanent magnet direct current motor

tromagnets of the armature always have the same poles as the permanent magnets (e.g., if the armature pole is south the matching permanent magnet pole will be south). Therefore, the armature will turn to try and align its south poles with the north poles of the permanent magnets around it. However, the commutator changes the poles before they are aligned. The alignment of the commutator with the armature, and the alignment of the electromagnets are critical to keep the motor spinning.

Motors are simply controlled reactions between magnets. The number of windings in the armature relates to the strength of its magnetic field. The strength of the permanent magnets, and the strength of the armature electromagnets per unit current determine the motor rating (i.e., horsepower or watts). The torque that a motor applies is dependent on the strength of the magnetic field between the permanent magnets and the electromagnets. The more current that is available to the electromagnets, the more torque the motor can apply. Current is limited by the batteries (i.e., how much current they can deliver), the armature windings (i.e., how much current they can withstand without being damaged), and the effectiveness of the motor in discharging heat (i.e., how well the motor keeps cool).

Permanent magnet motors are commonly used because they can be controlled with simple electronics, and they have high starting torque. High starting torque helps the wheelchair to perform the many tasks that require starting, stopping, and turning at low speeds. The greatest drawback of permanent magnet d.c.

motors is the need for brushes. Brushes wear during use, and also may cause arc across the commutator. This causes the surfaces of the brushes and commutators to deteriorate, and require periodic repair or replacement. Arcing is a source of electromagnetic radiation that can interfere with some electronic devices. However, this should not be a problem if the wheelchair is compliant with ANSI/RESNA or ISO standards.

A d.c. motor can be modeled by an electric circuit (see Figure 5.22). The voltage across the motor is described by a differential equation. The motor voltage ($v_{armature}$) is dependent upon the armature winding resistance ($R$), the armature winding inductance ($L$), and the voltage produced by the back electromotif force ($v_{b-emf}$),

$$v_{armature} = R(t) + L\frac{di(t)}{dt} + v_{b-emf} = Ri(t) + L\frac{di(t)}{dt} + k_b\omega(t) \tag{5.28}$$

The voltage produced by the back electromotif force (*emf*) is proportional to the motor's speed ($\omega(t)$). This proportionality is important because the voltage produced by the back *emf* is used in many power wheelchair controllers to measure the motor speed. The speed measured in this fashion is used to provide speed feedback for the controller's speed control algorithm.

Given equation (5.28) and a mathematical model describing the load on the motor produced by the wheelchair, one could show that a permanent magnet d.c. motor acts like a low-pass filter with the input being voltage and the output being wheelchair speed. This is exploited by engineers to use MOS-FETs to control electric-powered wheelchairs. Commonly, the voltage applied to the motors has a frequency of 20 kilohertz (i.e., 20,000 cycles per second). However, the wheelchair does not vibrate in response to these changes in the motor voltage.

**FIGURE 5.22** Model of a permanent magnet d.c. motor as an electric circuit

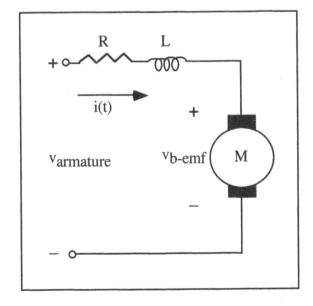

### 5.5.3 Speakers

Speakers are very similar to motors. In fact they operate on the same basic principles. Speakers can be thought of as linear motors. A speaker is made up of a series
of electromagnets. The core of the speakers moves to and fro. A membrane is
attached to the core on the inside and to the case along its outside. The membrane
moves like the surface of a drum as the core moves. This movement causes sound.
The pitch of the sound depends upon the material used to make the membrane,
and the size of the membrane. Small, stiff membrane is used to create high frequencies (i.e., a tweeter). In contrast, a large, flexible membrane is used to create
low frequencies (i.e., a woofer). Speakers are made to operate within frequency
bands. The frequency of the sound is controlled by vibrating the membrane with
the magnets that drive the core. At higher frequencies, a lightweight core is needed
so that it may be moved rapidly. At lower frequencies, very powerful magnets are
required to move the large amounts of air blocking motion of the membrane. In
movie theaters, sub-woofers that have diameters in excess of 60 centimeters are
used to move the air within the theater to create the feeling that one gets from low-
frequency mechanical sound. Speaker amplifiers use circuits similar to those
described to control motors. However, two important factors must be considered.
In order to obtain high fidelity sound, the frequency that the amplifier and
speakers produce must be closely controlled. Remember, a motor acts like a low-
pass filter and the frequency is not critical. Speakers produce sound and in some
applications (e.g., music, voice synthesis) frequency preservation or creation is
quite important. Speakers require a significant amount of power and it must be
delivered rapidly. The most power can be transferred with optimal efficiency when
the amplifier output impedance is the same as the speaker input impedance. This
concept is called *impedance matching*. This is why speakers and amplifiers list their
input and output impedances, respectively.

### 5.6 Basic Computers

The development of the computer and the associated discoveries have led to many
devices to assist people with disabilities. The wheelchair has also benefited in a number
of ways. Computers are used to design wheelchairs with computer aided design (CAD)
tools and computer aided engineering (CAE) tools. Computers are used to control
machines that make wheelchairs; this is commonly referred to as computer aided manufacturing (CAM) by engineers. Computers are also used to process orders, maintain
financial records, and maintain customer service records. Computers are intimately
involved in nearly all aspects of wheelchair ordering, design, and manufacture. Therefore, some degree of familiarity with computers is required.

Computers are commonly classified by their physical size and their computing
power. The hierarchy of computers ranges from palm tops to mainframes (see
Figure 5.23). However, specialized devices may fall in between common general
computers. Computers tend to get larger as they get more powerful for two reasons.
As computing power grows more transistors are used, which generate more heat.
Therefore as computers become more powerful they need to have cooling systems
to support continuous operation. Also, as computers grow more powerful they tend
to be used by multiple users, which requires the addition of more peripheral com-

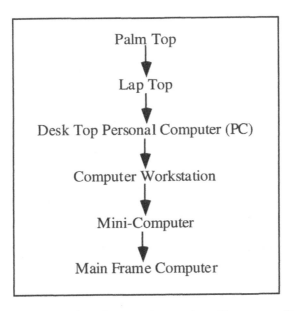

**FIGURE 5.23** Hierarchy of computers ordered by computing power

ponents. This also tends to increase their size. As computing technology evolves, engineers continue to find ways of making smaller logic devices and placing them more closely together. This helps to drive computers to become faster and faster.

To gain a basic understanding of computers some concepts need to be understood. Computers require some form of access device. The access device is the interface to the user which allows the user to transfer data to the computer. The most common form of access device is the keyboard. Keyboards come in a variety of styles to accommodate the environment in which the computer is used, and the abilities or comfort of the computer user. Another common form of access device is called a mouse. A mouse is commonly a set of potentiometers (i.e., variable resistors) that are turned as a ball is rolled across a mouse pad or desk top. The change in potentiometer resistance is used to determine a relative position in the computer display. Switches are incorporated into a mouse to assist with selecting commands. Some software uses the dwell time of the mouse position to select commands as well. A number of devices emulate a mouse to provide alternatives for computer users. Common devices for emulating a mouse include trackballs, mouse pads, mouse keys, head pointers, light pens, and digitizing pads. These devices all provide a means of positioning a pointer on the computer display and selecting a command.

A display provides information from the computer to the user. There are three common types of displays: cathode ray tubes, liquid crystal displays, and light emitting diode displays. Specialized displays exist that create Braille output or provide other forms of tactile feedback. Cathode ray tubes are the most common type of display used with most computers. Cathode ray tubes direct a beam of electrons onto a target. The location on the target is controlled by the computer to create a visual display. The beam and surface coating of the target allow red, green, blue, and yellow elements to be illuminated. The relative strength of the fundamental elements creates different colored images. The computer divides the screen into rows and columns. The beam moves across the columns and down the rows in a continuous sweep. Cathode ray tubes are capable of generating thousands of colors; however, they consume a substantial amount of power and they are heavy. This caused engineers to develop lightweight alternatives. The first lightweight low-power display was the light emitting diode display. The concept of a light emitting diode (LED) display is quite simple. Engineers developed an array of lights that were turned on and off to form images. LED displays are still used today where simple one- or two-color displays are acceptable. Some inexpensive calculators or instrument panels use LED displays to represent numbers or letters. LED displays commonly use red lights with a black background. Liquid crystal displays (LCD) represent a fundamental breakthrough in information technology. A liquid crystal display, used on most common lap tops, operates by using electric fields to orient polarized crystals that are immersed in fluid. When the electric field changes, the orientation of the liquid crystal changes and the amount of light transmitted changes. The original LCDs were black-and-white. A film of fluid containing an array of liquid crystals would be backlit, and through controlling the electric field light, would either be transmited or inhibited. Color was introduced as engineers learned to control the orientation of the crystals more precisely, and optimized the shape of the crystals. LCD technology allows them to be light, thin, and consume little power.

Computers can also be connected to each other or to other devices. This helps to make them extremely powerful tools. Computers operate by interpreting a series of ones and zeros. This means that computers are digital machines, although devices can be added to computers to allow them to receive continuously varying analog signals. The ones and zeros used by computers are represented as binary numbers (see Figure 5.24).

In order for computers to be able to generate and interpret text, computer engineers and scientists had to agree upon binary combinations that would be used to represent letters of the alphabet. The commonly agreed-upon format for text and number representation is based on an eight-bit word. Each bit represents a one or zero. Eight bits are called a byte. Most computers in use today use multiple byte words, but continue to use the standard definitions described in the American Standard Code for Information Interchange (ASCII) developed by the American National Standards Institute (ANSI). Table 5.1 provides a few examples of ASCII representations of common numbers and letters used by computers. Close examination of this table reveals that only seven binary bits are presented. This is because

**FIGURE 5.24** Comparison of binary and decimal number systems

| Binary Number | Decimal Number |
| --- | --- |
| 000 | 0 |
| 001 | 1 |
| 010 | 2 |
| 011 | 3 |
| 100 | 4 |
| 101 | 5 |
| 110 | 6 |
| 111 | 7 |

**TABLE 5.1  Comparison of binary code used by computer and ASCII definitions**

| Binary Code | ASCII Definition |
|---|---|
| 0110000 | 0 |
| 0110001 | 1 |
| 0110010 | 2 |
| 0110011 | 3 |
| 0110100 | 4 |
| 0110101 | 5 |
| 0110110 | 6 |
| 0110111 | 7 |
| 0111000 | 8 |
| 0111001 | 9 |
| 1000000 | @ |
| 1000001 | A |
| 1000010 | B |
| 1000011 | C |
| 1000100 | D |
| 1000101 | E |
| 1000110 | F |
| 1000111 | G |
| 1001000 | H |
| 1001001 | I |

the eighth bit is left as a control bit used by the computer to check errors and to represent its status. The ASCII standard is used throughout the world.

Computers communicate by sending ones and zeros, binary bits. Information is sent using one of two schemes: serial data or parallel data. With serial data only two wires are necessary to send information: one to transmit the binary data, and the other as a reference (commonly ground). When using serial communication all data are sent one after another. This is much like conversation between two people. One person speaks their entire sentence while the other person listens. Then the other person speaks while the original sender listens. This is a form of serial communication. Parallel communication is used within the computer and can be used between computers and other devices. Computers and printers often use parallel communication. Parallel communication sends each bit on a separate channel (wire), which requires more wires, but makes communication much faster. Serial communication is like saying hello one letter at a time h - e - l - l - o, whereas parallel communication is like holding up a sign that has "hello" written on it. The "hello" sign provides us with all of the letters at once, and their position on the sign provides the reader information as to the order in which the word should be interpreted.

Computers use several devices for communicating with one another and with other machines. Serial communication is accomplished using a serial port. A serial port is a device that contains all of the electronics (hardware) and software necessary to communicate with other devices that implement the same serial interface standard. There are several international serial interface standards. Parallel communication is accomplished using a parallel port. Like a serial port, a parallel port implements the hardware and software necessary to comply with a prescribed international standard. It is not unusual for serial and parallel ports to require some software to be installed on the computer in which the ports are used. This is because different devices, like printers, use different protocols, which must be communicated, or downloaded, to the serial or parallel port. A modem is a special type of serial port. A modem uses a telephone line to connect a computer to another device. Because telephone lines are used for communication, modems use special hardware and software to accomplish communication. A limitation of modems is that the rate of communication is sometimes limited by the quality of the telephone lines. Fiber optic telephone lines are designed for voice and data transmission. Hence, they permit much higher transmission rates.

Serial and parallel communication allows the creation of computer systems. A network is used to describe communication between two or more computers. The privileges, or degrees of access, each computer on the network has to the other computers on the network is determined by the computer software that governs the network. Connectivity is a term coined to describe the amount of software and hardware required to connect a computer to a network. In a global sense, computers that use electronic mail, the Internet, or the world wide web are all part of a network. Many offices use local area networks (LANs). A LAN is simply several computers in "close" proximity connected together.

A computer can be pictured in terms of hardware and software. Hardware is used to describe the electronics that make up the physical aspects of the computer. The actual electronics are made of chips and printed circuit boards. Chips are the small circuits designed to perform various functions. These circuits are placed on chips of silicon wafers. Complex techniques of selectively modifying the molecular structure of the silicon are used to make a wide variety of circuits that are very small, efficient, and powerful. The core of any computer is called the central processing unit (CPU). The CPU for a computer is embedded into a chip called the microprocessor or microcontroller, depending on the application. Pentium is the commercial name for a common microprocessor. The CPU controls calculations and manipulations with data, and transfers information to other chips. In order for hardware to be effective as a computer, it must have software to provide guidance. Software is a term used to describe the computer programs. Computers include programs at several levels. The most basic level software is called the basic internal operating system (BIOS). The BIOS is internal to the computer and programmed at the time of the computer's manufacture. The BIOS is stored in read only memory (ROM). Read only memory can only be programmed with special equipment, and its programs are stored permanently directly on the chip. The BIOS stored on ROM is necessary to start a computer. Once the computer is started then the CPU can use programs that are stored elsewhere in the computer. Most programs are stored in one of three locations: on floppy disc, hard disc, or compact disc. Floppy discs are magnetic wafers that a computer uses to store data or read programs. They are slow compared to other types of storage media, and are designed for temporary storage only. Hard discs are a more permanent form of magnetic media for storing programs and data. Hard discs are often built directly into the computer and are used as the primary storage space. Hard drives can easily store billions of bytes of data. They are faster than floppy discs, when computers sometimes have to pass through millions of bytes of data to get to the information a specific program needs. Compact discs are a means of storing data optically. They are portable, long-lasting, and have low cost per byte of storage. They are a popular medium for storing or transferring large amounts of information. The most common form of compact disc (CD) is the CD-ROM. A CD-ROM can only be programmed with special equipment, and cannot be erased. Thus a CD-ROM acts like a portable form of read only memory.

In order to prevent computers from being slowed down by having to access a floppy, hard, or compact disc drive, engineers have placed random access memory (RAM) on computers. The CPU can directly access RAM in only a few millionths of a second. With the addition of RAM the CPU copies the information from the floppy disc, hard disc, or CD-ROM into RAM where it can be accessed rapidly. This effectively makes the computer run faster. Computers commonly have 16 megabytes of RAM (i.e., 16 billion bytes of RAM). This permits the CPU to use this space for rapidly accessing programs or files. When more RAM is available the CPU can load more programs and files. This is useful with operating systems that allow multiple programs to be open simultaneously, especially with the memory requirements of many common programs. The amount of RAM a computer can effectively use is limited. The manufacturer's literature should be consulted prior to attempting to increase the amount of RAM in any computer.

## References and Further Reading

Adam J. A. (1995) Upgrading the Internet, *IEEE Spectrum*, 32, 9, 24–29.

American Standard Code for Information Interchange, American National Standards Institute, Standard No. X3.4-1968.

Aston R. (1990) *Principles of Biomedical Instrumentation and Measurement* Columbus, OH: Merrill Publishing Company.

Cook A. M., Webster J. G., eds. (1982) *Therapeutic Medical Devices Application and Design.* Englewood Cliffs, NJ: Prentice-Hall.

Cooper R. A. (1995) *Rehabilitation Engineering Applied to Mobility and Manipulation.* Philadelphia, PA: Institute of Physics.

Dorf R. C. (1989) *Introduction to Electric Circuits.* New York, NY: John Wiley & Sons.

Geddes L.A., Baker L.E., *Principles of Applied Biomedical Instrumentation*, 3rd ed. New York, NY: John Wiley & Sons.

Ghausi M. S. (1985) *Electronic Devices and Circuits: Discrete and Integrated.* New York, NY: Holt, Rinehart and Winston.

Grant D. A., Gowar J. (1989) *Power MOSFETS: Theory and Application.* New York, NY: John Wiley & Sons.

Kuo B. C. (1987) *Automatic Control Systems*, 5th ed. Englewood Cliffs, NJ: Prentice-Hall.

Larks M. M., Arzbacher R., Bailey J. J., Geselowitz D. B., Berson A. S. (1996) Recommendations for safe current limits for electrocardiographs: A statement for health care professionals from the committee on electrocardiography, American Heart Association, American Heart Association Medical/Scientific Statement, Special Report, *Circulation*, 93, 837–839.

Norman R. A. (1988) *Principles of Bioinstrumentation.* New York, NY: John Wiley & Sons.

*Test and Measurement.* (1995) Cleveland, OH: Keithley Instruments Inc.

Thacker J. G., Sprigle S. H., Morris B. O. (1994) *Understanding the Technology When Selecting Wheelchairs.* Arlington, VA: RESNA Press.

Waintraub J. L., Brumgnach E. (1989) *Electric Circuits for Technologists.* St. Paul, MN: West Publishing Company.

Wakerly J .F. (1981) *Microcomputer Architecture and Programming.* New York, NY: John Wiley & Sons.

Webster J. G., ed. (1992) *Medical Instrumentation Application and Design.* Boston, MA: Houghton Mifflin Company.

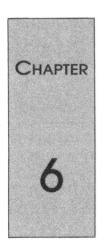

CHAPTER

6

# Wheelchair Standards and Testing

*Chapter Goals*

☑ To know basics of standards for wheelchairs
☑ To know state-of-the-art research and product development
☑ To understand the roles, constraints, and perspectives of manufacturers
☑ To understand the roles, constraints, and perspectives of regulatory agencies
☑ To understand the need for maintenance and repairs for wheelchairs

## 6.1 Introduction

The annual market for wheelchairs worldwide is approximately one billion dollars annually. Standards for wheelchairs have been and continue to be adapted by federal and private agencies that regulate or purchase wheelchairs. Wheelchair standards are very technical. However, when appropriately translated, they can help to ensure product quality, and they can provide assistance in selecting a wheelchair.

The proper selection of a wheelchair requires making several critical decisions, not the least of which is what type of wheelchair is appropriate. It is enticing to choose a wheelchair with which one is familiar or, as is often the case, a wheelchair that is least expensive. As with most things, initial purchase price is only one factor that should be considered. Since 1979, the American National Standards Institute (ANSI) and Rehabilitation Engineering and Assistive Technology Society of North America (RESNA) Wheelchair Standards Committee have been working to provide objective information about the characteristics and performance of wheelchairs. The committee membership includes rehabilitation engineers, manufacturers, representatives of regulatory agencies, wheelchair users, and clinicians.

The standards consist of a number of test procedures that apply to all wheelchairs, and some that apply specifically to power wheelchairs and scooters. Currently, there are 22 test procedures related to manual and electric powered wheelchairs. Some tests require exceeding some specified minimum performance level, whereas others provide a means for comparing results from various products.

Standards are designed and implemented to improve the quality of available wheelchairs, and to assist people in making informed selections of wheelchairs. The standards are voluntary in many instances. However, several federal agencies, such as the U.S. Department of Veterans Affairs and U.S. Food and Drug Administration, use wheelchair standards during their evaluations of wheelchairs and scooters. Consumers and clinicians must also be aware of wheelchair standards so that they can be used when making purchasing and prescription decisions.

Wheelchair and scooter products change constantly. The evolution of existing products and the development of new products necessitate the continual development and refinement of wheelchair standards. Wheelchair standards have, perhaps, had more positive impact on mobility for wheelchair users than any other research and development activity. Every major wheelchair manufacturer in the world has had its products tested using a version of the ANSI/RESNA or International Standards Organization (ISO) wheelchair standards.

The experience in wheelchair standards has shown the merits of taking a global viewpoint to standards development. To obtain the critical mass of knowledgeable people with access to testing laboratory resources requires effective coordination of global efforts to make essential progress. Working through the ISO facilitates harmonization between countries and develops world markets. ISO standards help to improve worldwide access to markets to assistive technology by reducing trade barriers.

## 6.2 Development of Standards

There are currently 22 international wheelchair standards that are either approved or in development (see Table 6.1). These standards address safety, durability, maneuverability, and transport. Some test procedures require exceeding some minimum performance specification, others provide guidance for documentation, and still others provide results for comparison with other products. Wheelchair and scooter products change constantly. The evolution of existing products and the development of new products necessitate the continual development and refinement of wheelchair standards.

Wheelchair standards must be proposed to ISO by a member organization representing one of the many countries involved in the standards process. Wheelchair standards are the responsibility of ISO Technical Committee 173 (TC-173), which is responsible for assistive devices. Sub-committee one (SC-1) is responsible for the development and revision of wheelchair standards. Under the umbrella of SC-1 are several working groups that address specific standards issues. Currently, there are six working groups developing or revising wheelchair standards. Working Group One addresses standards related to safety, durability, and stability for manual and power wheelchairs and scooters. Working Group Six is responsible for standards related to the safe transport of wheelchairs in personal motor vehicles and on public transit. Working Group Seven addresses standards for serial communication protocols to promote "plug-and-play" for assistive devices. Working Group Eight deals with standards related to stair-traversing wheelchairs and devices. Working Group Nine addresses standards for stand-up wheelchairs. Working Group Ten is responsible for standards for electromagnetic compatibility of electric-powered wheelchairs and scooters.

The Working Groups typically meet twice a year. Sub-Committee One meets about every 18 months. Some Sub-committees have enough work items to require breakout groups. Breakout groups work on specific tasks, in some cases components of standards. The process of developing a standard may require years, for

**TABLE 6.1  Current ISO standards for wheelchairs approved and in development**

| ISO Number | Document Title |
|---|---|
| 7176-00 | Nomenclature, Terms, and Definitions |
| 7176-01 | Determination of Static Stability |
| 7176-02 | Determination of Dynamic Stability of Electric Wheelchairs |
| 7176-03 | Determination of Effectiveness of Brakes |
| 7176-04 | Determination of Estimated Range of Electric Wheelchairs |
| 7176-05 | Determination of Overall Dimensions, Weight, and Turning Space |
| 7176-06 | Determination of Maximum Speed, Acceleration, and Retardation for Electric Wheelchairs |
| 7176-07 | Determination of Seating and Dimensions |
| 7176-08 | Static, Impact, and Fatigue Strength Testing |
| 7176-09 | Climatic Tests for Electric Wheelchairs |
| 7176-10 | Determination of Obstacle Climbing Ability of Electric Wheelchairs |
| 7176-11 | Wheelchair Test Dummies |
| 7176-13 | Determination of the Coefficient of Friction Test Surfaces |
| 7176-14 | Testing of Power and Control Systems for Electric Wheelchairs |
| 7176-15 | Guidelines for Information Disclosure |
| 7176-16 | Flammability Characteristics |
| 7176-17 | Serial Interface Compatibility (Multiple Master Multiple Slave) |
| 7176-18 | Stair Traversing Wheelchair Testing |
| 7176-19 | Wheelchair Tie-Downs and Occupant Restraints |
| 7176-20 | Stand-up Wheelchair Testing |
| 7176-21 | Electromagnetic Compatibiity for Electric Wheelchairs |
| 7176-22 | Wheelchair Set-Up Procedures for Testing |

three reasons: standards are very complex and far-reaching; standards require approval of 75% of the participating nations; and international standards remove regional or local trade restrictions. In order to develop a wheelchair standard, test procedures must be validated among laboratories and among various wheelchairs. This process often results in the refinement of the test procedures, and provides data for setting pass/fail criteria. Once a Working Group is satisfied with a standard it is submitted to SC-1 for voting by the participating countries. This process requires about six months, after which time the voting comments are compiled. All voting comments must be addressed, and a response prepared. Countries that vote "yes" to a draft standard (DIS) may make only editorial comments (i.e., comments that seek to clarify, or comments that correct syntax). Countries voting "no" may make substantive comments, but if the comments are accepted then the DIS must return to all countries for another vote. If a DIS fails to receive sufficient votes for approval, it must be revised or discarded. If discarded, a new draft must be prepared. Few standards are discarded. However, most must be voted on several times prior to acceptance.

International standards help to remove trade restrictions. Without an international standard, some countries insist on compliance with a national standard. Compliance with the national standard must be tested in an approved test laboratory within the country where the product is to be distributed. This may result in a product being tested in several countries in order to reach multiple markets. It is not unusual for a national standard to contain nuisances that require several efforts to obtain approval. Furthermore, some test laboratories provide information only as to whether the wheelchair passed/failed the tests, and not the specific test results or mode of failure. Therefore, companies must decide whether the effort to obtain approval is justified by the potential market. Unfortunately, consumers often suffer under these circumstances because superior products are discouraged from entering the marketplace.

Several wheelchair standards need to be developed, some of which have been proposed as work items. Wheelchair-related standards that may be forthcoming can be divided into the areas of safety, compatibility, and effectiveness. The current wheelchair standards that are either approved or in the draft stages provide a useful foundation for wheelchair standards, but they are not sufficiently comprehensive. Several issues must be addressed by Sub-Committee One, in order to ensure safe and effective products are provided to people with disabilities.

There are currently no standards that directly address cushion or upholstery for wheelchairs. This leads to several possible problems, some of which have already been identified by clinicians and consumers. Wheelchairs used in institutions are commonly cleaned with common household disinfectants between uses by different patients or residents. However, no standard addresses whether this is adequate protection against the transmission of infectious diseases (e.g., hepatitis B). Other medical/rehabilitation devices have such standards to prevent transmission of infectious diseases. In long-term care institutions it is common practice to use the same polyurethane foam or flexible honeycomb composite pressure-relief cushion for multiple residents. These cushions are exposed to urine and feces. When soiled the cushions are commonly washed in a washing machine with household detergent. However, cutting some brands or models of cushions reveals that urine or feces remains within the core of the cushion. Standards may help to improve the safety and quality of customized seating systems. In warm humid environments, maggots and cockroaches can infest custom seating systems. Standards could lead to the use of foams or coverings that prevent this from occurring. A test for the durability and pressure distribution of pressure-relief cushions is also required. This would allow cushions to be compared and contrasted.

Specialty wheelchairs and mobility devices require standards. Currently, there are no standards for standing frames (fixed or mobile). There are also no standards for tilt-in-space or reclining wheelchairs. These types of devices are commonly used, and are in need of means of ensuring quality. Standards need to be developed to determine the reliability of wheelchairs. This would allow consumers and clinicians to decide an acceptable rate of failure or repair. Currently, wheelchair fatigue tests provide only an estimated life of a wheelchair prior to replacement. They do not indicate whether a wheelchair is unavailable for use five days a year or 90 days per year. This standard should also apply to software. Currently, power wheelchair software is only peripherally tested. Requirements for software engineering and "whitebox" testing are also required. Software failures or glitches can produce hazardous situations for electric-powered wheelchair users.

Wheelchair batteries are not tested under current wheelchair standards. Future wheelchairs standards should provide test methods for determining the ampere-hour rating, charge characteristics, useful life, and safety. It would also be useful to provide consumers with information about the cost of operating a wheelchair with various batteries (i.e., cost per mile of operation).

## 6.3 Information Disclosure

Compliance with ANSI/RESNA or ISO wheelchair standards implies that the manufacturer will disclose specific test results in the owner's manual, and that additional information is available upon request (see Table 6.2). The results in the owner's manual pertain to the way in which the dimensions and weight of the wheelchair and its major components are reported. Before manufacturers used wheelchair standards, the reporting of dimensions and weight varied greatly from one manufacturer to another. The weight of one wheelchair may have been reported with legrests by one manufacturer, and without legrests by another manufacturer. Wheelchair standards specify how the weight of the wheelchair is to be recorded and reported. The overall weight of the wheelchair as reported, based on wheelchair standards, includes legrests, armrests, wheel locks, wheels, and casters.

Manufacturers are only required to test a single wheelchair from a specific model. Therefore, the results from an individual's wheelchair may vary from the data reported in the manufacturer's product literature. In some cases, the manufacturer may provide only a numerical result. To many clinicians and consumers, the number by itself may have little meaning. However, numerical results are useful for comparison purposes. A common example is where a number is reported in fatigue (durability) testing. In order to estimate the functional life of a wheelchair, manufacturers will test them on a machine called a double-drum tester. A double-drum tester simulates rolling the wheelchair over door thresholds, sidewalk cracks, and small potholes. If a manufacturer reports that their wheelchair can tolerate 200,000 cycles, this may have little meaning by itself. However, if another manufacturer claims that its product will tolerate 600,000 cycles, then the reader knows that the wheelchair from the second manufacturer is likely to last three times as long.

Standards are used to raise quality by setting a minimum threshold on some functions of the wheelchair, and providing a means of comparing other functions of the wheelchair. Manufacturers test new, unused wheelchairs. Only one of four sized standardized dummies is used. Therefore, it is difficult to extrapolate wheelchair standards information to the function of a specific wheelchair used by an individual consumer. Rather, standards provide a means of comparing products or product lines. Wheelchair manufacturers who claim compliance with ANSI/RESNA wheelchair standards must provide consumers with pass/fail results for all tests that have pass/fail criteria.

## 6.4 Performance Testing

Good clinicians understand that function is a very important factor for their patients. Consumers understand that function and reliability are important for their independent mobility. Engineers understand the importance of durability, reliability, and performance. Rehabilitation professionals have espoused the benefits of a team approach to design and assessment for many years. Bringing together a wide variety of perspectives is invaluable. However, professional teams require valid information in order to make wise decisions. From a clinical treatment perspective, this has led to the development of outcomes research, and from an engineering perspective has led to standards.

TABLE 6.2    Disclosure information required by ANSI/RESNA
             wheelchair standards

| ISO Standard Number | Information Available from Manufacturer upon Request |
|---|---|
| 7176-01 | • Static tip angle forward, laterally, and rearward with and without wheels looked |
| 7176-02 | • Response starting and driving uphill<br>• Response transitioning from ramp to flat, and flat to ramp<br>• Response during maximum speed and turn up and down hill |
| 7176-03 | • Wheel lock lever force<br>• Forward horizontal and sloped braking distance<br>• Reverse horizontal braking distance<br>• Force required to operate braking distance |
| 7176-04 | • Estimated range on a full battery charge<br>• Watt hours per kilometer |
| 7176-05 | • Dimensions and mass of each removable component<br>• Minimum turning radius<br>• Overall height with backrest in upright position<br>• Minimum volume (i.e., smallest box wheelchair can be put into)<br>• Minimum dimensions of largest component, usually the frame<br>• Dimensions of nonfolding wheelchair when prepared for storage<br>• Dimensions of a folding wheelchair for accommodation in an automobile |
| 7176-06 | • Maximum acceleration when driving forward<br>• Maximum acceleration when driving rearward<br>• Maximum retardation forward |
| 7176-07 | • Effective seat width<br>• Backrest width<br>• Headrest dimensions and location<br>• Footrest clearance<br>• Legrest length<br>• Footrest-to-leg angle<br>• Armrest width<br>• Armrest angle<br>• Vertical location of rear wheel axles |
| 7176-08 | • Double-drum cycles without failure<br>• Curb-drop drops without failure |
| 7176-14 | • Force necessary to operate joystick<br>• Force necessary to operate push-button, rocker, and keypad switches<br>• Force necessary to operate toggle switches<br>• Force necessary to operate pneumatic switches (sip-&-puff) |
| 7176-21 | • Pass/fail on whether wheelchair was able to meet 20 V/m field strength |

## 6.4.1 Classes of Failure

There are three classes of failure. (However, in many cases only one class is reported.) Class one failures include minor adjustments or repairs that may be accomplished by the wheelchair user or an untrained assistant, such as tightening a loose bolt or screw. Class one repairs may include making simple adjustments.

Class two failures include minor repairs that can be accomplished by a repair technician or in some cases by a bicycle mechanic. Class two failures include repairing or replacing flat tires, or making complex adjustments (e.g., camber, wheel alignment). Class three failures describe structural damage or repairs that would immobilize the wheelchair. If the wheelchair frame breaks it is an obvious class three failure. Not so obvious is when an axle or caster stem breaks; these are also considered class three failures. If an axle breaks, the ability to drive the wheelchair is significantly impaired. Class three failures provide information about the available life of the wheelchair. The specific type of class three failure must be ascertained to know whether the wheelchair can be repaired or whether the wheelchair must be replaced.

ISO wheelchair standards no longer require the three classes when reporting wheelchair test results. When applying ISO wheelchair standards, test laboratories and manufacturers are required only to report that length of time required to a class three failure or the second class one or class two failures. If during fatigue testing, which is described later in this chapter, a class three failure occurs prior to completing the prescribed number of cycles, the wheelchair is reported to have failed the test. Similarly, if a wheelchair experiences a class one failure or a class two failure, the test technician can make the necessary adjustment or repair. However, if another class one or class two failure occurs prior to completing the test, the wheelchair is reported to have failed the test. This can mean that one wheelchair fails because it developed two flat tires during the double-drum test, whereas another wheelchair failed because the frame broke. Therefore, people must be cautious when interpreting wheelchair test results.

### 6.4.2 Static and Impact Strength Tests

Wheelchairs undergo static loads during normal operation. Static loads can be described by applying a constant force to a component of the wheelchair. When a person sits in a wheelchair he/she applies a force proportional to their weight to the seat of the wheelchair. At the same time the wheels and axles are affected by forces of the person's weight. Other forces are applied to parts of the wheelchair when someone provides assistance to climb up or down a step, or to lift a person over an obstacle. Static strength tests are designed to evaluate whether a wheelchair can withstand the expectable forces that may be applied to it and its components. The static strength tests are performed only once; therefore, a *factor of safety* is applied. A factor of safety attempts to account for repeated forces by applying a larger force a single time. The amount of force varies by location and size of the wheelchair.

Static strength tests are performed to evaluate the strength of armrests, footrests, anti-tip levers, handgrips on the backrest canes, and push-handles on the backrest. For the armrests, forces are applied to each armrest that simulate a person doing a push-up (i.e., lifting the trunk upwards from the seat by pressing with the arms downwards on the armrests). After this test, the armrests must still retain all of their original functions. Armrests are also used to provide assistance to the user by others lifting the armrests to get over obstacles. A force is applied upward to the armrests. The armrests should either not permit lifting of the wheelchair and rider (i.e., lift out of their sockets or flip back) or they should allow the person to be lifted safely. Footrests are tested by applying a downward and then an upward force. The downward force is designed to simulate the force applied during a spasm, or when being assisted by someone who may place a foot on the footrest. After the downward force is applied, the legrests should function properly. An upward force is applied to the legrests because they are commonly used to lift persons when assisting them over physical obstacles. The legrests should either prevent using them for lifting the wheelchair (e.g., by lifting out of their sockets) or they should allow the person to be lifted safely. Tipping levers are tested with an applied force to ensure that they do not permanently deform when a person uses them, or when stepped on to provide assistance. Handgrips are tested by applying a force in an attempt to remove the handgrips from their handles. This is to prevent the handgrips from coming off or tearing while a person is providing assistance. The push-handle upward test is used to demonstrate that the wheelchair and occupant can be safely lifted using the push-handles.

Wheelchairs experience a variety of impacts during normal use. It is not uncommon for the footrests to experience impacts from hitting doors. The seat and backrest experience an impact when a person transfers into the wheelchair, especially if the person loses balance. Casters impact bumps, or in some cases may impact a curb in a failed attempt at hopping the curb. When going off a curb, the wheelchair may land with one wheel hitting the ground first; the wheel should not bend or break. The wheelchair or components may be dropped causing an impact. For these reasons and others, impact tests are performed. After each impact test, the wheelchair and the component being tested must continue to function properly and show no permanent sign of damage.

The impact tests are performed by either using a pendulum or actually dropping the component or wheelchair. The footrests, casters, and pushrims are tested using a ten-kilogram steel pendulum. The pendulum is released from various angles to strike the casters or pushrim in different ways. The angle of release varies with the mass of the wheelchair. The seat and backrest are tested with a compliant ball the size of a regulation soccer ball, with a mass of 25 kilograms. These tests help to ensure the quality of the wheelchair. Static and impact tests are pass/fail. Therefore, wheelchairs must meet the minimum level for all components of the static and impact strength standard in order to be in compliance with ANSI/RESNA standards.

### 6.4.3 Fatigue Strength Tests

The fatigue strength tests represent the teeth of the standards, as they are the most rigorous of all the mechanical tests. There are two fatigue strength tests: the curb-drop test and the double-drum test. The double-drum test is performed first. The double-drum test is used to simulate sidewalk cracks, door thresholds, potholes, and other road hazards (see Figure 6.1). The double-drum test consists of setting the wheelchair loaded with an appropriate-sized test dummy onto two drums. The drive wheels of the wheelchair are placed onto one drum while the caster wheels are placed onto the other drum. Both drums have two slats that are one centimeter high and two centimeters wide attached to them. The slats on a drum are transposed 180 degrees (i.e., the slats are on either side of the drum). The rear drum turns at one meter per second. The front drum turns 5% to 7% faster then the rear drum. This causes the impacts imparted by the slats to the wheels to change over time. This helps to prevent a wheelchair from being favored or unduly punished because of the

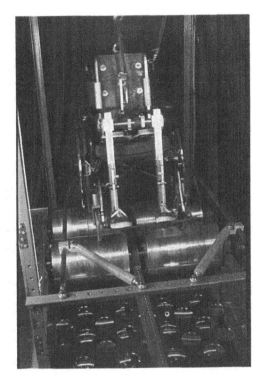

**FIGURE 6.1**  Photograph of a double-drum wheelchair fatigue testing machine (Photograph courtesy of VA Pittsburgh Health Care System)

orientation of the slats. The ANSI/RESNA standards allow wheelchair manufacturers to choose the number of cycles they wish to drive the wheelchair. In order to be in compliance with ANSI/RESNA wheelchair standards, the manufacturer must report the minimum number of cycles the wheelchair can withstand without a class three failure. ISO standards require that a wheelchair withstand 200,000 cycles without a class three or without two class one or class two failures.

The curb-drop test is used to simulate the repeated loads experienced by wheelchairs when going down small curbs (see Figure 6.2). Wheelchairs are loaded with a 100-kilogram test dummy. During the curb-drop test the wheelchair and dummy are lifted five centimeters and then dropped. In order to be in compliance with ANSI/RESNA or ISO standards, a wheelchair must be able to withstand one thirtieth (i.e., 1/30) the number of drops as the number of double-drum cycles the wheelchair withstood. This means that ISO standards require a wheelchair to withstand 200,000 double-drum cycles and 6,667 curb-drop drops. The ISO numbers were selected as being representative of between three and five years of active use.

### 6.4.4 Obstacle-Climbing Ability Test

People in both manual and electric-powered wheelchairs must negotiate obstacles during normal use. Curbs, separations in sidewalks, tree roots, and rough terrain must be negotiated. The obstacle-climbing ability test provides some insight into the height of obstacles an electric-powered wheelchair can safely negotiate. Manual

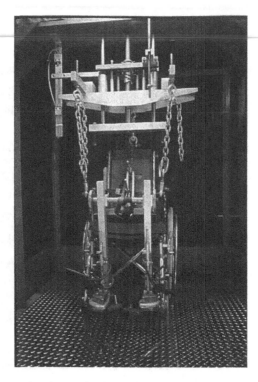

**FIGURE 6.2**   Photograph of a curb-drop wheelchair fatigue testing machine
(Photograph courtesy of VA Pittsburgh Health Care System)

wheelchairs are not subjected to an obstacle-climbing ability test. There is no obstacle-climbing standard for manual wheelchairs, because of the variability of obstacle-climbing ability based on the user's skill and the set-up of the wheelchair. This has hindered the development of a meaningful manual wheelchair obstacle-climbing standard.

The electric-powered wheelchair obstacle-climbing standard also relies on the skill of the user, but the variation in skill is acceptable to test engineers, and the test provides useful results for clinicians. The obstacle-climbing test is performed by determining the height of an obstacle that a wheelchair may be driven up onto with a run-up distance of one meter. The obstacle is typically made by stacking sheets of plywood higher than the base of the wheelchair. The wheelchair must be able to fit on top of the platform after having climbed up. The maximum obstacle-climbing ability is determined by stacking sheets of wood to build a higher and higher platform. The maximum height that a wheelchair can climb without tipping over or stopping is recorded.

The obstacle-climbing ability of power wheelchairs varies considerably. Power wheelchairs designed for indoor use may only be able to climb obstacles that are one to two centimeters in height. Lightweight power wheelchairs designed for indoor and moderate outdoor use are, typically, capable of climbing obstacles that are two to three centimeters high. Full-size electric-powered wheelchairs can often climb obstacles that are five centimeters high. Powered wheelchairs with front wheel drive are usually better at obstacle climbing than rear wheel drive wheelchairs.

### 6.4.5 Range

The range of a power wheelchair depends on many factors including battery type, battery state (whether charged or uncharged), wheelchair/rider weight, terrain, the efficiency of the drive train, and the driving behavior of the user. Various wheelchairs have different ranges. This variation in range may be related to the intended purpose of the power wheelchair or the settings selected by the user. Batteries are rated in ampere hours (amp-hours). The amp-hour rating and the current drawn by the power wheelchair will to a large extent determine the range.

Range is an important metric in power wheelchair selection and design. The range of a power wheelchair provides an estimate of the total distance that the wheelchair can be driven on a new, fully charged set of batteries. This estimate may vary depending on terrain and driving/maintenance habits. Determination of energy consumption for electric wheelchair standards is made on large external areas (e.g., parking lots, tennis courts).

Energy consumption is measured over a distance of 1500 meters over a level rolling surface. Using the proposed ISO standard tennis court range test the direction of driving (i.e., clockwise to counterclockwise) was changed at 750 meters. Wheelchairs are always driven in the forward direction. Each wheelchair is warmed up for 750 meters at or near maximal speed prior to data collection, to minimize the variation in current associated with heating electrical and electromechanical components. Hence each wheelchair is driven a distance of 2250 meters while loaded with the appropriate-sized test dummy or driver. The time required to complete the 1500 meters is recorded and later used to calculate maximum speed of each wheelchair while performing each experiment. A course is laid out around the perimeter of a tennis court and the distance measured with a steel tape. The pilot is instructed to follow the course as closely as possible, and must stay within specified boundaries.

Range is estimated to be the product of the nominal battery capacity and the speed traveled, divided by the amperes consumed (equation (6.1)).

$$range = \frac{nominal\ battery\ capacity \times speed\ traveled}{amperes\ consumed} \tag{6.1}$$

New batteries are installed in each power wheelchair prior to testing, and all batteries were fully charged (as determined from open circuit voltage and charging current) before each experiment. The state of charge for a new battery is somewhat subjective. Typically new batteries do not reach their full capacity until 30 to 40 charge/discharge cycles. This can add variability in range when driving to discharge. However, wheelchairs are driven only 2250 meters per test, which is well within battery capacity. Thus variations in state of charge will have minimal effect on the range estimates. In actual driving situations range will be less than the idealized estimates of range determined with the ISO test methods. This method is valuable for comparison purposes. The capacity (amp•hour) rating for batteries of the same size may vary considerably. For the ISO Range Test Standard (ISO 7176–04), the capacity reported by the battery manufacturer is used. The short distance actually driven minimizes the variability. Furthermore, ISO and ANSI/RESNA range tests are conducted in test laboratories around the world with various wheelchairs and batteries. One of the ISO and ANSI/RESNA objectives is that tests of similar wheelchairs will yield consistent results at each laboratory. Each wheelchair is configured per the manufacturer's specifications, and tires are properly inflated. Experienced test pilots (technicians) are used for the tennis court tests.

## 6.5 Sample Normative Values

Standards allow the objective comparison of products from various sources. This allows the consumer or clinician to assess wheelchairs with which they are not familiar by comparing test results. The use of standards permits a definition of quality based on fact and quantitative data to permeate clinical practice rather than a definition based on opinion and experience. While wheelchair manufacturers have conducted evaluations of their own and competitors' products for over 25 years, this information has been virtually inaccessible to the prescriber and consumer. More recently, some manufacturers have volunteered some test data for publication in comparison articles. However, much of this information is difficult to interpret because the reported results are typically similar. While it is comforting to learn that a minimum level of quality is being established through the standards process, it would be more useful to know, for example, which products last longer or require less maintenance.

Some comparison data are available. The National Rehabilitation Hospital in Washington, D.C. and ECRI gathered some data on rehabilitation technology and published a series of reports. Although these reports are helpful, continued effort is required. Several of the wheelchairs tested were unable to meet the requirements of one or more of the 18 ANSI/RESNA standards that were applied.

### 6.5.1 Testing for Durability

International Standards Organization static, impact, and fatigue strength testing standards require wheelchairs to complete 200,000 double-drum cycles followed by 6,666 curb-drop tester drops without a failure. This is equivalent to about 159 kilometers (100 miles) of moderately rough terrain. Peizer et al. studied the effects of destructive testing on a lightweight wheelchair. They weighted the chair with 200 pounds of lead shot and rolled it off a six-inch wooden platform repeatedly. Deformation of the frame was measured at regular intervals, and after 38 drops the crossbrace buckled.

National Rehabilitation Hospital and ECRI fatigue-tested ten electric-powered wheelchairs using ANSI/RESNA procedures. They used 200,000 double-drum cycles and 6,666 curb-drop drops as their pass/fail criteria. The same wheelchairs were used on both the double-drum and curb-drop tests. Using these criteria, two of the ten wheelchairs failed. The weld attaching the battery support frame to the wheelchair frame broke on the E&J Tempest after 203,135 double-drum cycles, and 3335 curb-drop drops. The welds on the seat frame broke on the Permobil Max 90 after 102,597 double-drum cycles and 3414 curb-drop drops. Testing was stopped if the pass criteria were met, therefore, the number of cycles to class three failure are unknown for the remaining wheelchairs. Several power wheelchair manufacturers did not participate in this study.

The Paralyzed Veterans of America publishes a list of wheelchairs and their ANSI/RESNA standards test results provided by the wheelchair manufacturers each year in *Sports 'N Spokes* magazine. Listing test results is optional, but the information contained in the articles is useful for comparing various wheelchairs. Most of the results reported in these articles use the 200,000 double-drum and 6,666 curb-drop cycles required by the proposed ISO standard for wheelchair-fatigue testing. This makes comparison of durability difficult because manufacturers either report the level proposed by the ISO standard or provide no test results at all.

Wheelchair test laboratories have existed in Europe for several years, and many countries have minimum performance standards, which all wheelchairs must meet. However, there has been no common test method for determining fatigue life. Some countries have used obstacles attached to the belts of treadmills, some obstacles attached to rollers, some eccentric rollers, some obstacles mounted to the floor and the chair pulled by a carousel, and even chairs pulled over a linear test track. Therefore, comparison data have not been reported. Moreover, most countries, including those in Europe, are adopting ISO 7176 wheelchair testing standards, which define using a double-drum tester and curb-drop tester for fatigue testing. Hence, there is little motivation for developing comparison methods for non-ISO standard fatigue tests that are being phased out. In the future, standardized testing methods and equipment should provide useful comparison data from test laboratories around the world. Some useful data on properties of wheelchairs are included in published reports sponsored by the European Community. European Community standards should help to produce a database of wheelchairs that meet the minimum performance standards.

Cooper and colleagues at the University of Pittsburgh tested 15 manual wheelchairs using both a double-drum tester and a curb-drop tester. Of the 15 wheelchairs, nine were considered rehabilitation wheelchairs and six were considered depot wheelchairs. Rehabilitation wheelchairs were defined as wheelchairs designed to be used as daily wheelchairs provided to an individual for personal mobility within the community. Depot wheelchairs were defined as those designed to be used in an institutional setting as part of a pool of wheelchairs available for temporary use (e.g., hospital-type wheelchair). The suggested retail price, provided by the manufacturers, for each depot wheelchair was about $450, while the suggested retail price for each rehabilitation wheelchair was about $1,700. The rehabilitation wheelchairs lasted on average 13.2 times longer than the depot wheelchairs. The total cycles before class three failure were significantly higher for the rehabilitation wheelchairs than for the depot wheelchairs. The three rehabilitation wheelchairs that were equipped with 8-inch pneumatic casters lasted on average 3.2 times longer than the six rehabilitation wheelchairs equipped with solid 8-inch casters. Pneumatic casters cause a significant increase in fatigue life.

Six of the nine rehabilitation wheelchairs experienced class three failures, while three successfully completed 2.05 million equivalent cycles (these three all had pneumatic caster tires). Two of the rehabilitation wheelchairs failed at the front right welds of the junction where the footrests connect to the vertical side tubes. The frame members may not have been properly preheated before welding and/or the joint may not have cooled slowly enough to prevent thermal expansion and stresses. One rehabilitation wheelchair failed due to the cross-brace fracturing on the rear bottom side next to the bolt location. Increasing the material thickness or cross-sectional area would increase its strength and fatigue life. Incorporating a bolt insert could also increase fatigue life since the fracture originated at the bolt hole. Three of the rehabilitation wheelchairs failed due to the right caster spindle bolts shearing off. These failures occurred at the bolt-thread junction due to the cyclic fatigue of the caster striking the ground. Using a thicker stem bolt or possibly using a higher grade bolt (SAE grade 5 was used for these tests) could increase the spindle bolt's fatigue life. Three rehabilitation wheelchairs did not suffer any class three failures. Rehabilitation wheelchairs tend to use higher quality materials and better manufacturing practices and to provide greater mobility for wheelchair users.

All six depot wheelchairs experienced class three failures during our testing. One depot wheelchair failed when the right front plastic caster spokes fractured. The spokes were made from nonreinforced polyvinylchloride (PVC) plastic which lacked suitable durability. Two depot wheelchairs experienced frame failures at the left front side weld vent holes located 12 mm (1/2 inch) behind the caster housing joint with the side frame. Stress concentrations built up at the vent holes and propagated through the frame tubing. Redesign of this frame member should exclude or relocate the vent holes. Two depot wheelchairs failed at the right upper-side horizontal tube weld at the junction of the side frame and the backrest tube (i.e., cane). One depot wheelchair failed at both side tube welds at the junction of the side frame and backrest tubes. Corrosion in the metal of the furnace-brazed welds could have caused the failure. Improper heating and cooling of the welds and the frame member could also have caused the failure.

Three of the rehabilitation wheelchairs could have been repaired by replacing the caster spindles. Our investigation was based on number of cycles to first class three failure as defined in the ANSI/RESNA wheelchair standards. Failure of a caster spindle, although repairable, is a class three failure. Therefore, testing was terminated on detection of a caster spindle failure, as it was with other class three failures. All of the wheelchairs could have been repaired if given appropriate technical assistance and materials (broken welds could have been rewelded, frame breakages could have been reinforced and welded, spindles could be replaced). In the case of the depot wheelchairs, cost of repair would likely exceed cost of replacement. The ANSI/RESNA definition of a class three failure was applied during this study to provide consistent and comparable data.

Rehabilitation wheelchairs tend to experience component failures (see Figure 6.3), whereas the depot wheelchairs tend to experience frame failures (see Figure 6.4). Testing indicates that the ISO–ANSI/RESNA standards can relate design features to fatigue test results and durability (i.e., differences are seen between depot and rehabilitation wheelchairs).

Test results indicate that there are several areas on wheelchairs where fatigue failures may occur. Hence, wheelchairs should be inspected regularly to detect damage before it becomes a problem. Caster forks and caster spindles may fail due to the repeated loading seen when hitting cracks, door thresholds, and surface irregularities (see Figure 6.5). The cross-brace is a critical component on both manual and electric-powered wheelchairs. When a cross-brace fails, the wheelchair may become inoperable and can trap the wheelchair user within the broken frame (see Figure 6.6). Cross-braces tend to fail because of riding over undulations, irregular surfaces, and going off curbs. Backrests may also break due to the forces applied while driving and other activities of daily living. The backrest experiences a cyclic force during each push, and can experience substantial loads while being used as a support structure during activities of daily living. In some wheelchairs, the backrest tubes are swedged and inserted into the frame of the wheelchair. The swedging can

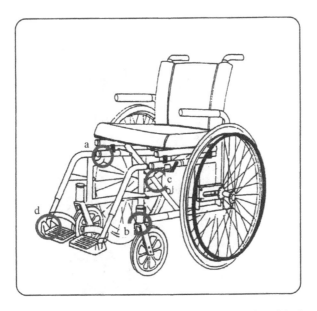

**FIGURE 6.3** Locations where rehabilitation wheelchairs tend to break: (a) the intersection of the legrest to the frame; (b) the caster spindles; (c) the joint between the two cross-braces; (d) the joint between the footrest and the legrest.

**FIGURE 6.4** Illustration of common fatigue failures experienced by depot wheelchairs: (a) the joint between the footrest and the legrest; (b) the side frame just near the weld for the caster bearing housing; (c) the joint between the cross-braces; (d) the joint between the side frame and the backrest cane.

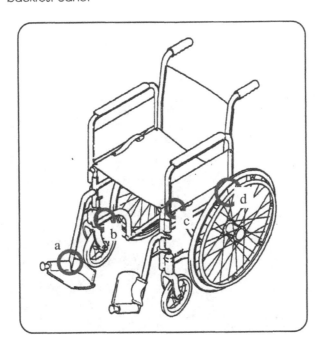

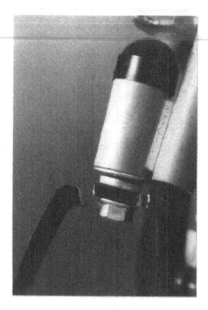

**FIGURE 6.5**   Photograph of a caster fork fatigue failure due to repeated loads
created by an ISO double-drum tester (Photograph courtesy of VA
Pittsburgh Health Care System)

lead to weakening the backrest leading to a failure (see Figure 6.7). Other wheelchairs have the backrest tubes integrated into the frame. Depot and lightweight-type
wheelchairs commonly use this type of design. If the frame is not strong enough or
the welding is not of high enough quality, the backrest may break. The problem
tends to appear most often in depot-type wheelchairs where lower-quality materials

**FIGURE 6.6**   Photograph of a depot-type wheelchair that has experienced a
cross-brace failure (Photograph courtesy of VA Pittsburgh Health
Care System)

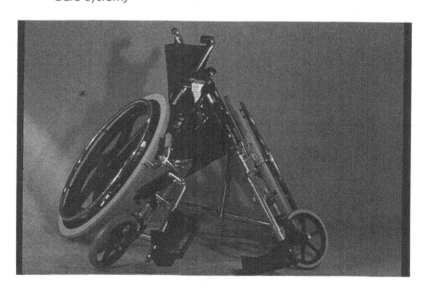

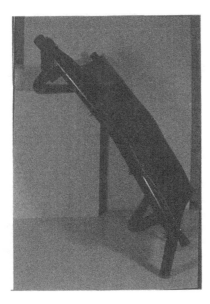

**FIGURE 6.7** Photograph of a backrest with swedged ends used on an electric-powered wheelchair. The failure can be seen at the rapid bend in the backrest tube near the bottom of the figure (Photograph courtesy of VA Pittsburgh Health Care System)

and lower-strength welding processes are used. These weaknesses are accentuated when the backrest is taller, as is common among depot and lightweight wheelchairs, because the forces applied to the backrest by the user or assistant create high moments at the joint between the backrest and frame. Figure 6.8 shows a backrest fatigue failure for a lightweight wheelchair. The batteries on scooters and electric-powered wheelchairs may also cause damage to the wheelchair frame. Batteries are typically quite heavy and when the wheelchair is subjected to repeated vertical bumps, the batteries may break the frame and/or casing (see Figure 6.9).

## 6.5.2 Impact and Static Strength

International Standards Organization (ISO) standard ISO 7176–08 specifies the procedures and test equipment specific to static, impact, and fatigue testing of wheelchairs. A section of this standard describes the pushrim impact pendulum. During normal wheelchair use it is not uncommon for the pushrims of the wheelchair to experience impacts due to hitting stationary objects (e.g., doorways, walls) while the user propels the wheelchair. The same is true for casters and footrests. Impact tests are designed to ensure that a wheelchair and its components can withstand reasonably large impacts infrequently. Impacts are tested by using a pendulum designed for that purpose. Use of the pushrim pendulum must be specified to yield consistent results from one laboratory to another. The mass, geometry, and point of impact affect the momentum imparted from the pendulum to the wheelchair. Therefore, these parameters must be specified. The wheelchair should make contact with the pendulum at the center of percussion to ensure consistent transfer of momentum.

Cooper et al. performed tests on five different wheelchairs loaded with an ISO 100-kilogram test dummy. Pendulum impact tests were performed using an ISO

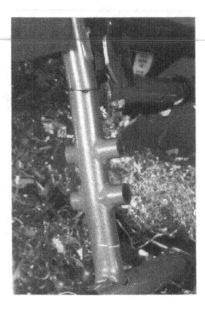

**FIGURE 6.8**   Photograph of a backrest fatigue failure at the joint with the wheelchair frame. This failure makes the wheelchair unsafe to use.
(Photograph courtesy of VA Pittsburgh Health Care System)

pushrim impact test pendulum. All impacts were at the center of percussion. The
pendulum was aligned to hit the caster or footrest squarely. The angle of the pendulum was measured to the nearest degree using a machinist protractor attached to
the test apparatus. The wheelchairs were elevated 4 inches from the floor so that the
pendulum could strike the casters properly. Wheelchairs were struck at 45 degrees
with respect to the frame, but in line with the right caster. Wheelchairs were struck
on the right footrest in the sagittal plane and in the frontal plane. Each wheelchair
completed three trials at each angle. Strikes were performed in order of increasing
angle. The rear axles of each of the chairs were placed in their most statically stable
position. The dummy was seated properly in the chair as per ISO 7176–07. The types
of chairs, their footrest types, and caster types are given in Table 6.3.

**FIGURE 6.9**   Photograph of a scooter where the batteries have broken through
the frame (Photograph courtesy of VA Pittsburgh Health Care
System)

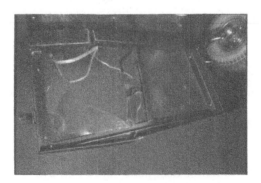

**TABLE 6.3  Description of test wheelchairs**

| Wheelchair Name | Caster Description | Footrest Description |
|---|---|---|
| E&J Catalina | 4 inch, solid rubber tire | steel, swing-away |
| Hoyer 1000 | 8 inch, solid tire, plastic rim | steel, swing-away |
| Kuschall 2000 | 8 inch, solid tire, plastic rim | reinforced plastic, flip-up |
| Quickie 1 | 5 inch, solid polyurethane | aluminum, rigid |
| Quickie 2 | 8 inch, pneumatic, plastic rim | plastic/aluminum, swing-way |

The raw data were converted to multiples of earth's gravitational constant (g). The resultant was calculated for each acceleration along the data stream. The maximum resultant acceleration was used to relate pendulum release angle to impact acceleration, and to compare accelerations by test and wheelchair manufacturer. The pendulum impact test mean of all the wheelchairs' maximum impact resultant accelerations are given in Table 6.4.

One factor analysis of variance (ANOVA) with Scheffe's post-hoc test did show significant differences (p = 0.0001) among wheelchair models for the pendulum impact tests with caster contact (p = 0.0001) and footrest frontal contact (p = 0.01). The Quickie 1, Quickie 2, Kuschall 2000, and E&J Catalina had significantly lower pendulum impact accelerations with caster contact than the Hoyer 1000 (p < 0.05). The caster impact results of the Quickie 2 were statistically significantly (p < 0.05) lower than for the Kuschall 2000. However, the accelerations differed by only a few g. The footrest frontal impact results showed significant (p < 0.05) differences between the Quickie 1 and Quickie 2 (the Quickie 1 had higher impact accelerations), as well as between the Quickie 2 and Hoyer 1000 (the Hoyer 1000 had higher impact accelerations). Differences in impact strength between wheelchairs can be detected by the pendulum impact tests, which is indication that these tests may be useful in evaluating wheelchair quality. They had one chair experience a footrest failure during the pendulum impact tests with a 60-degree release angle. All of the chairs tested can withstand 45 degrees, and the corresponding accelerations are larger than those for a curb impact measured at one meter per second.

### 6.5.3 Range Testing Results

Kauzlarich et al. examined battery performance of electric wheelchairs during indoor and outdoor conditions. Driving cycles were used to bench-test various types of batteries. A single instrumented wheelchair was used for all tests. The indoor test consisted of a 0.241-km test track including numerous obstacles and floor surfaces.

**TABLE 6.4  Mean of maximal resultant pendulum impact accelerations (g) for five different chairs loaded with ISO 100-kilogram test dummy**

| Impact Location | Pendulum Initial Angle | | |
|---|---|---|---|
| | 30 degrees | 45 degrees | 60 degrees |
| Caster Impact | 24.6 ± 6.29 g | 28.5 ± 7.00 g | 35.3 ± 5.73 g |
| Footrest Front Impact | 22.9 ± 6.47 g | 31.4 ± 6.72 g | 34.0 ± 7.39 g |
| Footrest Side Impact | 21.4 ± 7.14 g | 28.2 ± 7.22 g | 31.2 ± 11.30 g |

The wheelchair was driven continuously over the course for 11.1 km (3.85 hours) when the battery was depleted. The outdoor test route covered 2.75 km per lap, which included grades up to four degrees. A paved footpath and parking lot were used for this test. The wheelchair was driven for 15.6 km (2.74 hours) when the battery was depleted.

Cooper et al. performed range tests on seven different power wheelchairs loaded with an ISO 100-kilogram test dummy (see Table 6.5). A specially designed circuit was used to measure battery voltage and load current, which was interfaced to Motorola MC6811-based analog-to-digital computer interface attached to the serial port of a computer. Data were collected at 20 Hz per channel on a DOS-compatible 8088-based laptop. Current and voltage were monitored at the battery terminals. Each wheelchair was tested on a tennis court. New batteries were installed in each power wheelchair prior to testing, and all batteries were fully charged (as determined from open circuit voltage and charging current) before each experiment. The raw data were converted to voltages and amperes as appropriate. A program was written that used 20-point smoothing prior to calculating current, voltage, and power (see Table 6.6). Power was calculated as the instantaneous product of current and voltage. This is valid as the current and power were measured in phase. Using the same program, energy was calculated by integrating power using Simpson's Rule from the time the test was started until the power wheelchair completed 1500 meters. Range was estimated to be the product of the nominal battery capacity and the speed traveled, divided by the amperes consumed.

The data presented in Tables 6.5 and 6.6 were used in equation 6.1 to estimate the range of a wheelchair. The results of the study by Cooper et al. are presented in Table 6.7. The actual range will likely vary during actual use, but the data are useful for comparison. Since the tests are performed on a firm tennis court, the results are

**TABLE 6.5.  Description of power wheelchairs tested (all wheelchairs used deep-cycle lead acid batteries; * indicates type of battery used during testing)**

| Make & Model | Battery Size | Battery Type | Amp•Hour Rating | System Voltage |
|---|---|---|---|---|
| E&J Premier with 21st Century power components | Group 24 | Wet Cell* Gel Cell | 85 amp•hour 70 amp•hour | 24 volts dc |
| E&J Tempest | Group U1 | Wet Cell* Gel Cell | 48 amp•hour 32 amp•hour | 24 volts dc |
| E&J Marathon | Group 24 | Wet Cell* Gel Cell | 85 amp•hour 70 amp•hour | 24 volts dc |
| Quickie P100 | Group 22NF | Wet Cell Gel Cell* | 55 amp•hour 70 amp•hour | 24 volts dc |
| Quickie P110 | Group 22NF | Wet Cell Gel Cell* | 55 amp•hour 48 amp•hour | 24 volts dc |
| Quickie P300 | Group 24 | Wet Cell* Gel Cell | 85 amp•hour 70 amp•hour | 24 volts dc |
| E&J Scooter Premier 3-Wheeler | Group U1 | Wet Cell Gel Cell* | 48 amp•hour 32 amp•hour | 24 volts dc |

**TABLE 6.6   Electrical properties recorded during ISO range testing**

| Chair Number | Tennis Court Results | | | |
| --- | --- | --- | --- | --- |
| | Amps | Watts | kJ | m/s |
| Chair 1 | 19.1 | 466 | 304 | 2.3 |
| Chair 2 | 6.6 | 155 | 139 | 1.7 |
| Chair 3 | 8.8 | 198 | 126 | 1.8 |
| Chair 4 | 8.4 | 205 | 184 | 1.7 |
| Chair 5 | 19.8 | 545 | 327 | 2.5 |
| Chair 6 | 12.2 | 301 | 200 | 2.3 |
| Chair 7 | 6.0 | 146 | 101 | 2.0 |

amps=current in amperes, watts= power in watts, kJ = energy in kilojoules, m/s = average speed in meters per second.

more applicable to driving outdoors. Indoor driving in confined spaces or on soft surfaces such as carpet may reduce the range of a wheelchair. It is useful to ask manufacturers if they are aware of the estimated range indoors. Some wheelchairs may be more efficient outdoors than indoors or vice versa.

The predicted range for the tennis court test at maximum speed varied from a low of 23.6 to a high of 57.7 kilometers. The range of the power wheelchair can, normally, be improved by the use of wet lead acid batteries in place of gel lead acid batteries. However, wet batteries often require greater maintenance and care during transport. No alternative batteries were tested. All of the manufacturers specified lead acid batteries for their wheelchairs. The range at one meter per second was typically greater than it was at maximum speed. This information may be useful to consumers, who when warned of a low battery could extend their range by reducing speed. Current draw on an incline will be greater than the values indi-

**TABLE 6.7   Estimated range with 100-kilogram load at maximum speed and at approximately one meter per second (units are in kilometers)**

| Chair Number | 1 Meter Per Second | Full Speed |
| --- | --- | --- |
| *Gel Cells* | | |
| Chair 1 | 43.0 | 30.3 |
| Chair 2 | 76.6 | 44.5 |
| Chair 3 | 27.3 | 23.6 |
| Chair 4 | 46.7 | 35.0 |
| Chair 5 | 68.8 | 31.8 |
| Chair 6 | 75.3 | 47.5 |
| Chair 7 | 40.4 | 38.4 |
| *Wet Cells* | | |
| Chair 1 | 52.2 | 36.8 |
| Chair 2 | 87.8 | 51.0 |
| Chair 3 | 41.0 | 35.4 |
| Chair 4 | 53.5 | 40.1 |
| Chair 5 | 83.5 | 38.6 |
| Chair 6 | 91.4 | 57.7 |
| Chair 7 | 60.6 | 57.6 |

cated in this paper. Some wheelchairs incorporate regenerative braking (i.e., using the motors to charge the batteries and brake the wheelchair on downhills), which allows some of the energy expended while going up an incline to be regained through charging the batteries while driving down an incline. Range will also vary with driving habits.

## 6.6 Safety Testing

### 6.6.1 Flammability

Some parts of a wheelchair may burn when exposed to a cigarette or open flame. The upholstered parts are most likely to burn or melt when exposed to high heat or an open flame. Some people have died by falling asleep while smoking in their wheelchair. In such cases, either the upholstered parts of the wheelchair have started burning and produced smoke that has damaged the individual's lungs, or furnishings in the room that the wheelchair is occupying have caught fire. Fires are not a common occurrence among wheelchair users, and since most wheelchairs are made primarily of metal, standard precautions are suitable. Tires and casters may melt or smolder when exposed to extreme heat or fire. The tires of some wheelchairs may come in contact with the user, so the user should be aware of possible injury should a tire melt or smolder.

Cushions and seating systems are often susceptible to burning or smoldering when exposed to a cigarette or open flame for long periods of time (i.e., typically more than a few minutes). Cushions and seating systems present three types of risk once they begin burning: risk due to smoke inhalation; risk due to melting foam or plastic; and risk due to burning. Most materials used for cushions or seating systems will not burn freely unless exposed to substantial heat for prolonged periods. However, they can smolder, producing toxic gases and melting material. This can cause harm to the user. Cushions are not included in the ISO or ANSI/RESNA wheelchair standards for flammability. Therefore, it is important to request information from the cushion or seating system manufacturer regarding the flammability testing and certification of their products.

A few wheelchairs are made of wood or use wooden components. Until the 1940s wooden wheelchairs were quite common; today a few modern wooden wheelchairs are available. Although the recently developed wooden wheelchairs do not resemble their predecessors in design, they are susceptible to burning when exposed to an open flame. Extra caution should be observed when using a wooden wheelchair or wheelchair with wooden components near an open flame.

Electric-powered wheelchairs present a higher risk for flammability than do manual wheelchairs. This is because electric-powered wheelchairs are powered by electricity, which can cause burns if exposed to the skin of the user. Failures within the electric-powered wheelchair's electrical system can result in fire. Batteries must be charged, which requires the use of a battery charger plugged into a wall outlet. A fault in the battery charger or the electric-powered wheelchair while charging can result in fire. While lead-acid batteries are charging, small amounts of hydrogen gas may be emitted. Hydrogen gas is extremely flammable. The small amount of hydrogen gas that may be released with a properly operating and maintained wheelchair and battery charger does not present a risk. However, if a battery becomes cracked or damaged then there is risk if a spark occurs within the battery charger or the electric wheelchair. There may be some risk due to smoking around a charging electric-powered wheelchair that is poorly maintained or damaged. Gel cell batteries are closed and are much safer than wet cell batteries for use with electric-powered wheelchairs. Their flammability risk is substantially lower than that of wet cell batteries. Electric-powered wheelchair users should carefully follow the maintenance instructions for their wheelchair and battery charger.

The flammability characteristics of wheelchairs are tested according to ISO 7176–16. This standard applies to both manual and electric-powered wheelchairs. The safety of electric-powered wheelchairs and their battery chargers is further tested in ISO 7176–14. These standards, along with common sense, make a wheelchair reasonably safe from injury due to smoking or short-term exposure to an open flame.

## 6.6.2 Stability

Wheelchairs are subject to tips and falls. The majority of injuries that occur during wheelchair use are due to either tipping the wheelchair or falling out of the wheelchair. Tipping accidents can occur when driving on a slope, driving across a slope, or impacting an obstacle. Accidents can result in forward tipping, rearward tipping, or lateral tipping. Wheelchair standards have divided stability into static stability and dynamic stability. Static stability is measured with the wheelchair stationary. With a test dummy placed in the wheelchair, the wheelchair is tilted on an incline plane until the uphill wheels begin to tip. The rearward stability is measured with the wheelchair facing up the slope. The forward stability is measured with the wheelchair facing down the slope. The lateral stability is measured with the wheelchair facing across the slope.

Static stability testing is done for both manual and electric-powered wheelchairs. Static stability gives the user and clinicians an estimate of the maximum slope that the wheelchair can rest on without tipping. Manual wheelchair users may be able to develop the skill to negotiate steeper slopes by doing a "wheelie" or by shifting their weight. Normally, electric-powered wheelchair users or users of manual wheelchairs who are not highly skilled or are more severely impaired would be unsafe to drive on slopes equal to the static stability angle. The stability of the wheelchair can be influenced by altering the position of the center of gravity with respect to the wheels. Moving the center of gravity toward the rear wheels makes the wheelchair more likely to tip backwards. Moving the center of gravity toward the front wheels makes the wheelchair more likely to tip forwards. Reducing the width between the contact points of the wheels makes the wheelchair more likely to tip sideways.

Anti-tip casters may be used on the front and rear of a wheelchair. Anti-tip casters can help to prevent some tipping accidents. Figure 6.10 illustrates the effect of rear and forward anti-tip casters on the static stability angle of a wheelchair. Without anti-tip casters when the rear tip angle becomes large enough the front wheels lift off the surface. The wheelchair will tip over rearwards if the angle gets any steeper. In reality, with a skilled user the tip angle can be increased. However, not all users are capable of controlling a wheelchair once it begins to tip over. When rear anti-tip casters are in use and properly adjusted, when the wheelchair begins to tip over it is caught by the rear anti-tip casters. The rear anti-tip casters can pre-

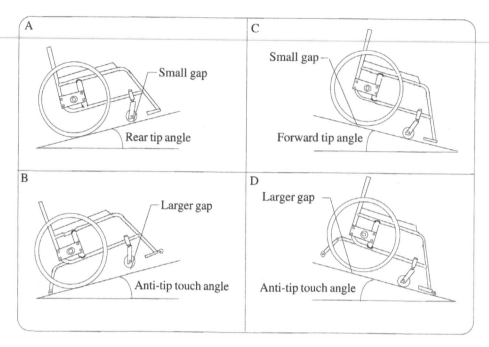

**FIGURE 6.10**   Static stability angles for wheelchairs. All static stability angles are measured using an ISO dummy in the wheelchair. Sub-figure (A) shows the rear tip angle. Sub-figure (B) shows the angle required to make the rear anti-tip casters touch. Sub-figure (C) shows the forward static stability angle. Sub-figure (D) shows the angle required to make the front anti-tip casters touch.

vent many rear tipping accidents. If the persons tips rearward too fast, then the wheelchair can continue to tip, pivoting around the rear anti-tip casters. Such cases are rare but when they do occur, the rider's only course of action is to lean forward and try to keep from hitting his or her head. Most wheelchairs are statically stable on upward slopes of ten degrees.

Forward tipping accidents can happen much like rear tipping accidents. When the wheelchair is driven down a slope that is too steep, the rear wheels begin to lift off the surface. If the wheelchair is rear-wheel driven, as most are, then the ability to control the wheelchair is lost. If the slope is steep enough, the wheelchair will continue to tip forward. Forward anti-tip rollers help to prevent forward tipping accidents by stopping the forward tipping once the wheelchair rotates forward enough for them to contact the surface. If the angle is too steep or the forward tipping too rapid, the wheelchair may continue to tip over the forward anti-tip rollers. It is uncommon for wheelchairs to tip over their forward anti-tip rollers. Most wheelchairs are statically stable on downward slopes up to 20 degrees.

Dynamic stability describes the behavior of a wheelchair as it is being driven over common obstacles (e.g., door thresholds, sidewalk cracks, curb cuts) and while being driven on slopes. The ANSI/RESNA and ISO wheelchair standards only address dynamic stability for electric-powered wheelchairs and scooters. The dynamic stability of manual wheelchairs is not evaluated because it is too dependent on the skill of the rider. For example, very skilled riders can safely climb and descend six-inch curbs. Some people can ride manual wheelchairs down stairs, and up 20-degree slopes. Therefore, it becomes impossible to measure the dynamic stability of manual wheelchairs. This can only be done with the actual user, and should be a part of each person's wheelchair assessment and training process.

The dynamic stability of electric-powered wheelchairs is also dependent on the skills of the rider. However, there is much less variability than with manual wheelchairs. Dynamic stability of electric-powered wheelchairs is tested by driving the wheelchair over a variety of obstacles and ramp angles. The ANSI/RESNA and ISO 7176 parts two require the wheelchair to be driven on a three-, six-, and ten-degree slope. At each slope the wheelchair is driven up and down at full speed. Any lifting of the wheels or difficulty in driving the wheelchair is noted. If a wheelchair is unstable at one of the lower ramp angles it is not tested at the higher ramp angles. The wheelchair is also driven up and down a transition from level to a ramp. Again, the three ramp angles (i.e., three, six, and ten degrees) are used. Ramp transitions, especially downward, can be very difficult for power wheelchair users to negotiate (see Figure 6.11). This section of the dynamic stability standard also examines whether the anti-tip casters (both front and rear) will hit while per-

**FIGURE 6.11** Electric-powered wheelchairs and scooters require extra caution when making ramp transitions.

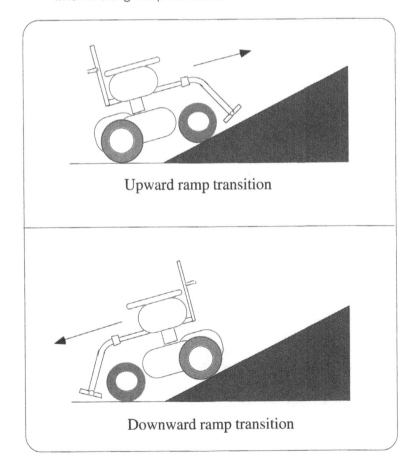

Upward ramp transition

Downward ramp transition

forming this maneuver. The wheelchair is also driven over a five-centimeter (2-inch) obstacle with only one side of the wheelchair impacting the obstacle. This test illustrates whether the wheelchair will remain stable when the user unexpectedly drives the wheelchair into an obstacle.

Some electric-powered wheelchairs are capable of doing a "wheelie"; this has been designed into them so that they may climb obstacles better or may be more mobile. Power wheelchairs that perform "wheelies" may do so by using six wheels: two front casters; two center drive wheels; and two rear wheels. When accelerating over obstacles the power wheelchair user rapidly accelerates the wheelchair. This causes the chair to move onto the center and rear wheel sets. When the driver lowers the acceleration or the wheelchair reaches full speed, it returns to driving on the front casters and center drive wheels. This type of electric-powered wheelchair allows some maneuvers to be performed like a manual wheelchair. This provides a wider range of obstacles that can be negotiated.

Some specialty wheelchair use clusters of wheels to negotiate obstacles (see Figure 6.12). Clusters are usually made of three wheels that are connected by a triangular linkage centered about an axle. The wheels normally rotate about their own axles, but when climbing an obstacle, the driver can command them to rotate about the center axle (i.e., cluster axle). This allows the wheelchair to climb a step. Cluster-type obstacle-climbing wheelchairs require a special control system that controls the cluster and maintains the balance of the wheelchair while climbing obstacles with the cluster. Such wheelchairs may only be stable when the power is active. This is a different type of dynamic stability that requires an active control system to maintain stability while negotiating an obstacle.

### 6.6.3 Standards for Wheelchairs and Transportation

Personal mobility for wheelchair users is often dependent on access to a private automobile or to public transportation. There are two standards that address the wheelchair aspect of transportation. The first is concerned with a standard for wheelchair tiedowns and occupant restraints. This standard is addressed by the Society of Automotive Engineers (SAE) and ISO. The second standard is concerned with test procedures and values to deem a wheelchair suitable for use as a seat in a motor vehicle. The standard to determine the suitability of a wheelchair for use as a seat in a motor vehicle is the responsibility of the ANSI/RESNA committee for Standards on Wheelchairs and Transportation (SOWHAT). To provide access to automobiles and public transportation, wheelchairs, tiedowns, and occupant restraints must be compatible. Standards help to ensure that design specifications include compatibility.

In the United States, the Wheelchair Tiedown and Occupant Restraint Standard (WTORS) is under the auspices of the Adaptive Devices Committee of the SAE. The SOWHAT is under the auspices of the ANSI/RESNA Technical Guidelines Committee. Internationally, both standards are under the auspices of Working Group Six of Technical Committee 173, Sub-Committee One. In ISO language this is written TC173/SC-1/WG-6, and this code is added to all documents related to wheelchairs and transportation.

Three fundamental issues are involved with people remaining in their wheelchairs or scooters while in motor vehicles, if people are to maintain safety and accessibility equivalent to non–wheelchair users. Wheelchairs must be designed and marketed that incorporate features which facilitate use as a seat in transportation

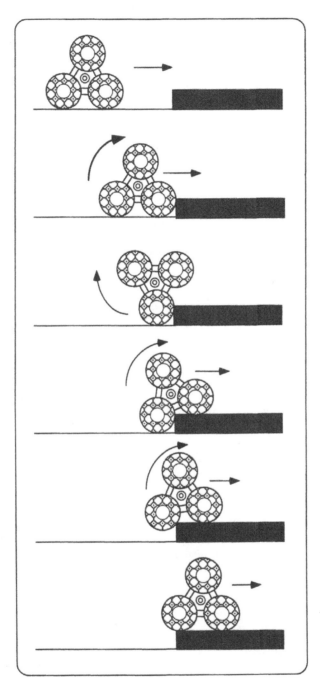

**FIGURE 6.12** Illustration of cluster obstacle-climbing ability. From the top to the bottom the cluster-type obstacle-climbing wheelchair rolls along on four or more wheels during normal driving. When the user switches the wheelchair to obstacle-climbing mode, the wheels cluster around their common axle, as well as rotate about their individual axles. This allows the wheelchair to climb over obstacles. However, the wheelchair requires a sophisticated control system to prevent it from tipping while climbing obstacles.

vehicles. There must be compatibility between the wheelchair or scooter, the occupant restraint, and the wheelchair tiedown technology. Standards must be available that wheelchair and vehicle accessory manufacturers can follow to ensure safety and compatibility requirements.

Wheelchair geometry and mass/inertial properties affect its response in a crash. For this reason, wheelchair transportation research has divided wheelchairs into categories based on frame characteristics in addition to division by whether the wheelchair is manually propelled or uses electric power. Features such as mass (weight), center of gravity, frame structure/design, and physical dimensions all affect the response of a wheelchair and occupant in a transportation vehicle crash.

## 6.7 Cost Analysis

Pressures experienced by clinicians and cost-conscious third-party payers have changed the face of the wheelchair marketplace. Manufacturers are producing and more consumers are receiving depot-type wheelchairs designed to meet cost constraints imposed by third-party payers. Some of these wheelchairs may be appropriate for some consumers, while others clearly are not. Rehabilitation wheelchairs typically last significantly longer than depot wheelchairs. Perhaps more important to third-party providers, clinicians, and consumers is that rehabilitation wheelchairs cost approximately four times that of depot wheelchairs yet may last more than ten times as long on average. It may be more cost effective for hospital systems to purchase rehabilitation wheelchairs and not depot wheelchairs, as is the current practice for in-hospital use and some community use. Rehabilitation wheelchairs are certainly more appropriate and cost effective for people who are moderately active.

When evaluating wheelchairs, the initial purchase price can be misleading. Therefore, the suggested retail price for each wheelchair can be divided by the total number of cycles until a class three failure occurred to yield the dollars per equivalent cycle. Table 6.8 presents the results of cost to first class three failure analysis from Cooper and colleagues. This gives a simple measure of how much it costs to operate a wheelchair until it needs to be replaced (i.e., the wheelchair has some retail value when new and no value once destroyed). The depot wheelchairs cost about 3.4 times as much to operate per cycle or per meter than the rehabilitation wheelchairs. The costs per cycle are significantly higher for the depot wheelchairs than for rehabilitation wheelchairs. The six rehabilitation wheelchairs that were equipped with solid 8-inch casters cost 3.2 times as much per cycle than the three identical rehabilitation wheelchairs equipped with pneumatic 8-inch casters. The effect of tires' cost is insignificant in this analysis as only one rehabilitation wheelchair experienced a leak in the tube of a front caster tire at a cost of less than $5.00 for repair. No other repairs were performed. Costs per cycle were significantly higher for the rehabilitation wheelchairs equipped with solid casters than for the rehabilitation wheelchairs equipped with pneumatic casters.

The simple change from a solid front caster to a pneumatic front caster has a dramatic effect on fatigue life. This simple change may extend the wheelchair life by over three times without a significant increase in cost (i.e., the increase in cost was a total of about $5 amortized over three wheelchairs in this example). This result is

**TABLE 6.8**   Dollars per equivalent (i.e., combined double-drum and curb-drop) cycle during fatigue tests

| | Wheelchair Type | | Rehabilitation Wheelchairs Caster Tire Type* | |
| --- | --- | --- | --- | --- |
| | Rehabilitation (n=6) | Depot (n=6) | Pneumatic (n=3) | Solid (n=6) |
| Dollars per cycle | 0.0038 ±0.0032 | 0.0128 ±0.0061 | 0.0008 ±0.0000 | 0.0038 ±0.0032 |

*NOTE: Only rehabilitation wheelchairs with solid casters were used in these calculations.

particularly timely in light of the current trend by rehabilitation professionals to order manual wheelchairs with solid casters to reduce maintenance expenses.

The quality of manual wheelchairs varies from manufacturer to manufacturer and within the models produced by each manufacturer. Initial purchase price is only one factor to consider when selecting a wheelchair. Quality must be defined from user, clinical, and engineering perspectives. Purchasers and prescribers of wheelchairs should consider the life-cycle cost and not just the purchase price for wheelchairs. Clinical factors related to the use of wheelchairs (e.g., adjustability, postural support, maneuverability) may further impact costs. The prevention of carpal tunnel syndrome or rotator cuff tendinitis or tears may negate the cost of the wheelchair.

The ISO–ANSI/RESNA standards do provide useful information and can be used to assure a minimum quality level. It should be a goal of all people intimately involved with wheelchairs to understand and apply wheelchair standards and to work toward a quality definition. One step in this process is to systematically investigate the effect of wheelchair components and design features on durability. Another step is to investigate user perceptions of rider comfort and how these perceptions are related to wheelchair design. A third step is to examine means of reducing the incidence of secondary disability due to wheelchair use. Eventually comprehensive selection guidelines could be developed which incorporate product evaluation information.

## 6.8 Reliability and Failure Modes

Electrical and mechanical components are used in wheelchairs and scooters. It is essential that wheelchairs operate reliably during all common activities. Failure of a key component could result in serious harm to the user or people in the vicinity. The reliability of a wheelchair is dependent on the reliability of its components. Some wheelchairs are becoming more complex, and are dependent on more parts. The reliability of the wheelchair can only be improved by improving the reliability of the parts or by reducing the number of parts. Reliability also influences cost. For example, if an electric-powered wheelchair breaks down, the user may incur costs for a rental wheelchair, cost of repair, and potentially lost income. These factors can have a significant impact on the cost of failure to the user. Often higher performance is associated with higher cost. Among wheelchairs, part of the higher cost for performance wheelchairs is associated with improving or at least maintaining high reliability.

Reliability is achieved by solid design, sound production practices, and well-planned testing. The available time of use for a wheelchair is dependent on reliability and maintainability. Reliability is the amount of time that a wheelchair is able to perform all of its functions during normal use, without the need for repair. Maintainability is defined by the amount of time required to detect, diagnose, and correct a failure or part in need of repair.

Reliability does not account for human error, which can be the cause of an accident or breakdown. Engineers attempt to anticipate and test for failures that may result from misuse, and to design safeguards into the system. Safeguards provide the user some additional degree of safety, but are no substitute for common sense. Owners and service manuals provide information about the safe operation and maintenance of wheelchairs. The manuals are developed from engineering design criteria, testing, consumer feedback, the records of wheelchair repairs, and accident reports. Consumers should work with clinicians and wheelchair suppliers to understand their wheelchair user's manual. They should also receive some training in the safe and effective operation and maintenance of the wheelchair.

### 6.8.1 Types of Failures

Failures are typically classified into two categories: misuse failure and inherent weakness failure. Misuse failures are due to stressing the wheelchair or one of its components beyond the capabilities for which it was designed. Inherent weakness failures are attributable to the wheelchair or a part exceeding its normal life expectancy. Failures are also classified by time. Sudden failures cannot be anticipated by prior examination, whereas gradual failures can be detected by prior examination. Failures are also defined as partial or complete. Partial failures are used to describe parts that are damaged, but retain some portion of their ability to function. A flat tire can be considered a partial failure of the wheel. The wheel retains its function, but does not perform well. A complete failure describes when a part or the entire wheelchair loses its ability to function. A broken axle would be described as a complete failure. Failures are also categorized by their impact on the function of the person and wheelchair. Catastrophic failures are both sudden and complete. When the bolt connecting the cross-braces fails, it usually results in a catastrophic failure. Degradation is used to describe failure that is both gradual and partial. Wheelchair bearings typically degrade. As wheelchair bearings are used, their resistance gradually increases making the wheelchair harder to push.

Engineers use two common measurements to characterize wheelchairs and other products. The *mean time between failures* (MTBF) is used to describe the average time expected between repairs. If a manual wheelchair user must tighten the spokes on the rear wheels after two months, then again after six months, and again at nine months within a one-year period, than the MTBF is three months. The *mean time to failure* (MTTF) is used to describe the average time between repairs. If a user of an electric-powered wheelchair must replace the rear tires after six months, then again after thirteen months, and again after 24 months, then the MTTF is 8.33 months.

Wheelchairs can be described as failing during one of three time periods. The *early failure period* is when the wheelchairs can be considered new, and something fails due to a faulty part or flaw in manufacturing. This period is sometimes called "infant death" among electronic product manufacturers. Wheelchair manufacturers work to keep the number of *early period failures* to a minimum as this is usually the period covered by the full manufacturer's warranty. Most wheelchairs function into a time described as a *constant failure period*. This period covers most of the product's life, and is characterized by the infrequent repairs that are necessary to maintain the wheelchair in proper working order. As a wheelchair lasts longer, the planned life of its components begins to pass. As this happens, the number of failures begins to increase. It is during this time that the wheelchair should be retired. This typically takes about three years for active manual wheelchair users, and about five years for active electric-powered wheelchair users. The period beyond the wheelchair's planned life is called the *wear-out failure period*. Wheelchair users should pay careful attention to their owner's manual for maintenance and warranty information. Using a wheelchair beyond its planned life can result in injury, and will result in poor performance.

## References and Further Reading

Axelson P., Minkel J., Chesney D. (1994) *A Guide to Wheelchair Selection.* Washington, DC: Paralyzed Veterans of America.

Axelson P., Phillips L. (1989) Wheelchair standards: Pushing for a new era. *Homecare Magazine*, October.

Axelson P., Wood Z. (1992) Wheelchair standards and you. *Paraplegia News*, 46(10):54–55.

Axelson P. Chairs (1994) Chairs, everywhere! *Sports 'n Spokes*, 19(6):15–63.

Axelson P. (1993) Wheelchair comparison. *Sports 'n Spokes*, 18(6):34–70.

Axelson P., Chesney D., Goodman S. (1994) Lightweight choice. *Mainstream*, 18:22–23.

Aylor J. H., Thieme A., Johnson B. W. (1992) A battery state-of-charge indicator. *IEEE Transaction on Industrial Electronics*, 39(5):398–409.

Baldwin J. D., Thacker J. G. (1993) Stress response of wheelchair frames to front caster impact. *Proceedings RESNA 16th Annual Conference*, Las Vegas, NV, 321–323.

Baldwin J. D., Dee L. S., Thacker J. G. (1992) Dynamic structural response of a cross-tube wheelchair frame. *Proceedings RESNA International '92*, Toronto, Canada, 622–623.

Baldwin J. D., Thacker J. G., Baber T. T., Aylor J. H. (1990) Simulation of a random fatigue process applied to wheelchair structures. Washington, DC: RESNA Press, June, 63–64.

Baldwin J. D., Thacker J. G. (1991) Structural reliability techniques applied to tubular wheelchair frames. *Proceedings RESNA 14th Annual Conference*, Washington, DC, 237–239.

Baldwin J. D., Thacker J. G., Baber T. T. (1991) Estimation of structural reliability under random fatigue conditions. *Reliability, Stress Analysis and Failure Prevention*, T.H. Service, American Society of Mechanical Engineers, 43–48.

Baldwin J. D., Thacker J. G. (1993) Characterization of the dynamic stress response of manual and powered wheelchair frames. *Journal of Rehabilitation Research and Development*, 30(2):224–232.

Barnicle K. (1993) *Evaluating powered wheelchairs*. Request evaluating assistive technology, The Rehabilitation Engineering Center at The National Rehabilitation Hospital, May.

Bode H. (1977) *Lead-Acid Batteries*. New York, NY: John Wiley & Sons.

Bryant L. (1991) Wheelchair standards ready to roll. *Team Rehab Report*, May/June, 44–45.

Cooper R. A., (1995) *Rehabilitation Engineering Applied to Mobility and Manipulation*. Bristol, UK: Institute of Physics Publishing.

Cooper R. A., Brienza D.M., Brubaker C. E. (1994) Wheelchairs and seating. *Current Opinion in Orthopedics*, 5(6):101–107.

Cooper R. A. (1991) High tech wheelchairs gain the competitive edge. *IEEE Engineering in Medicine and Biology Magazine*, 10(4)49–55.

Cooper R. A., Ster J. F., Myren C., Pettit D. J. (1992) An improved design of a 100 kilogram ISO/RESNA wheelchair test dummy. *Proceedings 15th Annual RESNA Conference*, Toronto, Canada, 210–212.

Cooper R. A., Myren C., Ster J. F., VanSickle D. P., Stewart K. J., Reifman G., Heil T. A. (1993) Design of an anthropomorphic ISO-RESNA/ANSI wheelchair test dummy. *Proceedings 16th Annual RESNA Conference*, Las Vegas, NV, 283–285.

Cooper R. A., Ster J. F., Heil T. A. (1991) Development of a new ISO wheelchair two-drum tester. *Proceedings 13th Annual IEEE/EMBS International Conference*, Orlando, FL, 13:1867–1868.

Cooper R. A., Stewart K. J., VanSickle D. P., Albright S., Heil T. A., Robertson R. N., Flannery M., Ensminger G. (1994) Manual wheelchair ISO-ANSI/RESNA fatigue testing experience. *Proceedings 17th Annual RESNA Conference*, Nashville, TN, 324–326

Dummer G. W. A., Winton R.C. (1990) An *Elementary Guide to Reliability*, 4th ed. Oxford, England: Pergamon Press.

*European Report on Wheelchairs Testing* (1992) I. Johnson and R. Andrich (editors). Milano, Italy: Edizioni Pro Juventute (publishers).

Fisher W. E., Garrett R. E., Seeger B. R. (1988) Testing of gel-electrolyte batteries for wheelchairs. *Journal of Rehabilitation Research and Development* 25(2):27–32.

Ford M. R., Kauzlarich J. J., Thacker J. G. (1992) Powered wheelchair gearbox lubrication. *Proceedings RESNA International '92*, Toronto, Canada, 316–318.

Ford M. R., Thacker J. G., Kauzlarich J. J. (1991) Improved wheelchair gearbox efficiency. *Proceedings RESNA 14th Annual Conference*, Kansas City, MO, 146–147.

Hekstra A. (1993) Simulation models for test evaluation and product development of wheelchair. *Proceedings Second European Conference on the Advancement of Rehabilitation*, 3.3.

Hekstra A. C. (1991) Human factors in wheelchair testing. *Proceedings of Workshop Ergonomics of Manual Wheelchair Propulsion: State of the Art*, Amsterdam, Vrije University, 25–35.

Hekstra A., Hull D., Harris J., Herbert H. (1993) Energy Consumption ISO 7176/4—Break Out Group Minutes, WG1-620, Santa Cruz, California.

Horn J. (1991) U.S. committee adopts wheelchair standards. *P.T. Bulletin*, 6(6):4, 34.

International Standards Organization (ISO), Committee Draft ISO/CD 7176-8(E) Wheelchairs—Part 8: Requirements and test methods for static, impact, and fatigue strength, Technical Committee 173, Sub-Committee 1, N 200, Zurich, Switzerland, December, 1994.

ISO Standard 7176/7: *Wheelchairs—Determination of Seating Dimensions-Definitions and Measuring Methods*, RESNA Press, Washington, DC, 1991.

Johnson I., Andrich R. (1991) European Report on Wheelchair Testing, Commission of the European Communities (COMAC BME) Mobility Restoration for Paralyzed Persons, Edizioni Pro Juventute, Milano.

Junkman B. C., Aylor J. H., Kauzlarich J. J. (1988) Estimation of battery state-of-charge during charging using the charge recovery process. *Proceedings RESNA 11th Annual Conference*, 280–281.

Kauzlarich J. J. (1990) Wheelchair batteries II: Capacity, sizing, and life. *Journal of Rehabilitation Research and Development* 27(2):163–170.

Kauzlarich J. J., Thacker J. G., Ford M. R. (1993) Electric wheelchair drive train efficiency. *Proceedings RESNA 16th Annual Conference*, Las Vegas, NV, 310–312.

Kauzlarich J. J., Dwyer M. A. (1982) Test of nickel-zinc battery for wheelchairs. *Proceedings RESNA 5th Annual Conference*, 110.

Kauzlarich J. J., Ulrich V., Bresler M., Bruning T. (1983) Wheelchair batteries: Driving cycles and testing. *Journal of Rehabilitation Research and Development*, 20(1):31–43.

Kauzlarich J. J., Thacker J. G. (1985) Wheelchair tire rolling resistance and fatigue. *Journal of Rehabilitation Research and Development*, 22(3):25–41.

Klinger C. (1991) Pruefplaene fuer die Programmierbare Rollende Strasse. Technical Report, Technische Universität Berlin, September.

Lavanchy C. (1990) Comparative evaluation of major brands of lead-acid batteries. *Proceedings 15th Annual RESNA Conference*, 541–543.

Lawrence B. M., Cooper R. A., Gonzalez J., VanSickle D. P., Robertson R. N., Boninger M. L. (1996) The effect of shape factors on wheelchair cross-brace strength. *Proceedings 19th Annual RESNA Conference*, Salt Lake City, Utah, 501–503.

Lawrence B. M., Cooper R. A., Robertson R. N., Boninger M. L., Gonzalez J., VanSickle D. P. (1996) Manual wheelchair ride comfort. *Proceedings 19th Annual RESNA Conference*, Salt Lake City, Utah, 223–225.

Marathon Owner's Manual, Everest & Jennings, 3601 Rider Trail South, Earth City, MO, 63045, 1990.

Marlowe D. E. Assessing Wheelchair Performance: The Role of Regulations and Standards, Wheelchair IV. Report of a Conference on the State-of-the-Art of Powered Wheelchair Mobility, RESNA Press, December, 61–63, 1988.

Mauger-Cote D., Audet J., Nolet J. (1993) Wheelchair emergency repair services. *Proceedings Second European Conference on the Advancement of Rehabilitation*, 5.3

McFarland S. R. (1990) Seeking information about wheelchair evaluation: A call for action, choosing a wheelchair system. *Journal of Rehabilitation Research and Development—Clinical Supplement No. 2*, 86–87.

McLaurin C. A. (1986) Wheelchair development, standards, progress, and issues: A discussion with Colin McLaurin. *Journal of Rehabilitation Research and Development*, 23(2):48–51.

McLaurin C. A., Axelson P. (1990) Wheelchair standards: An overview, choosing a wheelchair system. *Journal of Rehabilitation Research and Development—Clinical Supplement No. 2*, 100–103.

Molino L., McAnany J. (1993) Technique for positioning an ISO test dummy in a wheelchair, Rehabilitation Technology Assessment Service, U.S. Department of Veterans Affairs, Baltimore, MD, April.

Molino L. (1993) Determination of pendulum swing angle for ISO 7176–08 footrest and caster impact tests, Rehabilitation Technology Assessment Service, U.S. Department of Veterans Affairs, Baltimore, MD, July.

Pettit D., Cooper R. A., Bennet P. (1992) Design and evaluation of a simple, inexpensive, ultralight wheelchair. *Proceedings 14th Annual IEEE/EMBS International Conference*, Paris, France, 14(4):1515–1516.

Premier Scooter Owner's Manual, Everest & Jennings, 3601 Rider Trail South, Earth City, MO, 63045, 1990.

Pronsati M. P. (1991) Standardization will bring better products to wheelchair consumers. *Advance for Physical Therapists*, 2(36):22–23.

Quickie P100 Owner's Manual, Quickie Designs, 2842 Business Park Ave., Fresno, CA, 93727, 1993.

Quickie P110 Owner's Manual, Quickie Designs, 2842 Business Park Ave., Fresno, CA, 93727, 1993.

Quickie P300 Owner's Manual, Quickie Designs, 2842 Business Park Ave., Fresno, CA, 93727, 1993.

Roebroeck M. E., van der Woude L. H. V., Rozendal R. H. (1987) Methodology of Consumer Evaluation of Hand Propelled Wheelchairs, Commission of the European Communities (COMAC BME) Evaluation of Assistive Devices for Paralysed Persons, Edizioni Pro Juventute, Milano.

Schnoll L. (1991) The ISO 9000 Series: Worldwide Standards for Quality, Medical Design and Materials, February, 36–40.

Stout G. (1979) Some aspects of high performance indoor/outdoor wheelchairs. *Bulletin of Prosthetics Research*, 10(32):330–332.

Tam E. W. C., Chiu E. Y. M., Evans J. H. (1992) Using ISO standards for manual wheelchair testing: the Hong Kong experience. *Proceedings RESNA International '92*, Toronto, Canada, 625–626.

Tempest Owner's Manual, Everest & Jennings, 3601 Rider Trail South, Earth City, MO, 63045, 1993.

Thacker J. G., Todd B. A., Disher T. D. (1985) Stress analysis of wheelchair frames. *Proceedings RESNA 8th Annual Conference*, Memphis, TN, 84–86.

Thacker J. G., Gorman S. F, Todd B. A. Evaluation of rider comfort with front caster suspension. *Proceedings RESNA 8th Annual Conference*, Memphis, TN, 87–89.

Ulerich P. L., Demcyzk B. G., Buzzelli E. S. Battery-in-vehicle analysis of the iron-air battery system. Technical Report#: 81-9J22-EVMOT-P1, Westinghouse R&D Center, Pittsburgh, PA.

Ulrich V., Bresier M., Kauzlarich J. J. (1990) Wheelchair battery testing. *Proceedings RESNA 3rd Annual Conference*, 132–133.

Vanderby R., Patwardhan A. G. (1983) A CAD approach for optimal design of a wheelchair frame—A preliminary report. *Proceedings 6th Annual Conference on Rehabilitation Engineering*, San Diego, CA, 115–117.

VanSickle D. P., Cooper R. A., Robertson R. N. (1993) A 2-dimensional wheelchair dynamic load history using accelerometers. *Proceedings 16th Annual RESNA Conference*, Las Vegas, NV, 324–326.

VanSickle D. P., Cooper R. A., and Robertson R. N. (1993) A 2-dimensional wheelchair dynamic load history using accelerometers. *Proceedings 16th Annual RESNA Conference*, Las Vegas, NV, 324–326.

VanSickle D. P., Cooper R. A. (1993) Demonstration of a methodology for wheelchair acceleration analysis. *Proceedings 15th Annual IEEE/EMBS International Conference*, San Diego, CA, Vol. 15, in print.

Wheelchair Standards, *RESNA Press*, Washington, DC, 1994.

# Manual Wheelchairs

*Chapter Goals*

☑ To know features of manual wheelchairs
☑ To know state-of-the-art research and product development
☑ To understand person-to-device interface and access
☑ To know how to select manual wheelchairs for consumer use

## 7.1 Introduction

Manual wheelchairs have developed rapidly in recent years. Only a few years ago there was one style of wheelchair and it came in one color: chrome (see Figure 7.1). Now there are numerous types of wheelchairs to choose from and they come in a wide range of colors. Wheelchairs have moved from being chairs with wheels designed to provide some minimal mobility to advanced orthotics designed to meet the mobility demands of the user. The proper selection and design of a wheelchair depends on the abilities of the user and on the intended use. Thus, specialized wheelchairs have been and continue to be developed to yield better performance for the user.

### 7.1.1 Depot and Attendant-Propelled Wheelchairs

The depot or institutional wheelchair is essentially the same wheelchair that was produced in the 1940s. Some depot wheelchairs may be a bit lighter than the 1940s models, but the basic frame design is unchanged. Depot wheelchairs are intended for institutional use where several people may use the same wheelchair. These wheelchairs are typically used in airports, hospitals, and nursing care facilities. Generally, they are inappropriate for active people who use wheelchairs for personal mobility (see Figure 7.1). Depot wheelchairs are designed to be inexpensive, to accommodate large variations in body size, to be low maintenance, and to be attendant-propelled. Hence, they are generally heavier and their performance is limited.

Many depot wheelchairs are manufactured in developing countries. Low labor costs make the manufacture of inexpensive depot wheelchairs possible. A typical depot wheelchair will have swing-away footrests, removable armrests, a

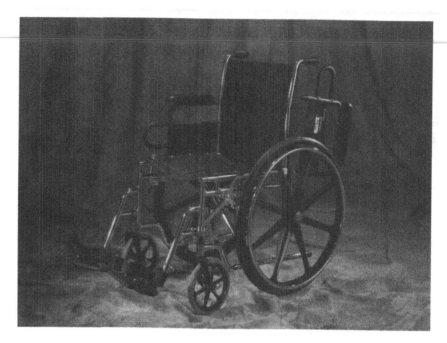

**A**

**FIGURE 7.1**   Classic chrome cross-brace manual wheelchairs (Photographs courtesy of (a) Everest & Jennings; (b) Lumex)

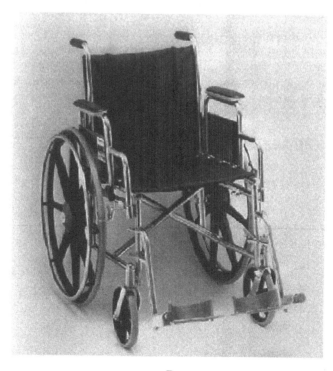

**B**

single cross-brace frame, and solid tires. Swing-away footrests add weight to the wheelchair. However, they make transferring in and out of the wheelchair easier. Armrests provide some comfort and stability to the depot wheelchair user, and they can aid in keeping clothing off the wheels. Depot chairs typically fold to reduce required storage area, so that the chair will fit into the automobile of the borrower. Solid tires are commonly used to reduce maintenance. Solid tires dramatically reduce ride comfort and add weight; pneumatic tires are recommended for outdoor usage. Very little if anything can be adjusted to fit the user on a depot chair. Typically, only the legrest length is adjustable. Depot chairs are available in various seat widths, seat depths, and backrest heights. These dimensions must be specified to the manufacturer or distributor.

Not all wheelchairs are propelled by the person sitting in the wheelchair. In many hospitals and long-term care facilities wheelchairs are propelled by attendants (see Figure 7.2). The design of these wheelchairs requires special consideration. If the wheelchair is to be propelled solely by attendants with no assistance from the rider, there may be no need for the larger drive wheels.

**FIGURE 7.2**  Photograph of an attendant-propelled wheelchair designed for elderly persons (Photograph courtesy of Homecrest Industries, Inc.)

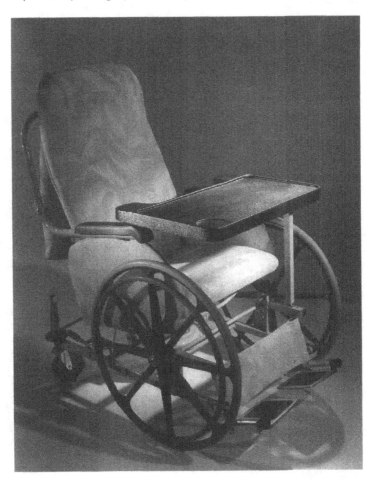

Attendant-propelled wheelchair designs must consider the rider and the attendant as users. The rider must be transported safely and comfortably. The attendant must be able to operate easily and maneuver safely with minimum physical strain. The design of the wheelchair must be such that the attendant can assist the rider with transfers and maneuver around the chair in restricted spaces. The push handles should be such that the attendant experiences no undue stress to the hands, arms, and back. Consideration must be given for how the chair will be maneuvered over obstacles. The primary consideration is that the wheelchair has two users: the rider and the attendant. Attendant-propelled chairs are most commonly used by people who are elderly. Sometimes these chairs are called "Gerry" chairs in reference to geriatric users. This type of attendant-propelled wheelchair is typically designed to minimize the independent mobility of the rider. The rider is seated in a large recliner-type wheelchair. The soft padding, reclined position, small wheels, and large size make it impossible for the rider to move the wheelchair and difficult for most riders to exit the wheelchair. This helps long-term care facilities to exercise control over their clients. There has been considerable discussion about the appropriate use of attendant-propelled chairs that significantly impair the rider's mobility.

Children's wheelchairs may also be attendant-propelled (see Figure 7.3). With children's chairs the philosophy is that the parents of an assistant can propel the chair until the child is capable of doing so on his/her own or until

**FIGURE 7.3**  Photograph of attendant-propelled children's wheelchairs (Photograph courtesy of Otto Bock Orthopaedic Industry, Inc.)

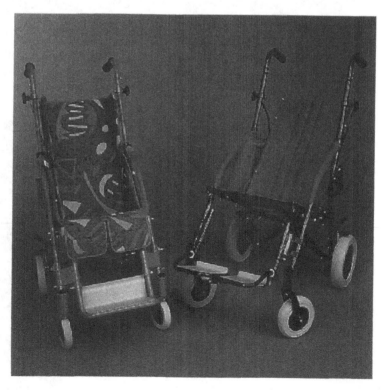

the child is ready for a powered wheelchair. Children's wheelchairs may also allow them to be either attendant-propelled or rider-propelled (see Figure 7.4). Children's chairs are semi–custom fit for children without severe orthopaedic impairments. If necessary, specialized seating can be adapted to most children's wheelchairs.

### 7.1.2 Rehabilitation Wheelchairs

The rehabilitation wheelchair is designed to be used by an individual as a mobility device. The selection and configuration of a rehabilitation wheelchair involves understanding the needs of the individual intending to use the wheelchair. Some rehabilitation wheelchairs can be assigned to a category by their intended use or intended user.

People with lower limb amputations typically have a different center of gravity location than do people who have their lower limbs. When seated in a wheelchair the center of gravity of the person with lower limb amputations may be close enough to the rear axles of the wheelchair to require some modification to the wheelchair axle position. The amputee wheelchair came about because wheelchairs were originally designed for people who were anatomically intact. Thus the center of gravity of the wheelchair and amputee was too close to the

**FIGURE 7.4**  Photograph of children's wheelchairs that can be propelled by an attendant or the rider (Photograph courtesy of Otto Bock Orthopaedic Industry, Inc.)

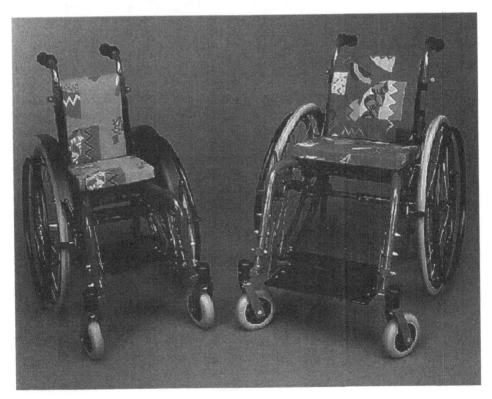

rear axles. This caused the wheelchair to have too great a tendency to do a "wheelie." Hence, amputee wheelchairs had the rear axle positions extended rearwards on the frame. The frame of an amputee wheelchair has to be designed to accommodate the offset between the back of the seat and the rear axle housings. Not all people with lower limb amputations require the more stable axle mountings, and the abilities of the user must be evaluated before the wheelchair is specified or designed.

People who have a single arm amputation with a mobility impairment or brain-related motor impairments often require specialized wheelchairs that permit operation with a single arm. Typically a one-arm-drive wheelchair consists of a linkage connecting the rear wheels. This allows the user to push on the pushrim of one wheel and to propel both wheels. To effectively turn the wheelchair the user must have the ability to disengage the drive mechanism and to propel a rear wheel independently. One-arm-drive wheelchairs are modified versions of standard wheelchairs. Most models of rehabilitation wheelchairs can be modified to accommodate one-arm-drive mechanisms. The proper fit of the wheelchair to the user is most critical with one-arm-drive wheelchairs because of the user's reduced physical strength. The wheelchair must fit such that the user can get maximal leverage for pushing and controlling the wheelchair.

### 7.1.3 Foot-Drive Wheelchairs

Some people have weakness of the upper and lower extremities and can gain maximal benefit from wheelchair propulsion by combining the use of their arms and legs or by using their legs. The design and selection of a foot-drive wheelchair depends greatly on how the user can take greatest advantage of his motor abilities. The strength and coordination of the user's legs must be determined to decide whether it is best to pull or to push with the legs. When pushing, the user moves with the back toward the direction of motion. The design of the chair is affected by whether the user pushes or pulls.

Typically, if the user pulls the chair along with the leg(s), then a wheelchair with footrests removed is effective. If the person pushes the wheelchair, modifications are required from the design of standard wheelchairs. Placing the casters at the back of the seat helps to make the wheelchair easier to control (see Figure 7.5). For wheelchairs propelled solely with the feet, the wheels at the front edge of the seat do not swivel. The casters should lead the rear wheels for the most common direction of travel. This will help to reduce the possibility of the user flipping over when hitting an obstacle and will make the chair more directionally stable. The wheelchair should be set up so that the user/wheelchair center of gravity is well within the footprint of the wheelchair. This will require some consideration when positioning the large wheels.

### 7.2 Frame Styles

Presently all common wheelchair frames center around tubular construction. Manual wheelchairs are generally made out of some lightweight tubing (e.g., aluminum, aircraft steel). The tubing can either be welded together or bolted together using lugs. There are two basic frame types—folding and rigid—and

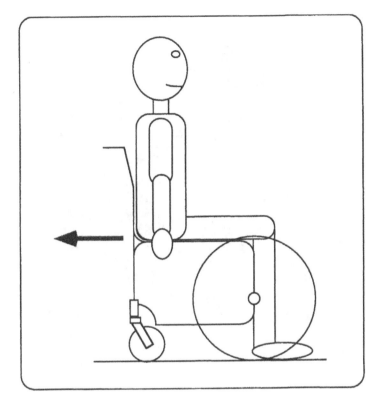

**FIGURE 7.5**   Schematic of a foot-drive wheelchair. The casters are placed under the backrest to make it simpler to control the chair while driving backwards. This is the most efficient direction for propulsion for many people.

three common frame styles: the box frame (Figure 7.6), the cantilever frame (Figure 7.7), and the T or I frame (Figure 7.8).

The box frame is named such because of its rectangular shape and the frame tubes that outline the edges of the frame to form a "box." Box frames can be very strong and very durable. A cantilever frame is so named because the front and rear wheels, when viewing the chair from the side, appear to be connected by only one tube; this is similar to having the front wheels attached to a cantilever beam fixed at the rear wheels. Both of these frame types require cross-bracing (i.e., tubes that connect the two halves) to provide adequate strength and stiffness. The T or I frame uses a minimal number of tubes. The T frame uses a single tube called an axle tube to mount the rear wheels. Another tube is welded or mounted to the axle tube that extends forward to the front caster(s). The frame appears like a T if the wheelchair has only one front caster. The caster of a T-frame is mounted at the end of the tube that extends forward from the axle tube. The frame appears like an I if another tube is mounted at a right angle to the front of the center tube. The front cross tube holds a caster at either end (see Figure 7.9).

Box frames, cantilever frames, and T-I frames stem from slightly different design philosophies. The box frame provides great strength and rigidity; thus, the wheels are mounted to a fairly rigid framework. If designed and constructed properly, the frame

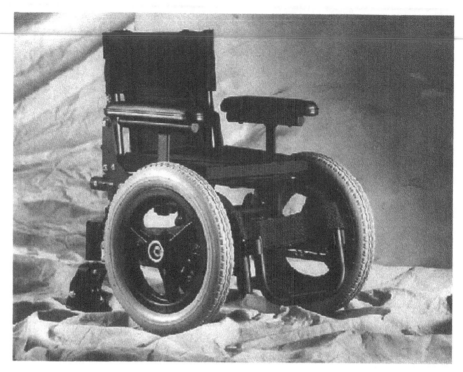

**A**

**FIGURE 7.6** Photographs of box frame wheelchairs: (a) shows a wheelchair designed for active children; (b) shows a wheelchair designed for adults. (Photographs courtesy of Quickie Designs, a division of Sunrise Medical)

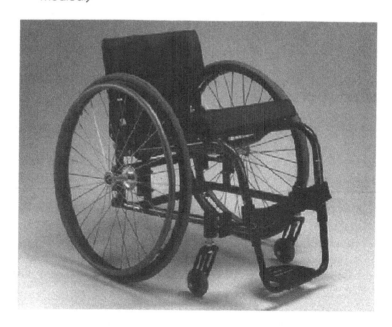

**B**

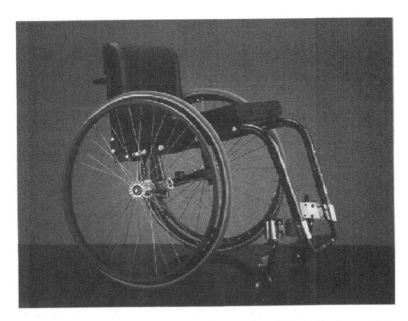

**FIGURE 7.7** Photograph of a cantilever frame wheelchair (Photograph courtesy of Kuschall of America)

**FIGURE 7.8** Photograph of an I frame manual wheelchair (Photograph courtesy of Top End by Action, a division of Invacare)

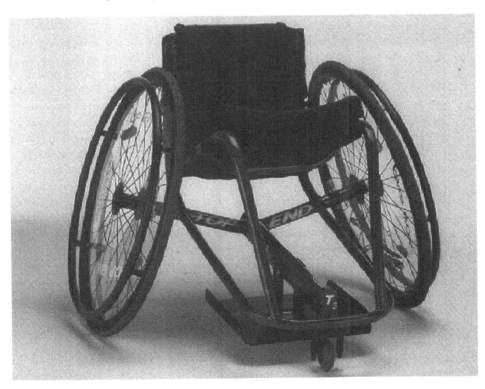

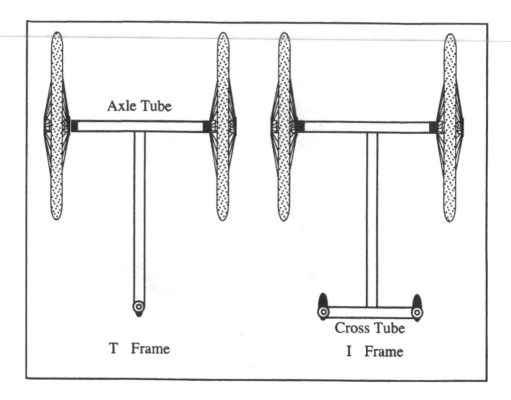

**FIGURE 7.9** T and I frame styles as viewed from above. Seats and footrests are not shown.

deflects minimally during normal loading, and most of the suspension is provided by the seat cushion and the wheels. Many manufacturers do not triangulate, or have tubes crisscrossing the frame, in their box frame designs. This allows some flexibility in the frame. A few manufacturers have taken this concept one step further by adding suspension elements to the frame. Hinges are placed at the front of the seat while elastic elements are placed at the back of the seat (see Figure 7.10). The elastic elements act to provide some suspension. The flexible element for the suspension can use either metal springs or polymer dampeners (elastomers). The cantilever frame is based on a few basic principles: (1) the frame can act as suspension (i.e., there is some flexibility purposely built into the frame); (2) there are fewer tubes and they are closer to the body, which makes the chair less conspicuous; and (3) there are fewer parts and fewer welds, which makes the frame easier to construct. The T-I frames are designed to make the frame as light and small as possible. In some cases durability is sacrificed in order to provide a very lightweight and unobtrusive design. The T-I frame is popular among active wheelchair users who enjoy a wheelchair suitable for both daily use and sports. All of these basic frame types are very functional and have their merits.

### 7.2.1 Folding Mechanisms

There are three commonly used folding mechanisms for wheelchair frames: (1) cross-brace, (2) parallel-brace, and (3) forward-folding. Most common folding wheelchairs use variations on the cross-brace design. Each of these folding mech-

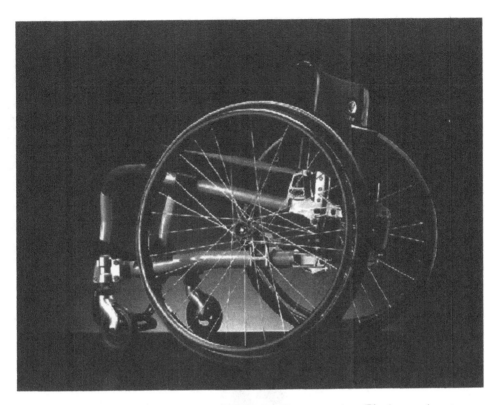

**FIGURE 7.10**  Box frame manual wheelchair with suspension (Photograph courtesy of Vision, a division of Everest & Jennings)

anism designs have their relative advantages and their selection depends on the
user's preferences.

Cross-brace folding wheelchairs are available with either single or double
cross-brace mechanisms. Double cross-brace designs add some stiffness to the
frame. A cross-brace folding mechanism consists of two frame members connected
in the middle, attached to the bottom of a side frame member on one side of the
chair and to the seat upholstery above the top side frame member on the opposite
side (Figure 7.11). The cross members are hinged at the bottom and pinned
together in the middle. When viewed from the back of the frame the cross members form an X. The chair is folded by pulling upwards on the seat upholstery.
When the seat is lifted the cross members move upward, pulling the frame
together. The user's weight keeps the frame from folding when the wheelchair
frame is extended. Cross-member folding mechanisms are simple and easy to use.
However, the wheelchair may collapse when tilted sideways, and the frame
becomes taller when folded. Some chairs incorporate snaps or over-center locking
mechanisms to reduce the problem of frame folding while on a side slope. Folding
cross-brace type wheelchairs are available from every major manual wheelchair
manufacturer. There are several variations of this basic design (see Figure 7.12).

The parallel-brace folding mechanism lets the frame fold sideways by having
the frame cross member hinge forward. Each cross member is hinged in the center
and at each end (Figure 7.13). When in the extended position the center hinge is
locked. The user releases the lock and pulls forward. The chair folds as the user

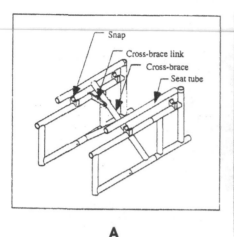

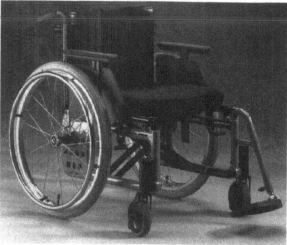

**A**

**B**

FIGURE 7.11   Folding cross-brace design wheelchair frame. Schematic of frame design is shown in (a). Photograph (b) shows a cross-brace folding wheelchair ready for use. Photograph (c) shows the same wheelchair in its folded position (Photograph courtesy of Otto Bock Orthopaedic Industry, Inc.)

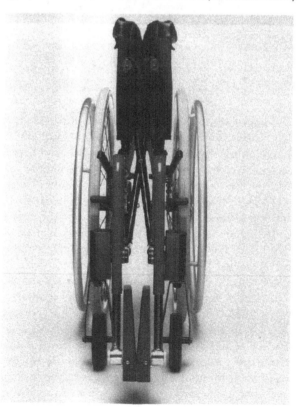

**C**

pulls forward. The cross members can be locked with a pin or a cam mechanism. The advantages of this design are that the frame behaves like a rigid frame in the extended position, and that the chair can be folded some with the user in it. This could permit negotiation of some narrow entrances. Parallel-brace mechanisms are more difficult to operate and maintain.

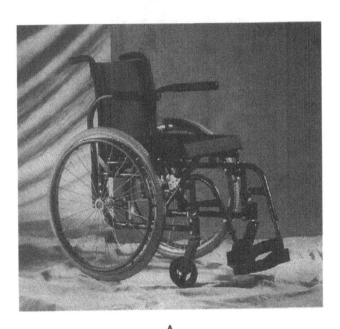

A

**FIGURE 7.12** Cross-brace folding wheelchairs (Photographs courtesy of (a) Quickie Designs, a division of Sunrise Medical; (b) Kuschall of America; and (c) Otto Bock Orthopaedic Industry, Inc.)

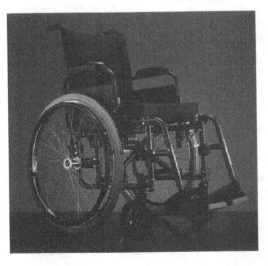

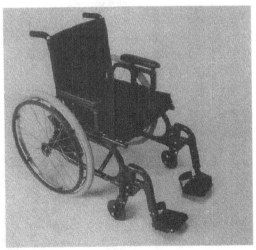

B                                                                   C

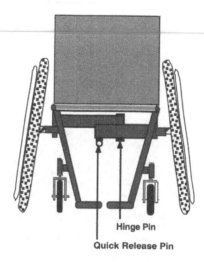

Hinge Pin

Quick Release Pin

**FIGURE 7.13** Illustration of wheelchair with parallel-brace design (front view)

Forward-folding wheelchairs have some nice features. Many ultralight wheelchairs incorporate forward-folding backrests. The forward-folding wheelchair extends this concept. The design of a forward-folding wheelchair involves hinging the front end of the wheelchair and the backrest (Figure 7.14). The backrest folds onto the seat and the front end folds under the seat. Forward-folding wheelchairs can be made very compact if the rear wheels are quick release. However, front-folding wheelchairs require more operations and latches to fold them.

**FIGURE 7.14** Photograph of a forward-folding wheelchair (Photograph courtesy of Rory Cooper)

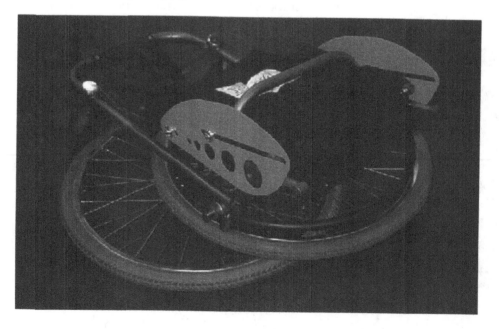

## 7.3 Wheels and Casters

### 7.3.1 Wheels

The wheels have a profound effect on the performance of the wheelchair. Wheels are available in a wide range of styles and sizes. Rear wheels come in three common sizes: 22, 24, and 26 inches. They come in two styles: spoked and MAG (see Figure 7.15). MAG wheels are typically made of fiber-reinforced ABS or PVC plastics and are die cast. MAG wheels require minimal maintenance and wear well. However, spoked wheels are substantially lighter, more active, and are generally preferred by active wheelchair users. Rear tires can be two types: pneumatic or puncture-proof (see Figure 7.15). Pneumatic tires can use either a separate tube and tire or a combined tube and tire (i.e., sew-up). Commonly, a belted rubber tire with a Butyl tube (65 psi) is used. However, people who desire higher performance prefer sew-up tires or Kevlar-belted tires with high-pressure tubes (180 psi). Puncture-proof tires are heavier, provide less suspension (i.e., shock absorption), and are less lively (i.e., tend not to grip as well) than pneumatic tires. Pneumatic tires are preferred by most manual wheelchair users.

**FIGURE 7.15**  Rear wheels and tires come in many types. Spoked wheels can be strong and lightweight. MAG wheels are low maintenance. Tires can be made of expanded rubber (A), tubular with pneumatic pressure (B), semi-pneumatic foam and rubber with valveless insert (C), and solid rubber tires (D). (Adapted from *Wheelchairs: A Prescription Guide*, A. Bennett Wilson, Jr., Demos, New York, NY, 1992)

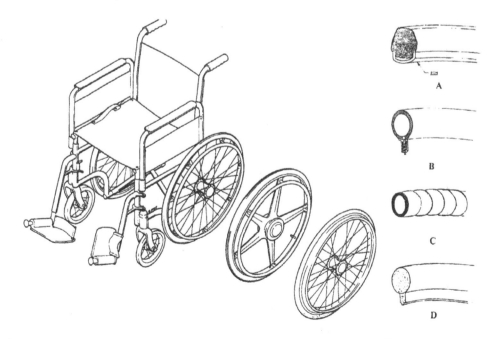

### 7.3.2 Casters

Casters can range from 50 to 200 millimeters in diameter for manual wheelchairs designed for daily use. Smaller casters provide greater foot clearance, which helps to prevent the casters from striking the rider's heels when turning. Casters are either pneumatic or polyurethane. Pneumatic casters offer a smoother ride at the cost of durability, whereas polyurethane casters are very durable. Most active users prefer 125-millimeter polyurethane casters for daily use. However, 200-millimeter polyurethane casters offer better ride comfort at the expense of foot clearance. Caster foot clearance is maximized with 50-millimeter "Roller Blade" casters often used for court sports (e.g., basketball, tennis, and racquetball). Smaller casters are more apt to get stuck in bumps or cause forward falls. Riders who prefer small casters for daily use typically have little weight on the front casters and will float the casters over most bumps. The styling of the casters often reflects a personal statement by the user (see Figure 7.16).

### 7.3.3 Pushrims

Pushrims are metal or plastic rings attached to the drive wheels (i.e., rear wheels) used to propel a manual wheelchair. Plastic pushrims are mostly used on inexpensive wheelchairs as a means of cost savings. Pushrims are commonly polished aluminum or steel tubing bent into circles a few centimeters smaller in diameter than the wheels. Pushrims can also be coated or have protrusions attached (i.e.,

**FIGURE 7.16**   Wheelchair casters come in a variety of styles and sizes. They can be pneumatic, solid, and without tread. The width of casters also varies. (Adapted from *Wheelchairs: A Prescription Guide*, A. Bennett Wilson, Jr., Demos, New York, NY, 1992)

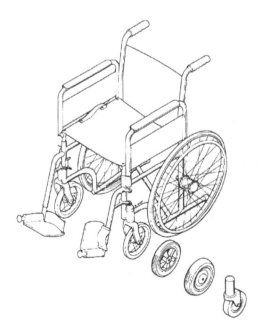

protruding pushrims) by people with limited grasp (see Figure 7.17). The most common coatings are vinyl and foam. Foam is not very durable as a pushrim coating and is rarely used except for people with very poor hand function or people with severe upper extremity pain. Vinyl-coated pushrims are quite useful for increasing the friction between the hand and the pushrim. This helps to reduce the forces necessary for propelling the wheelchair. The major drawbacks are that the increased friction causes increased heat while going down a hill or ramp, and the vinyl coating is poor at dissipating heat. Some wheelchair riders will bring gloves with them for use when going downhill. Others will use metal pushrims and push using the pushrim and tire when more friction is needed. This is effective, but it causes the hands to become soiled. Gloves can be helpful to prevent chafing and in keeping the hands clean. Protrusions are useful for people with very poor hand function. The protrusions eliminate the need to rely on friction for propelling the wheelchair. However, protrusions are more awkward to use because force can only be applied to the pushrim at locations where a protrusion is placed. At higher speeds the task of hitting the protrusions becomes very complicated. Moreover, protrusions reduce the maneuverability of the wheelchair.

The diameter of the pushrim tubing can also vary. Most manual wheelchair pushrims use tubing about 1 cm (1/2 inch) in diameter. This size was chosen for the cost and convenience of wheelchair manufacturers. It has become a *de facto* standard. Larger diameters are available on a custom order basis. Larger diameter

**FIGURE 7.17**  Pushrims are used to protect the hands and propel the drive wheels. Normally aluminum or steel tubing is used to construct pushrims. Pushrims can be used with the natural metal finish or coatings can be added. Protruding pushrims can be used by people with limited hand function. (Adapted from *Wheelchairs: A Prescription Guide*, A. Bennett Wilson, Jr., Demos, New York, NY, 1992)

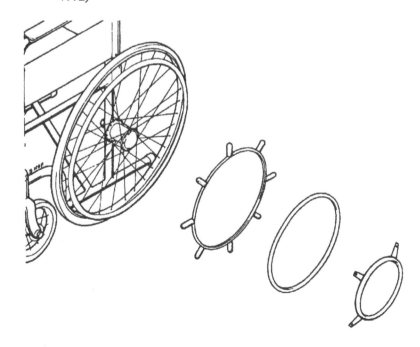

tubing (e.g., up to 1 inch) may be easier to grasp and turn. For some individuals, larger diameter tubing should be considered when other alternatives appear impractical.

### 7.3.4 Performance of Wheels

Five critical performance factors need be considered: (1) caster flutter, (2) caster float, (3) tracking, (4) alignment, and (5) trail. Caster flutter is the shimmy (i.e., rapid vibration of the front wheels) that may occur on some surfaces above certain speeds. Caster flutter results when there is not enough trail (see Figure 7.18). Trail determines the tendency of the front wheels to follow the path of the caster housing. It is desirable to have enough trail as to prevent caster flutter for the maximal speed expected for the chair, yet not have the front wheels interfere with the placement of the rider's feet. This has become a rather complex trade-off as many active riders prefer to have their feet tucked in nearly directly below the knees. In order to achieve a long enough wheelbase to yield reasonably stable support, and have enough trail to minimize caster flutter, caster size, trail, and foot placement all have to be evaluated. Generally, trail of 63 to 75 millimeters will prevent noticeable flutter; however, this is dependent on the size and type of wheel, weight distribution of the chair and rider, and frame geometry. Simple alternatives to reduce caster flutter include using a viscous silicon-based grease in the caster housing bearings, or to place an oversized washer between a bearing and the shaft of the caster fork (i.e., add a small amount of friction).

When one of the casters does not touch the floor while on level ground, the wheelchair has caster float. Caster float decreases the stability and performance of the wheelchair. If the wheelchair has caster float, a few items should be checked. Unequal rear wheel camber will cause caster float (i.e., most of the weight of the rider/chair system is over the rear axles). Thus correcting the camber may eliminate the problem. If both caster housings are not vertical, caster float will result. Setting the orientation of both housings to vertical with a level should eliminate

**FIGURE 7.18**   Caster trail (T) is required for a manual wheelchair to be capable of turning. Commonly, the caster stem is adjusted to be vertical and the axle of the caster follows the center of the caster stem by about 50 mm. The size of the caster and the amount of trail determine the area swept out by the caster when turning. A large area decreases maneuverability and heel clearance.

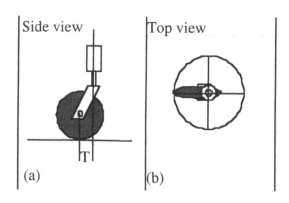

caster float. One caster may be excessively worn more than the other; replacing the casters will solve the problem. Otherwise, placing a spacer under the floating caster will solve the caster float.

As manual wheelchairs use rear-wheel steering via differential propulsion torque (i.e., pushing unequally on each wheel), tracking is the tendency of the wheelchair/rider to maintain its course once control has been relinquished (i.e, once the rider has stopped pushing). Tracking is important as the rider propels the pushrims periodically (e.g., about every second). If the chair does not track well, it will drift from its course between pushes and force the rider to correct heading. This will waste valuable energy and reduce control over the chair. In sports like basketball, tracking is extremely important. To ensure tracking does not present a substantial problem, all four wheels must be pointing in the forward direction when in their natural (resting) position. If the caster housings are tilted, such that they have a tendency to rest in an other than forward-pointing direction, tracking will be affected. If the rear wheels are misaligned, tracking can present a problem. Tracking can be easily checked by rolling through a puddle of water and allowing the chair to coast. The chair should maintain its heading.

Alignment generally refers to the orientation of the rear wheels with respect to each another. Typically, it is desirable to have the rear wheels parallel to each another without any difference between the distance across the two rear wheels at the front and back. Misalignment on the order of 2 millimeters can cause a noticeable increase in the effort required to propel the wheelchair. Alignment is adjusted in various ways depending on how the rear wheels are mounted to the frame.

## 7.4 The Wheelchair User Interface

The user wheelchair interface is the most critical design factor, and it is the least understood. The rider and the wheelchair must act as one. The chair is to be selected such that the user's potential is maximized. The chair should not limit the user. Experience tells us that there is a great deal of variability among individual preferences. The chair must become an extension of the user's body, much like an orthosis. This requires carefully matching critical chair dimensions to body dimensions, user ability, and intended use.

To specify a wheelchair properly it is important to understand the intentions and abilities of the user. The best wheelchair will not be successful if rejected by the user. Therefore the needs, desires, and abilities of the user must be ascertained and incorporated into the wheelchair selection. The selection of a wheelchair depends on the intended use of the wheelchair. It is no longer acceptable to stock a particular model of wheelchair and to provide it to all new wheelchair users. Manufacturers who do not follow the intended uses of the consumer will soon find themselves wanting for business. The intentions of the user must be ascertained *a priori*. The activities and the environment of the wheelchair and the user must be determined. This will assist with defining the geometry, components, and durability of the wheelchair.

The abilities of the user must be matched with the intended use of the wheelchair. For some users many of the desired tasks may be simply accomplished with existing technology; others will require custom products, and still others will not be able to achieve their goals with existing components. The type of chair and how it is set up depend on the interaction between the user and the intended use (person, place, task). The real abilities of the user as related to the intended uses must be assessed.

Financial and physical resources are required to select and purchase wheelchairs. The limits of the available resources must be weighed against the abilities and desires of the user. Resources are always limited, and new technology can be costly. The user should be provided the best possible product with the available resources. Assistive technology is considered to be medical equipment and thus caution must be taken to ensure the safety of all potential users.

The assistive technology clinician must remain current with respect to new product developments. There is no sense in reinventing the wheel. Often an existing product can be adapted to meet the user's needs. Caution must be observed when modifying existing technology for applications not intended by the manufacturer. A rehabilitation engineer should evaluate possible problems that could result from any modifications. Often products in other areas may provide help in the selection and development of wheelchairs.

There are several critical seat dimensions to be considered during wheelchair selection: seat height, seat angle, seat depth, seat width, back height, and backrest angle . The seat base should be made of some stiff material to provide a rigid base of support for the cushion. Either a pliable material (i.e., canvas, nylon) stretched tightly across the side frames or a rigid base (i.e., plastic, aluminum, composite) works well. Seat height varies based on desired use. In general, while sitting upright with the hands resting on the top of the wheels, the elbow angle should be between 100 and 120 degrees for optimal mobility (see Figure 7.19).

Seat heights vary from about 300 to 600 millimeters. The seat height is also dependent on the total body length of the user. Users with longer lower leg lengths will require higher seat heights to achieve sufficient clearance for the footrests. There is some flexibility when selecting seat height even for taller individuals, because most active users prefer some seat angle. By tilting the seat toward the backrest the user fits more securely into the chair, and the chair becomes more responsive to the user's body English. Seat angle also gives the user some pelvic tilt, which provides greater trunk stability. Seat angle can be as little as zero degrees and as much as 20 degrees. Seat depth is determined from the length of the upper legs. Generally no more than a 75-millimeter gap should be between the front of the seat and the back of the knees when the person is in the wheelchair. This will help to ensure broad distribution of the trunk weight over the buttocks and upper legs, without placing undue pressure behind the knee. Some gap is required to allow the user some freedom to adjust position. Seat width is determined from the width of the person's hips, the intended use, and whether the person prefers to use side guards (pieces of plastic, aluminum or steel sheet placed between the seat and rear wheels to prevent clothing from rubbing on the rear wheels) or not. Generally, the wheelchair should be as narrow as possible. Thus a chair about one inch wider than the user's hips is desirable. Side guards or armrests can help to keep clothing clean, and have the user and chair mesh better. Seat widths for adults typically range from 250 to 500 millimeters.

Backrest height, one of the most critical dimensions, is dependent on the user's disability etiology, intended use, and wheelchair skills. The comfort, stability, and control of the wheelchair are influenced by backrest height. Generally, the

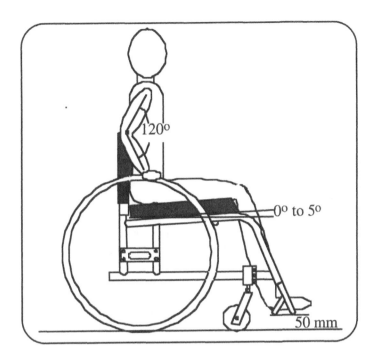

**FIGURE 7.19** Sagittal plane illustration of seat height and angle for proper posture and efficient propulsion. Safe and effective propulsion can be
assisted by placing the elbows at about 120 degrees of flexion
when grasping the pushrim at top dead center, placing the seat
angle between zero and five degrees, and setting the footrest
ground clearance to 50 millimeters. The user's cushion must be in
place when all measurements are taken.

lower the mobility impairment, the lower the desired backrest height. Commonly,
backrest height is made to be adjustable so that the user can tune it to his/her
liking. A lower backrest height permits greater freedom of motion (e.g., leaning,
turning) and is less restrictive (i.e., does not interfere with arms when pushing),
but provides less support than a high backrest. Backrest heights may vary from 200
to 500 millimeters. The backrest should be made of a padded pliable material, or
when made of rigid material it should not only be padded but also be mounted
such as to conform to the user's changing body position. It is sometimes desirable
to taper the backrest to provide for comfortable support of a user's well-developed
upper torso. The backrest angle is often set so that the backrest is vertical with
respect to a level floor.

The wheelbase and width affect handling and performance. The wheelbase
affects caster flutter, rolling resistance, stability, controllability, and obstacle performance. A longer wheelbase chair becomes more stable, but less controllable.
Therefore, a long chair may be less apt to tip over, but the user may not be able to
negotiate common terrain. Typically, active use rehabilitation wheelchairs are very
controllable and maneuverable and hence less stable. This is because users prefer
control over the chair to stability. A longer wheelbase makes negotiating obstacles
like curbs easier as the angle of ascent for the center of gravity is reduced. This is
an important consideration. A short wheelbase is more maneuverable, and can get

the user closer to furnishings. However, a short wheelbase may move more weight over the front wheels, which may increase rolling resistance and reduce the speed of onset of caster flutter. This could also increase the risk of a forward fall. Obviously, trade-offs need to be made. Typically, the wheelbase of wheelchairs is between 250 and 500 millimeters. The width of the footprint of the wheelchair is also an important design variable.

Often camber is variable. Camber has several advantages: the footprint of the chair is widened, creating greater side-to-side stability; camber allows quicker turning; camber helps to protect the hands by having the bottom of the wheels scuff edges, preventing them from hitting the area where the hands are in contact with the pushrims; and camber positions the pushrims more ergonomically for propulsion (it is more natural to push down and out). Camber angle can either be fixed or adjustable, depending on the frame design. The width of the chair depends on the width of the frame and the camber angle. Frame widths for adults range from 300 to 500 millimeters, and camber angles are usually between 0 and 15 degrees, mostly between 7 and 12 degrees. Thus wheelchair widths vary from about 550 to 750 millimeters. Generally, for daily use the chair should be as narrow as possible without substantially diminishing the handling characteristics. The wheels should be offset enough from the seat to avoid rubbing against the clothing or body. Narrow chairs are easier to maneuver in an environment made for walking. Some suspension can be gained through the use of wheel camber. By adding camber to the rear wheels the effective stiffness between the rolling surface and frame is reduced.

## 7.5 Legrests

Most wheelchair users require support for their feet and lower legs. This support is provided by footrests. Footrests may be fixed, folding, or swing-away (see Figure 7.20). The footrest must provide sufficient support for the lower legs and feet and hold the feet in proper position to prevent foot drop or other deformities. The feet must remain on the footrests at all time during propulsion and therefore some type of cradle is recommended. Some wheelchairs (i.e., primarily those with swing-away footrests) use foot stirrups behind the heels of each foot. However, for other wheelchairs it is best to use a continuous strap behind both feet as the rider's feet sometimes come over stirrups during active use, which is not possible with a strap. The feet should not be permitted to be pinched or trapped or scratched by the footrests during normal driving activities or when transferring. The frame should be selected and configured so that the feet sit firmly upon the footrests with shoes on without lifting the upper legs from the seat cushion. Care must be taken that sufficient ground clearance is maintained. The footrests are commonly placed between 25 and 50 millimeters from the ground. Often the footrests are the first part of the chair to come in contact with an obstacle (i.e., door, wall, another chair), so they must be durable.

Rigid wheelchairs often use simple tubes across the front of the wheelchair. By using a tubular rigid footrest, the wheelchair becomes stiffer and stronger. Rigid footrests are used during sports activities, and work well for people who are very active in their wheelchair. Forward anti-tip rollers can be mounted to rigid footrests. This is helpful for playing court sports and reduces the risk of some for-

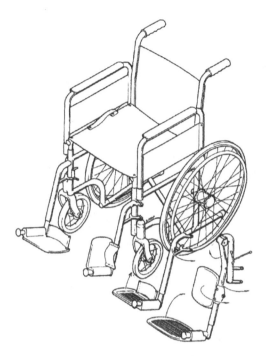

**FIGURE 7.20** Many different types of leg- and footrests are used on manual wheelchairs. (Adapted from *Wheelchairs: A Prescription Guide*, A. Bennett Wilson, Jr., Demos, New York, NY, 1992)

ward tipping accidents. Rigid footrests may be used on folding wheelchairs. This prevents them from folding. However, for people who like to use one wheelchair for daily use and recreational use, two sets of legrests (e.g., one rigid and one split) may help to accomplish this. Folding wheelchairs often use footrests that fold up and legrests that swing out of the way to ease transfers. Most people use this type of footrest. Swing-away legrests are not as durable as rigid legrests. In some cases manufacturers design swing-away legrests so that they will bend upon impact. This helps to absorb the energy of the impact by bending, possibly preventing serious injury to the wheelchair rider. Elevating legrests can be used for people who cannot maintain a 90-degree knee angle or who need their legs elevated for venous return. Elevating legrests make the wheelchair longer. This has the effect of making the wheelchair less maneuverable by increasing the turning radius.

## 7.6 Armrests and Clothing Guards

Armrests provide a form of support and are convenient handles when the rider leans to one side or the other. Armrests are also helpful when attempting to reach higher places. Some people even use their armrests as a tool to nudge items off high shelves. Armrests are commonly used to assist with pressure relief by performing a "push-up." By placing an arm on each armrest and pushing upward, some wheelchair users are capable of lifting their buttocks from the seat. This helps to improve blood flow to the lower extremities and reduce the risk of developing a pressure ulcer. There are three basic styles of armrest: wrap-around, full-length, and desk-length. Wrap-around armrests mount at the back of the wheelchair to the frame below the backrest in most cases. The armrest comes up along the back of the backrest canes and wraps around to the front of the wheelchair. This is how the wrap-around armrest gets its name. The major advantage of this design is that the armrest does not increase the width of the wheelchair like other types of armrest. Wrap-around armrests are popular among active wheelchair users. The most significant drawback of this design is that the armrest does not serve as a side guard to keep the rider's clothing away from the wheels.

Full-length and desk-length armrests are similar in design, the main difference being the length of the armrest. Full-length armrests provide support for nearly the entire upper arm. They are popular on electric-powered wheelchairs because they make a convenient and functional location for a joystick or other input device. Full-length armrests provide good support for the arms, but they make it difficult to get close to some tables and desks. This is why manufacturers produce desk-length armrests. Both of these types of armrests include clothing guards to protect clothing from the wheels. These types of armrests are mounted to the side of the wheelchair and may add as much as 5 cm (2 inches) to the width of the wheelchair.

Armrests can be fixed or adjustable. Adjustable armrests may move up and down to accommodate the length of the rider's trunk and arms. Most armrests can be moved in order to provide clearance for transferring in and out of the wheelchair, and to allow a person to lean over the sides of the wheelchair. Armrests are either removed or flipped back. Both styles commonly use a latch operated by the user. It is important to have latches on armrests because armrests form convenient places for people to grasp when attempting to provide assistance. If the armrests and latches are designed properly, two people can lift the rider and wheelchair using the armrests. In some cases, armrests are designed to pull out if any upward force is applied to them. They are not intended to be used for lifting.

## 7.7 Wheel Locks

Wheel locks act as parking brakes and assist when transferring to other seats, or when the rider wishes to remain in a particular spot. They allow the rider to push things, and to be more stable when desired. There are a variety of wheel locks used to restrain wheelchairs when transferring or parked. High-lock brakes are most common. They require the least dexterity to operate. Extension levers can be added for people with limited reach and or minimal strength. Some wheel locks are over-center and are either engaged or disengaged. Other wheel locks allow selection of the braking force; these are sometimes called sweeper brakes as the wheelchair can still be pushed in some positions, allowing the user to push and then sweep a broom to clean a floor. Wheel locks are standard equipment on wheelchairs. They are simple to mount if the wheelchair does not come so equipped from the manufacturer.

Wheel locks may be pushed to lock or pulled to lock. Most people prefer push-to-lock because wheel locks are more difficult to engage than to disengage, and riders often find it easier to push with the palm than pull with the fingers. High wheel locks are often mounted to the upper tube of the wheelchair's side frame. Low wheel locks are usually mounted to the lower tube of the wheelchair's side frame. Low wheel locks require more mobility to operate. They also alleviate the common problem of hitting the thumb that plagues high wheel lock users. This problem can be addressed for high wheel lock users by selecting retractable (i.e., scissors or butterfly) wheel locks. This type of wheel lock helps to prevent jamming the thumbs and can accommodate a wide variety of camber angles. The major drawback of retractable wheel locks is that they are more difficult to use than other types of wheel locks. The wheel lock must be positioned properly with respect to the wheel in order to operate effectively. If the wheels are repositioned, then the wheel locks must be repositioned. Tire pressure will also affect the grip of the wheel locks.

## 7.8 Propulsion and Performance

Simplicity of form and function are the key guidelines to the design of a desirable wheelchair. The handling of a wheelchair is primarily dependent on a few factors: the location of the center of gravity of the person and chair; the stiffness of the frame, wheels, and components; and how well the pilot and chair mesh together.

### 7.8.1 Center of Gravity (COG) Location

Figure 7.21 illustrates the location of the COG for a hypothetical wheelchair with rider. The COG is typically located along the midline of the person and chair; generally bilateral symmetry is assumed. The COG in the sagittal plane (fore and aft) should be located slightly forward of the rear axles. This depends on the user, as having the COG located near the rear axles makes the person and chair more likely to flip backwards (wheelie). However, having the COG near the rear axles has certain advantages: the downhill turning moment due to crown (slope for drainage on roadways and sidewalks) is minimized as the turning torque is related to the mass of the individual/wheelchair and their location relative to the pivot point (the rear axles); the tendency for caster flutter is also reduced; the rolling resistance is reduced as most of the weight is borne by the larger rear wheels; and the user-initiated turning ability is increased. The farther the COG gets from the midpoint between the front and rear wheels and the closer it gets to the rear axles, the greater the control effort and ability required to maintain balance. Thus, in general, the greater the functional ability of the user, the closer the COG can be to the rear axles. There is going to be some variability due to personal preference and intended use. For most chair/user systems the mass of the system is dominated by the user. Thus the COG can be adjusted by adjusting the position of either the rear wheels with respect to the seat or vice versa. Generally this is an option left to the user. However, if the desired location of the COG is known, then the frame can be made lighter by designing fixed axle and seating structures.

### 7.8.2 Ride Comfort and Durability

Ride comfort is primarily a function of the following: frame, wheel and component stiffness, frame geometry, seat and cushion design, and compliance. Ride comfort is an important issue because people must sit in the chair from 12 to 18 hours per day every day. Because some chairs are used by active users they may be used nearly

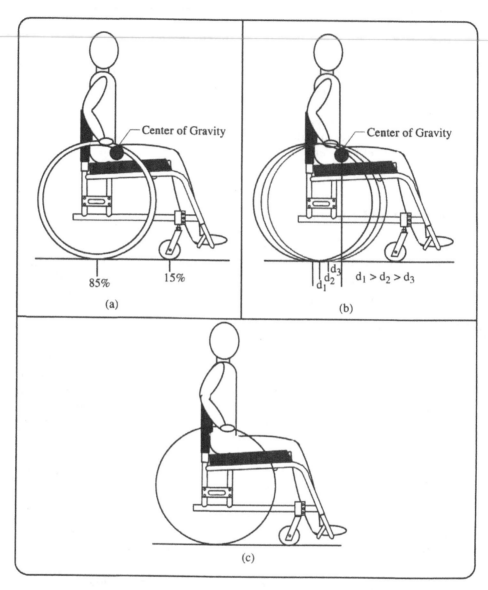

**FIGURE 7.21** The location of the COG for a hypothetical wheelchair with rider. (a) The location of the COG affects the distribution of mass on each of the wheels. Front casters typically exhibit higher rolling resistance than the larger rear drive wheels. A depot wheelchair may have 40% of the total weight placed on the front wheels whereas a sports chair may have only 15%. Shifting the COG may reduce stability in some directions. (b) The downhill turning tendency is related to the COG location with respect to the contact point of the rear drive wheels. The downhill turning moment commonly increases with d. (c) If the user sits too far forward or too low, the shoulders will be excessively elevated, extended, and internally rotated, which may lead to rotator cuff injury. When the user is seated properly (a), the shoulder position is more neutral and the propulsion phase is more balanced between horizontally and vertically directed motion.

ten miles per day over a variety of terrain (i.e., grass, carpet, gravel, concrete, asphalt, etc.). The frame design must be durable but should have sufficient flexibility to withstand dropping off curbs (up to 35 centimeters high), and also not to break after several thousand miles of road vibration. Most wheelchair suspension comes from the cushion and the tires. Typically, wheelchairs will use pneumatic tires, and will have a foam, gel, or air cushion. The frame geometry can be used to reduce the effects of the impact observed when going off a curb, or to minimize road vibration.

Durability is also a very important issue in wheelchair design. Wheelchairs may be used by demanding riders and/or receive little maintenance. The same wheelchair is often used for work, school, and recreation. Therefore the chair must be designed to meet these demands. Typically, a wheelchair will be used all day every day for all major life activities (i.e., activities of daily living, work, school, recreation, sport) over a period of three to five years. The wheelchair must be designed to regularly withstand obstacles (i.e., rocks, curbs, bumps, dips, impacts) encountered during a variety of activities. Making the frame too flexible will cause it to absorb the energy of the rider and make it inefficient. Making the chair too stiff may cause it to fracture due to shock, and will reduce ride comfort.

## References and Further Reading

Brubaker C. E., McLaurin C. A., McClay I. S. (1985) A preliminary analysis of limb geometry and EMG activity for five lever placements. *Proceedings RESNA 8th Annual Conference*, Memphis, TN, 350–352.

Brubaker C. E. (1986) Wheelchair prescription: An analysis of factors that affect mobility and performance. *Journal of Rehabilitation Research and Development*, 23, 4, 19–26.

Collins T. J., Kauzlarich J. J. (1988) Directional instability of rear caster wheelchairs. *Journal of Rehabilitation Research and Development*, 25, 3, 1–18.

Cook A. M., Hussey S. M. (1995) *Assistive Technologies: Principles and Practice.* St. Louis, MO: Mosby.

Cooper R. A. (1995) *Rehabilitation Engineering Applied to Mobility and Manipulation.* Bristol, England: Institute of Physics.

Cooper R. A. (1991) High-tech wheelchairs gain the competitive edge. *IEEE Engineering in Medicine and Biology Magazine*, 10, 4, 49–55.

Cravotta D. (1991) Mobility for the masses. *Mainstream*, July, 11–17.

Denison I., Shaw J., Zuyderhoff R. (1994) *Wheelchair Selection Manual: The Effect of Components on Manual Wheelchair Performance.* Vancouver, BC: British Columbia Rehabilitation Society.

Department of Veterans Affairs. (1990) Choosing a wheelchair system. *Journal of Rehabilitation Research and Development*, Clinical Supplement No. 2, March.

Flippo K. F., Inge K. J., Barcus J. M. (1995) *Assistive Technology: A Resource for School, Work and Community.* Baltimore, MD: Paul H. Brookes Publishing.

Gaines R. F., La W.H.T. (1986) Users' responses to contoured wheelchair handrims. *Journal of Rehabilitation Research and Development.* 23, 3, 57–62.

Galvin J. C., Scherer M. J. (1996) *Evaluating, Selecting, and Using Appropriate Assistive Technology.* Gaithersburg, MD: Aspen Publishers.

Gordon J., Kauzlarich J. J., Thacker J. G. (1989) Tests of two new polyurethane foam wheelchair tires. *Journal of Rehabilitation Research and Development*, 26, 1, 33–46.

Heil T. (1992) Design of a dynamic wheelchair brake. *Proceedings RESNA International '92.* Toronto, Canada, 643–645.

Hotchkiss R. D., Pfaelzer P. (1992) Measuring success in third world wheelchair building. *Proceedings RESNA International '92.* Toronto, Canada, 618–620.

Hotchkiss R. D. (1993) Ground swell on wheels. *The Sciences,* July/August, 14–19.

Kauzlarich J. J., Thacker J. G. (1991) Antiskid wheelchair brake design. *Proceedings RESNA 14th Annual Conference,* Kansas City, MO, 143–145.

Kauzlarich J. J., Thacker J. G. (1987) A theory of wheelchair wheelie performance. *Journal of Rehabilitation Research and Development,* 24, 2, 67–80.

Kauzlarich J. J. (1990) A new maintenance-free wheelchair tire. *RESNA Press,* June, 67–68.

Kauzlarich J. J., Bruning T., Thacker J. G. (1984) Wheelchair caster shimmy and turning resistance. *Journal of Rehabilitation Research and Development,* 20, 2, 15–29.

Lemaire E. D., Lamontagne M., Barclay H., John T., Martel G. (1991) A technique for the determination of center of gravity and rolling resistance for tilt-seat wheelchairs. *Journal of Rehabilitation Research and Development,* 28, 3, 51–58.

Masse L. C., Lamontagne M., O'Riain M. D. (1992) Biomechanical analysis of wheelchair propulsion for various seating positions. *Journal of Rehabilitation Research and Development,* 29, 3, 12–28.

McLaurin C. A., Brubaker C. E. (1985) A lever drive system for wheelchairs. *Proceedings RESNA 8th Annual Conference,* Memphis, TN, 48–50.

Nashihara H., Shizukuishi K. (1992) Development of indoor wheelchair mainly made of wood. *Proceedings RESNA International '92,* Toronto, Canada, 533–535.

Pettit D., Cooper R. A., Bennet P. (1992) Design and evaluation of a simple, inexpensive, ultralight wheelchair. *Proceedings 14th Annual IEEE/EMBS International Conference,* Paris, France, vol. 14.

Quickie Designs Inc. (November 1989) *The perfect fit:. An adjustments guide to your manual wheelchair.*

Szeto A. Y. J., White R. N. (1983) Evaluation of a curb-climbing aid for manual wheelchairs: Considerations of stability, effort, and safety. *Journal of Rehabilitation Research and Development,* 20, 1, 45–56.

Trefler E., Hobson D. A., Taylor S. J., Monahan L. C., Shaw C. G. (1993) *Seating and Mobility for Persons with Disabilities.* Tucson, AZ: Therapy Skill Builders.

Veeger D., Van der Woude L. H. V., Rozendal R. H. (1989) The effect of rear wheel camber in manual wheelchair propulsion. *Journal of Rehabilitation Research and Development,* 26, 2, 37–46.

Veenbaas R. (1993) A method for choosing the main measures of a hand propelled wheelchair system, based on anthropometric sources and multivariate statistics. *Proceedings Second European Conference on Advancement of Rehabilitation Technology,* Stockholm, Sweden, 3–4.

Wilson Jr. A. B. (1992) *Wheelchairs: A Prescription Guide,* 2nd ed. New York, NY: Demos.

# CHAPTER

# 8 | Powered Mobility

*Chapter Goals*

- ☑ To know features of powered wheelchairs
- ☑ To know state-of-the-art research and product development
- ☑ To understand person-to-device interface and access
- ☑ To know how to select powered wheelchairs

## 8.1 Introduction

Electric-powered wheelchairs were first invented around the turn of the century. The first U.S. patent describing an electric-powered wheelchair was approved around 1940 (see Figure 8.1). However, the very early designs were impractical and did not receive significant attention. There was also little demand for powered wheelchairs. This is because powered wheelchairs are most beneficial to people with severe disabilities, and the long-term prognosis for people with severe disabilities was poor at that time.

Medical advances that occurred and were implemented during World War II enabled more people with severe disabilities to survive. Moreover, the emphasis changed from acute treatment to long-term rehabilitation. These changes created a demand for better wheelchairs and, more specifically, for powered wheelchairs. The first practical electric-powered wheelchairs used starter motors and batteries from automobiles. These early wheelchairs provided limited mobility for some people with upper extremity impairments. Relays were soon used to provide greater control over electric-powered wheelchairs. Next, the transistor provided much better control and allowed for the development of specialized control interfaces for the user. The number of electric-powered wheelchairs expanded during the 1960s and 1970s. However, powered wheelchairs still suffered from being bulky, inefficient, and unreliable. The 1980s saw the implementation of microprocessors and metal-oxide-semiconductor-field-effect-transistors (MOS-FETs). These both helped to improve reliability. The microprocessor provided improved control and greater ability to match the characteristics of the chair to the abilities of the user. The MOS-FETs improved efficiency. Because of their low-cost, extra MOS-FETS have been used to provide some redundancy.

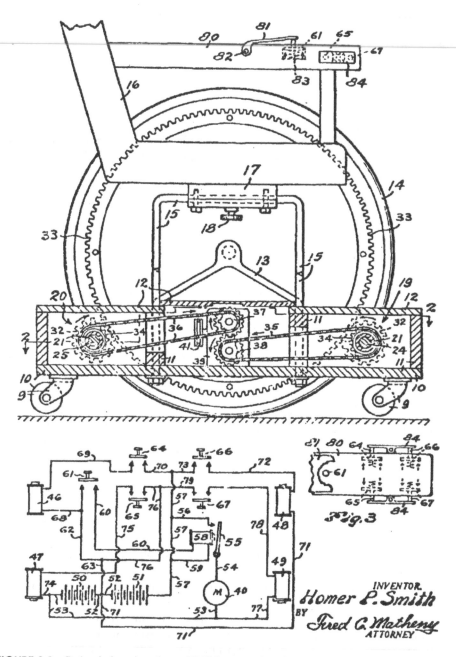

**FIGURE 8.1** Patent drawing from 1940 for an electric-powered wheelchair (Reprinted from *Wheelchairs: A Prescription Guide*, 2nd Edition, A. Bennett Wilson, Jr., Demos, New York, NY, 1992)

The 1990s have brought about changes in frame design. Manufacturers began to develop frames designed specifically for electric-powered wheelchairs. The most significant change was separating the seat from the frame. This is referred to as a powered wheelchair base design. With the introduction of this concept, other innovations such as rear-wheel suspension developed.

## 8.2 Differentiation of Powered Wheelchairs

Twenty years ago there were very few differences between the designs of powered wheelchairs. Most powered wheelchairs were simply iterations of manual wheelchair design (see Figure 8.2). As the powered wheelchair market grew and products developed, powered wheelchairs began to evolve. Eventually, consumers, clinicians, engineers, and manufacturers began recognizing the need for product differentiation. Moreover, as more manufacturers of electric-powered wheelchairs emerged to address the specialized needs of the consumer, manufacturers began to desire to have their products be distinguishable from those of other manufacturers.

Powered wheelchairs can be grouped into several classes or categories. The most common groupings are based on the functions provided by the wheelchair and the intended use. A convenient grouping by intended use is primarily indoor, both indoor/outdoor, and active indoor/outdoor. Indoor wheelchairs have a small footprint (i.e., area connecting the wheels). This allows them to be maneuverable in confined spaces. However, they may not have the stability or power to negotiate obstacles outdoors. Indoor/outdoor powered wheelchairs are used by

**FIGURE 8.2**   Photograph of a classic electric-powered wheelchair (Photograph courtesy of Gendron)

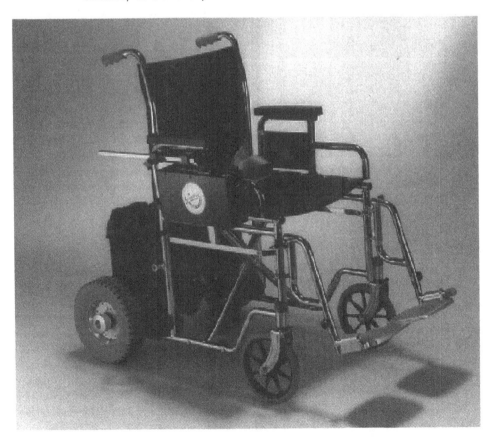

people who wish to have mobility in the home, school, office, and community, but who stay on finished surfaces (e.g., sidewalks, driveways, flooring). Both indoor and indoor/outdoor wheelchairs conserve weight by using smaller batteries. This often results in reduced range.

Some wheelchair users want to drive over unstructured environments, travel long distances, and move fast. Active indoor/outdoor wheelchairs may be best suited for these individuals. The active indoor/outdoor-use wheelchairs include those with suspension, and use of a power base design is increasing. A power base separates the seating system from the main chassis of the wheelchair. With power bases, the main chassis consists of the motors, drive wheels, casters, controllers, batteries, and frame. The seating system (e.g., seat, backrest, armrests, legrests, footrests) is a separate integrated unit. Often, seating systems from one manufacturer are used on a power base from another manufacturer.

Indoor/outdoor powered wheelchairs can be further divided into categories by the design of the seating system. The simplest form of seating system is a linear seating system. A linear seating system refers to a planar seat and back with fixed angles and orientations. For people who have low sitting tolerance or who need to change posture to perform some activities of daily living, a reclining seating system may be beneficial. A reclining seating system allows the angle of the backrest to be changed (i.e., from upright to reclined). For people with very low sitting tolerance, severe spasticity, or hemodynamic problems, a tilt-in-space seating system may be appropriate. Tilt-in-space systems allow the backrest, seat, and legrests to tilt as a unit, without changing their orientation with respect to each other, but as a unit change with respect to the wheelchair's chassis. Changing the user's position in space has other advantages besides assisting with posture and sitting tolerance. Stand-up wheelchairs assist users in performing many activities of daily living. Stand-up wheelchairs may have some physiological benefits due to upright posture, and have been reported to provide psychological benefits to the user. Some people cannot use a stand-up wheelchair because they do not have the range of motion or their bones may be too fragile. Some of the benefits of a stand-up wheelchair can be obtained by using a variable seat height wheelchair. The most common function of variable seat height wheelchairs is to provide seat elevation. Some wheelchair models come with seat elevation and seat lowering. Lowering may extend to a few inches from the floor, while raising can be as high as three feet from the floor to the base of the seat.

### 8.2.1 Power Wheelchairs

People with severe disabilities might need a power wheelchair for mobility purposes. Individuals who have a moderate level of trunk control can use a conventional power wheelchair. Conventional power wheelchairs contain a standard seat system (see Figure 8.3). Alternative seating systems have been designed to provide customized seating in the standard power wheelchair seat. Power wheelchairs are distinguishable by their integrated frame and seat. Their appearance is most similar to that of a conventional wheelchair. Power wheelchairs may use a range of drive wheels from 8 inches to 20 inches in diameter. The drive wheels may be driven by either belts or gear boxes. All powered mobility systems are generically lumped under the title powered wheelchair.

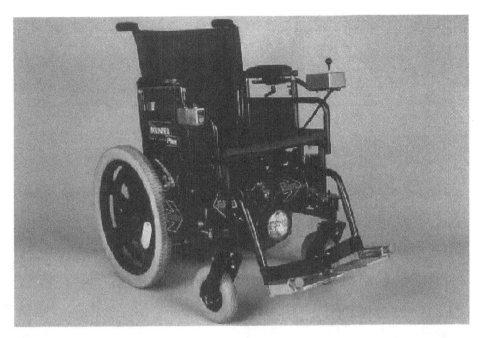

**FIGURE 8.3**   Photograph of an electric-powered wheelchair with an integrated seat (Photograph courtesy of 21st Century Scientific America)

### 8.2.2 Power Bases

Power bases are simply powered wheelchairs consisting of the power drive system on a mobile platform (see Figure 8.4). Power bases are developed for those people with minimal trunk control who need a customized seating system mounted to the base. The conventional powered wheelchair seating system does not fulfill their needs as individuals. Power bases also tend to offer higher performance (i.e., faster, more torque). A significant advantage of some power bases is that the position of the wheels with respect to the seat can be changed. This permits adjustment of the handling of the wheelchair without losing some of the power. The power base includes all wheels, the motors, the batteries, and most often the controller. This allows seating systems to be developed without modifying the power base. Power bases provide locations suitable for mounting seating hardware.

### 8.2.3 Scooters

Scooters are designed for people with limited walking ability and substantial body control. They are power bases with a mounted seat and usually a tiller (e.g., handlebar) steering system (see Figure 8.5). Scooters are characterized primarily by the upholstered seat, which is often similar to that used on a lawn tractor or fishing boat. Most scooter seats swivel to ease ingress and egress. The seats are often removable to simplify transport in a personal automobile. From an engineering and clinical perspective, one of the most important distinguishing features of a scooter is that speed is controlled electronically and direction is controlled manu-

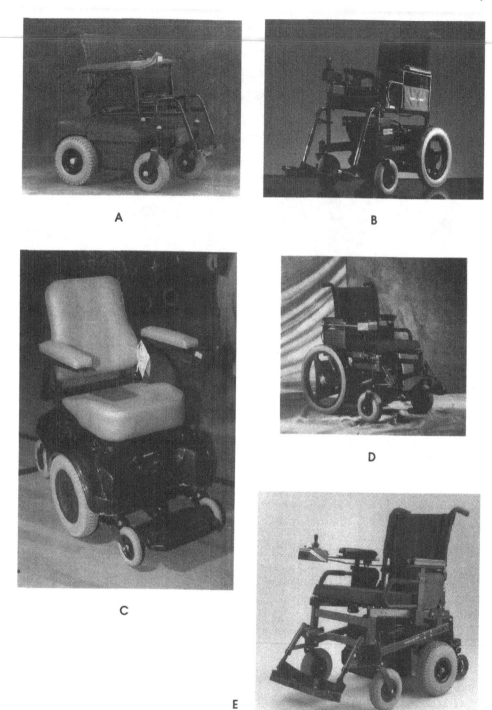

**FIGURE 8.4**  Photographs showing common styles of power bases used to provide electric-powered mobility (Photographs courtesy of (a) Invacare Corporation–Action Division, (b) Everest & Jennings Corporation, (c) VA Pittsburgh Health Care System, (d) & (e) Sunrise Medical Incorporated–Quickie Designs)

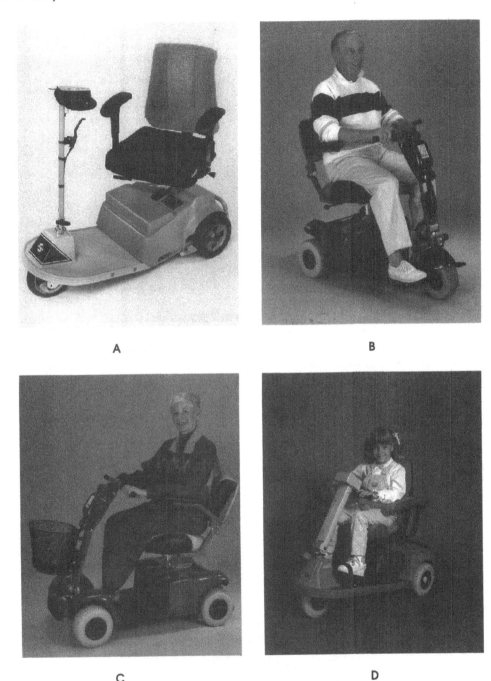

**FIGURE 8.5** Common styles of scooters used to provide electric mobility: (a) shows a lightweight three-wheel scooter with tiller steering and hand brake, (b) shows an active duty three-wheel scooter with handlebar steering, (c) shows an active duty four-wheel scooter with handlebar steering and carrying basket, (d) shows a pediatric three-wheel scooter. (Photographs courtesy of (a) Amigo International Incorporated, (b-d) Bruno Incorporated)

ally. Most scooters allow the steering column to fold or be removed without tools in order to make the scooter easier to transport in a personal motor vehicle. There are products that use electronic steering by using a motor to change the direction of one or both front wheels. Technically, such products should be considered wheelchairs. Scooters use either front- or rear-wheel drive. Rear-wheel drive scooters are usually best for active drivers.

### 8.2.4 Add-on Units

Some people do not require electric-powered mobility all of the time. They may have sufficient arm strength to use a manual wheelchair for shorter distances or on finished surfaces (e.g., tile, linoleum). However, traveling longer distances becomes strenuous. Power add-on units allow a manual wheelchair to be used as a lightweight electric-powered wheelchair for some activities. The most common type of power add-on unit attaches to the frame of the wheelchair and uses small rollers to drive the rear wheels of the wheelchair (see Figure 8.6). Because this type of drive relies on friction between the rollers and the wheelchair tires, it may cause premature tire wear. Proper adjustment can help to minimize tire wear. The battery to operate the add-on unit may be integrated into the motor-controller-roller unit or it may be in a separate case, permitting mounting at a more stable location on the wheelchair frame. Add-on units are typically controlled using a joystick or switches. Not all wheelchairs are suitable for power add-on units, and the setup of the wheelchair will be affected by the add-on unit. Therefore, one should consult an expert prior to installing an add-on unit.

### 8.2.5 In-wheel Motors

Another means of providing powered mobility to a manual wheelchair is to use in-wheel motors. In-wheel motors are wheel hubs made from a motor. The hub is much larger than that of a standard manual wheelchair in order for the motor to

**FIGURE 8.6**   Friction drive electric-powered add-on unit to provide assistance on a manual wheelchair (Photograph courtesy of Damaco)

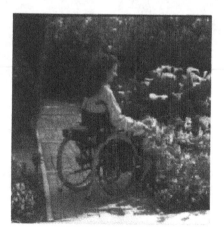

be of sufficient size to provide function power. In-wheel motors use a battery pack that attaches to the frame. The most common means of attaching the battery is to use a small bag slung under the wheelchair. In-wheel motors are commonly made with quick-release axles in order to simplify transport. Either a joystick or switches can be used to control the motors (i.e., right and left side) to provide electric-powered mobility for a manual wheelchair. One must exercise some caution when converting a manual wheelchair to an electric-powered wheelchair. Manual wheelchairs are not designed to accommodate the additional weight. This may reduce the stability, durability, and ease of propulsion when in the manual mode. The speeds possible with a powered unit are also likely to be greater than the rider is capable of with a manual chair. Moreover, powered wheelchairs drive much differently than manual wheelchairs. A skilled manual wheelchair rider may pop the casters over small bumps without noticing. However, when the chair is converted to being electrically powered the caster may be damaged in short order. When used properly with appropriate training and awareness of the trade-offs, power conversion units can provide valuable assistance.

## 8.3 Assessment and Selection

When selecting the most appropriate wheelchair, it is important to involve a multi-disciplinary team of support personnel in the decision-making process. This assessment team will examine the needs of the wheelchair user, the environments they will encounter, the activities they will perform in the chair, and the amount of training or instruction they might require to use the chair safely and effectively. The decision to accept the chair should ultimately be made by the person spending the most time in it—the wheelchair user. The family and caregiver should also provide input, as they will be the next most affected by the choice of chair.

The assessment team usually consists of a variety of rehabilitation professionals. A physician usually signs the prescription for the wheelchair. An occupational or physical therapist is also helpful. A rehabilitation engineer or a professional certified in rehabilitation technology by RESNA (Rehabilitation Engineering and Assistive Technology Society of North America) is crucial to include on the assessment team. Such an individual will have the skills to assess the needs of the user, and will take into account the environment the chair will be used in and the activities that will be performed.

Those involved in the wheelchair selection process should learn about the many powered wheelchairs available on the market. Magazine articles and commercial database sources such as ABLEDATA are good places to begin your research. Wheelchair manufacturers can be contacted directly or through the Internet for additional information.

The funding agency or third-party payer for the wheelchair should be contacted early to determine the amount and kinds of costs that will be covered. In addition to the purchase price, the chair's long-range maintenance costs should also be considered. This may be an important factor in making the final decision.

Once the model and pricing options have been investigated, the needs of the individual should be assessed by examining the environment and regular activities of the wheelchair user. Most people's activities can be placed into one of three categories: daily living, vocational/educational, and leisure. Activities of daily living include those activities done in the home environment, such as transferring in and out of bed, bathing and other toilet activities, and cooking. Access to a range of heights might be important to reach objects in the home and other environments. Other daily living activities include running errands, performing chores, shopping for groceries, and stopping by the post office. Vocational/educational activities can involve maneuvering in an office, outdoor construction site, agricultural setting, or school environment. People's professions are often highly specialized and specific requirements may exist for mobility within a laboratory, operating room, courtroom, clean room, or machine shop. Leisure activities, pursued in such places as community centers, restaurants, movie theaters, and recreational environments, often place the most demands on the wheelchair.

The wheelchair model chosen should also be compatible with the public and/or private transportation options available to the wheelchair user, such as a bus, car, or van. If the wheelchair user plans to travel by air, only modular wheelchairs that operate on sealed gel batteries should be considered; chairs using other power sources are not permitted on commercial planes. In other countries, access to buses and trains can be an important requirement.

In all environments, the surface conditions will impose the greatest restrictions on the type of wheelchair that is most appropriate. The regularity of the surface and its firmness and stability are important in determining the tire size and wheel diameter. The performance of the wheelchair is often dictated by the need to negotiate grades, as well as height transitions such as thresholds and curbs. The clearance widths in the environment will determine the overall dimensions of the wheelchair. The climate the chair will be operated in, and the need to be able to operate in snow, rain, changing humidity and temperature levels, and other weather conditions, are important considerations.

Overall, a variety of performance characteristics of the wheelchair should be considered with regard to the environment and activities that the individual is trying to perform. The maximum speed of the wheelchair is important when using the wheelchair to travel longer distances, such as across campus or across town. The obstacle-climbing ability of the chair will help determine the rider's access to environments that do not meet ADA accessibility guidelines. Static and dynamic stability characteristics (the "tipsiness" of the chair) will determine how safely the rider will be able to negotiate many of these nonideal environments.

The overall dimensions of the chair will determine how well the wheelchair user can maneuver in tight quarters. The range of the wheelchair will indicate how long and far the user can go in a given day without having to recharge the batteries. The maximum overall weight of the chair can be an important consideration if the wheelchair user does not have access to mass transit, or a van equipped with a lift or ramp. For all users, regardless of functional ability, skills need to be developed and tuned to enable safe operation of a particular wheelchair, with its given performance characteristics, in specific environments.

With an understanding of the individual's need or desire to perform different activities, you should now examine the most important factor in the wheelchair selection process—the user. Since you have inventoried the different kinds of activities important to the user, you will have gained an idea of that person's level of independence or dependence on others. You will also have gained a sense of their physical abilities. To verify this, you can perform some simple tasks with the person to determine the lateral and frontal stability of their trunk, their hand and arm strength, and the fine motor skills of their fingers.

Many powered wheelchair users brace some portion of their hand against the control box and use their hand and arm coordination to operate the joystick. Gross arm function, in many cases, can be used to operate a joystick. If the user does not have the hand function or coordination to operate a joystick input device, other options are available. Other parts of the body such as the chin or foot can operate a modified joystick, or a sip-&-puff control can be used.

Be aware, however, that as the physical and functional abilities of the user decrease, the cognitive abilities required to operate an alternative control typically increase. You can obtain a sense of an individual's cognitive function by assessing verbal and visual skills, the rate and accuracy with which they can perform various tasks, their spatial problem-solving abilities, and their understanding of their body's position in space. Visual skills, including sight accuracy and depth perception, are also important for safe operation of a powered wheelchair. Programmable wheelchair controllers allow reduction of the maximum velocity, and acceleration and deceleration rates of the wheelchair. To assist persons with more severe cognitive or visual limitations, technologies are being developed that enable the wheelchair to follow walls, navigate through doorways, and stop when other objects are contacted.

It is also important to assess whether persons have spasticity in their hands or arms. For persons with spasticity, particularly tremor in the hand, modern controllers have filters that can be adjusted to give smooth wheelchair control. A magic arm or similar positioning technology will enable positioning the joystick in numerous places to optimize the user's joystick operating function. Finally, once the appropriate choice and technologies in powered mobility have been made, you will want to spend a lot of time optimizing the seating setup to maximize the rider's function.

Before individuals ride away in their new powered mobility, they should go through a wheelchair training program. This is particularly important for younger children. Wheelchair users can first practice basic maneuvers in controlled environments that meet ADA accessibility guidelines. They should practice negotiating uneven surfaces, slope transitions (i.e., level to sloped surfaces) in both the uphill and downhill directions, and maneuvering through tight environments. Once these skills are mastered, they should gradually tackle more challenging environments, such as steep grades and step transitions that exceed ADA accessibility guidelines. The rider should always practice with an appropriate lap belt and chest support in place, as well as spotters standing by to assist if needed. The wheelchair user should also be given an opportunity to experience the limits of the technology they are using. By setting up and practicing in safe environments users can experience the limits of the lateral stability, as well as the front and rear stability of their chair, so that they have a better understanding of its performance limits.

## 8.4 Access Devices

The primary function of an access device is the control of the powered mobility system (see Figure 8.7). Secondary applications are for use with environmental control systems and computer access. By using the same control interface for both

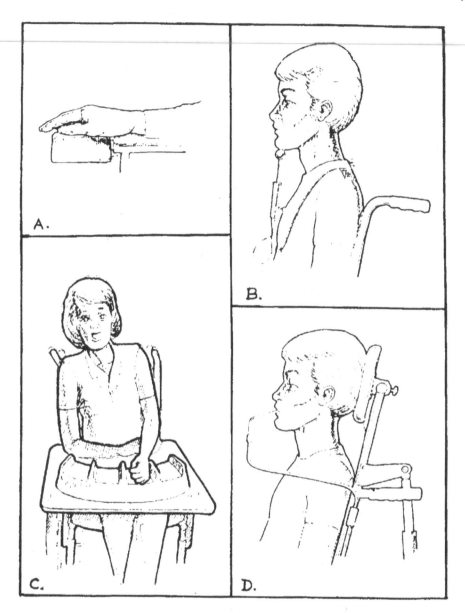

**FIGURE 8.7**   Illustration of common access devices used to control electric-powered wheelchairs (Reprinted from *Wheelchairs: A Prescription Guide*,
2nd Edition, A. Bennett Wilson, Jr., Demos, New York, NY, 1992)

the powered wheelchair and the secondary systems, the seating position and control selection can be optimized for multiple purposes. A critical consideration
when selecting or designing a user interface is that the ability of the user to accurately control the interface is heavily dependent on the stability of the user within
the wheelchair. Often custom seating and postural support systems are required
for a user interface to be truly effective. The placement of the user interface is also
critical to its efficacy as a functional access device (Figure 8.8).

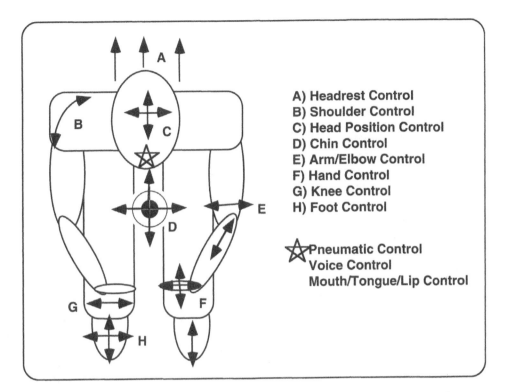

**FIGURE 8.8** Access site locations that can be evaluated for use in controlling an electric-powered wheelchair

### 8.4.1 Joysticks

Joysticks are the most common access device for powered wheelchair systems. When a powered wheelchair is ordered and nothing is specified, a joystick is almost always supplied by the powered wheelchair manufacturer. Joysticks can either be switched or proportional. Switched joysticks respond to discrete positions of the joystick. Usually four switches are implemented. There are eight discrete states with four positions being defined by the activation of a single switch and four positions being defined by the activation of two switches together. Proportional joysticks get their name because the control output sent to the wheelchair from the joystick is in proportion to how far the joystick is pushed from the center position.

The control output can be one of several electrical signals. A change in electrical resistance can be used to indicate the position of the joystick. This type of joystick is called a resistive joystick. As the joystick is moved left, the electrical resistance is increased, and as the joystick is moved to the right, the electrical resistance is decreased. Another independent change in resistance is used to indicate the position of the joystick fore and aft. A change in inductance can also be used to signal the position of the joystick. Two independent inductors (i.e., coils) vary with the position of the joystick in the same manner that the resistance does with resistive type. Digital joysticks based on a new standard called M3S are being introduced, especially in the European market. These joysticks may offer improved immunity to interference from sources such as police radios, cellular phones, ham radios, and even the electric motors of the wheelchair itself.

### 8.4.2 Sip-&-Puff

Sip-&-Puff switches are used primarily by people with tetraplegia who do not have functional use of their arms or hands. A Sip-&-Puff access device consists of a replaceable straw located near the mouth. The wheelchair is controlled by a sequence of pulling and pushing air through the straw with the mouth. These systems can be set up in a variety of configurations. Generally, the user will sip a specific number of times to indicate a direction, and puff to confirm the choice and activate the movement of the wheelchair. It is common for an auxiliary display to be used with Sip-&-Puff to provide feedback to the user. This display is often an LCD flat panel which is capable of displaying about 20 characters.

### 8.4.3 Switches

An array of switches can be used for the directional input of a wheelchair. The control scheme is similar to that of a switched joystick, except a combination of switch activations are rarely used for directional input. Switches are indicated for individuals who have good control over an anatomical site not usually used to control a wheelchair. An individual with a disability might, for example, have better motor control over a foot than a hand. An array of large switches mounted to the footrest could then be used as a direction input. Switches are also a primary means for computer access. Often one switch is used to toggle between the functions of computer access and powered wheelchair control. In computer access mode, the switches are used with any number of coding schemes.

These coding schemes include International Morse Code, automatic scanning, step scanning, inverse scanning, array scanning, and multi-level scanning. Morse code has the advantage of only requiring one switch (although two switches can be used), but generally places the highest cognitive demands on the user of all of the different types of coding schemes. The common feature of the scanning methods is that the selection choices proceed until the user chooses the correct function or types the correct character. The act of selection can be through a time delay or the activation of a switch. In automatic scanning, the choices are presented to the user on a computer screen or LCD panel with a preset time delay between each choice. When the desired choice is presented, the user must activate a switch before the next choice is shown. With step scanning the user switches from one choice to the next with each press of the switch. A delay on any one choice indicates acceptance of that function or character. Inverse scanning is the reverse operation of automatic. The switch is held down until the desired choice is reached, and then released to finalize the selection. All three of the scanning methods can be further modified to mixed use. One such modification would be to use one switch to step through the choices and a second switch to accept the choice.

Array scanning uses four switches to guide a cursor through an x-y grid of choices; a fifth switch with a time delay is used for the selection process. The switch arrangement in array scanning is highly applicable to both powered wheelchair control and computer access. This is due to the similarity in skills necessary to master each task.

Multi-level scanning is similar to the above methods, but after the selection of a choice, a new menu is presented. The final function or character is entered from this new menu. The number of levels can also be increased. With all of the possibilities for computer access and the ability to use unusual access sites, switches provide one of the most versatile powered wheelchair control inputs. The disadvantage is the same as for a switched joystick—there is no proportional control of the wheelchair's speed with switched control.

### 8.4.4 Ultrasonic and Infrared

Many of the input devices described in this section can be used for more than the control of powered wheelchairs. Two common additional uses are environmental control and computer access. In some cases, the computer is mounted to the wheelchair, but often it is at a fixed site. In this case, there must be a method for the linkage of the computer to the control device. Older systems that were used primarily for environmental control used ultrasonic signals to transmit information. Newer designs are based on infrared for both environmental control and computer access.

## 8.5 Integrated Controls

Many powered wheelchair users require multiple assistive devices (e.g., wheelchair, environmental control unit, communication device, computer access device). Integrated controls allow the user to control more than one assistive device through a single input device. Typically, this is the device chosen to control the powered wheelchair. If the powered wheelchair is optimized to the driver as described previously, then the appropriate hardware and software protocol can be used to interconnect various devices. This would provide the user effective control of a variety of electronic assistive devices. *Integrated controls* is the term used to describe plug-and-play for assistive devices. Ideally, all electronic assistive devices would use compatible communication protocols and interconnect hardware. The need for integrated controls is illustrated by the walking/talking problem. Many powered wheelchair users who use augmentative communication devices cannot operate both systems simultaneously (i.e., the walking-and-talking problem). Neither of these systems requires constant vigilance, but they are limited by their input structure and inability to communicate over a common communications bus. If the powered wheelchair and augmentative communication system both could be controlled with the same input device and communicate over a common data bus, then shared control would permit the user to toggle between driving and talking states. The two subsystems maintain speech and safe driving while the other subsystem is being controlled by the user. This case and others like it have prompted work on a worldwide assistive device electronic communications standard.

The RESNA Serial Interface Standards Committee and Trace Center have made significant advances toward developing a worldwide serial interface communications standard between powered wheelchairs and other devices. This work and the work of European groups has formed the basis for a draft ISO standard (TC 173/SC-1/WG-7). The Multiple Master Multiple Slave (M3S) initiative is a European Economic Community (EEC) effort to develop a standard interface between various electronic assistive technologies. M3S is based on the CAN (controller area network) protocol used in many modern automobiles.

Many assistive devices include at least one input device (e.g., joystick, head-operated switch, extremity-operated switch, or voice recognition system) and at least one actuator (e.g., wheelchair, environmental control unit, robot, voice synthesizer). The M3S bus is suitable for general purpose applications with the proper systems and subsystems (see Fig. 8.9). The M3S standard is essentially the CAN bus with additional lines used to increase margins of safety and reliability. The advantage of M3S over current technology is the ability to simply interface multiple assistive devices and other technical products within the user's environment. The M3S bus permits control of multiple actuators with a single input device. This allows the input device to be optimized to the user's abilities, and subsequently used to control a number of actuators.

The M3S standard would specify a basic hardware architecture, a bus communication system, and a configuration method. A basic M3S bus consists of 7 wires: 2 power lines, 2 CAN lines, 2 safety lines, 1 shield, and 1 special support line

**FIGURE 8.9**  Illustration of multiple master multiple slave (M3S) architecture. Multiple input devices and multiple actuators can be on the M3S bus simultaneously. A system navigator works with the command and configuration module (CCM) to set priorities, perform handshaking, and for device identification. The CCM monitors and controls communication between various components of the system.

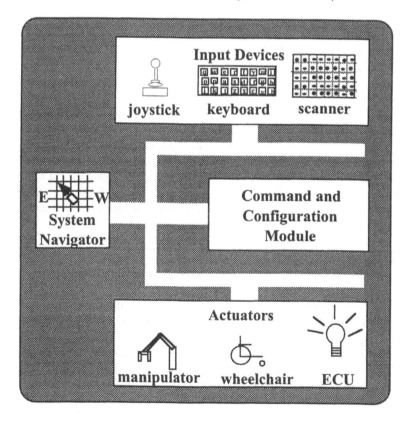

(harness number). The M3S bus is intelligent in that it is easily configured to meet each user's individual needs. The intelligence in the system exists in the controllers of the individual input devices, actuators, and control and configuration module (CCM). The CCM deals with the processing necessary to configure the system and the ongoing need to monitor the safety of the system. The CCM is linked to a simple display that allows the user to select and operate each actuator. The CCM processor itself contains the master menu used to select individual actuators. The M3S system possesses the capability to access a wide range of devices via wireless link (infrared or radio) to a home bus.

## 8.6 Batteries

The battery energy storage system is recognized as one of the most significant limiting factors in powered wheelchair performance. Battery life and capacity are important. If battery life can be improved, the powered wheelchair user will have longer, reliable performance. An increase in battery capacity will allow powered wheelchair users to travel greater distances with batteries that weigh and measure the same as existing wheelchair batteries. Most importantly, increases in battery capacity will enable the use of smaller and lighter batteries. Because batteries account for such a large proportion of both the weight and volume of current powered wheelchair systems, wheelchair manufacturers must base much of their design around the battery package.

Powered wheelchairs typically incorporate 24-volt d.c. energy systems. The energy for the wheelchair is provided by two deep cycle lead-acid batteries connected in series. Either wet cell or gel cell batteries are used. Wet cell batteries may require greater maintenance, but can have the ability to store greater energy than gel cells at temperatures from freezing to room temperature. Wet cell batteries also cost less than gel cell batteries. Gel cells may be required for transport by commercial air carriers.

Battery technology for wheelchair users remains unchanged despite the call for improvements by powered wheelchair users. This may be in part due to relatively low number of units purchased, about 500,000 per annum, when compared to automotive applications, about 6.6 million per annum by a single manufacturer. Wheelchair batteries are typically rated at 12 volts and 30–90 ampere-hours capacity at room temperature. A powered wheelchair draws about 10 amps during use. The range of the powered wheelchair is directly proportional to the ampere-hour rating for the operating temperature.

Batteries are grouped by size. Group size is indicated by a standard number. The group size defines the dimensions of the battery (Table 8.1). The ampere-hour rating defines the battery's capacity.

It is important that the appropriate charger be used with each battery set. Many battery chargers automatically reduce the amount of current delivered to the battery as the battery reaches full charge. This helps to prevent damage to the battery from boiling. The rate at which wet and gel cell batteries charge is significantly different. Some chargers are capable of operating with both types of batteries. Many require setting the charger for the appropriate battery type. Most wheelchairs contain two 12-volts batteries connected in series, and are charged simultaneously with a 24-volt battery charger.

**TABLE 8.1  Standard powered wheelchair battery group sizes (units are in inches)**

| Group Number | Length | Width | Height |
|---|---|---|---|
| U1 | $7^3/4$ | $5^3/16$ | $7^5/16$ |
| 22NF | $9^7/16$ | $5^1/2$ | $8^{15}/16$ |
| 24 | $10^1/4$ | $6^{13}/16$ | $8^7/8$ |
| 27 | $12^1/16$ | $6^{13}/16$ | $8^7/8$ |

## 8.7 Electrical Systems

### 8.7.1 Electromagnetic Compatibility

Electric-powered wheelchairs may be susceptible to electromagnetic interference (EMI) present in the ambient environment. Some level of EMI immunity is necessary to ensure the safety of powered wheelchair users. While there are many advantages to digital and microcontroller based designs, these components can be sensitive to electromagnetic radiation and electrostatic discharge (ESD). Many people attach accessories (e.g., car stereos, computers, communication systems) to their powered wheelchairs, which share the batteries. Such interconnection may increase the susceptibility of other system components to EMI. A number of companies make electric-powered devices designed to operate on powered wheelchairs to provide postural support, pressure relief, environmental control, and motor vehicle operation. These devices may alter the EMI compatibility of powered wheelchairs as provided by the original equipment manufacturer.

There have been some cases of powered wheelchairs behaving erratically for unexplained reasons. Field strengths have been measured at 20 V/m from a 15 W hand-held cellular telephone, and 8 V/m from a 1 W hand-held cellular telephone. Picofarad capacitors are currently being used on wheelchair motors to filter EMI. The U.S. Food and Drug Administration (FDA) has begun to require that a warning sticker be placed on the wheelchair. The FDA Center for Devices and Radiological Health (CDRH) has investigated several powered wheelchairs and scooters and have found them to exhibit some degree of susceptibility to EMI. The CDRH found some wheelchairs to be susceptible to field strengths as low as 5 V/m, which is equivalent to a 4 W hand-held radio transmitter at a distance of 2 m.

EMI testing is expensive and complicated. Standards are required to ensure that test results are valid and consistent among test laboratories. Some wheelchairs have sheet metal components or enclosures that may affect the field strength around critical components (e.g., controller, joystick, significant portions of loom). The wheelchair must be exposed in the frontal and lateral planes. The wheelchair must be irradiated from the sides that provide maximum exposure to electronic components and the wiring harness. No part of the wheelchair should be closer than one meter from the floor and ceiling when testing in a shielded environment or anechoic chamber. The supports for the wheelchair must be nonconductive.

When the wheelchair is exposed to EM radiation, the brakes must not release. Nonelectrical contact methods (e.g., audio sensing, optical sensing) of measuring brake release or wheelchair movement are preferable. The percentage change in wheel speed during exposure to EM interference should be referenced to the nominal wheel speed for that test interval. The variation in absolute forward speed is to be within 30% of the nominal forward speed. The differential speed between the two wheels is to be within 30% of each other.

### 8.7.2 Motors

The electric motors are the heart of any powered wheelchair system (Figure 8.10). They convert the electrical energy of the batteries to mechanical work. There are several types of electric motors. Most powered wheelchairs use armature controlled, permanent magnet direct current motors. However, other electric motors have been used in prototypes and may eventually be used in production.

## 8.8 Drive Trains

The efficiency of a powered wheelchair is affected by the drive system. An efficient drive system can extend the distance covered on the energy stored in the batteries. Pulse width modulated servo-amplifiers can be designed to have high efficiencies, in excess of 80%. The motors of the wheelchair are often connected to the wheels through a gear box or pulley set. The pulley set or gear box decreases the speed of the motor and increases the torque seen at the wheels. This allows the motor to

**FIGURE 8.10** Schematic diagram for an electric-powered wheelchair

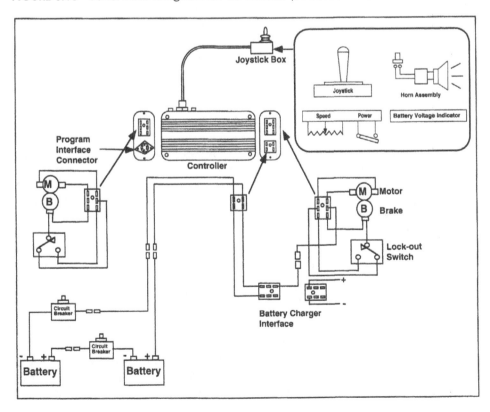

operate at about its rated speed, where it is more efficient. However, mechanical losses in the gear boxes or pulley set are also causes of inefficiency.

Three common methods are used to reduce the speed of the motor and to increase the torque at the wheel: a worm gear right angle drive, a spur gear reducer, and a belt-pulley system. The worm gear drive, although compact, is not very efficient because the sliding contact between the worm and the worm gear creates high friction forces. A spur gear uses a small pinion, driven by the motor, and a larger gear. Involute cutting of the gear teeth permits the pinion and gear combination to turn with rolling friction, rather than the constant sliding friction of the worm gear. However, the spur gear arrangement requires the motor to be orthogonal to the gears, which restricts folding the wheelchair frame. Efficiency of a gear train is affected by speed. The efficiency of a powered wheelchair worm gear drive is about 70% compared to 80% for a spur gear drive. Belt drives vary from about 60% to 90%. Helical timing drive (HTD) belt systems, though not commonly used on powered wheelchairs, have been shown to be about 90% efficient on motorcycles and other electric vehicles.

Lubrication is also an important factor to consider when studying gear box efficiency. Many wheelchair gear boxes are designed for other applications and are filled with high viscosity grease by the factory. This is because the gear drives are often designed for higher speed and load applications. At the relatively low speeds of wheelchair use, this high viscosity grease can cause excess drag. A polytetrafluoroethylene (PTFE) can be used to improve the efficiency of powered wheelchair drives because of its good lubrication properties at low speeds. PTFE is a solid lubricant; very small solid particles slide over one another with a very low coefficient of friction. As two surfaces slide over one another the PTFE particles act as microscopic ball bearings. Only small amounts of PTFE are required for lubrication, in contrast to total immersion used with standard grease. About a 5% improvement in performance can be gained using PTFE.

## 8.9 Performance Characteristics

The capabilities of electric-powered wheelchairs are continually expanding. Since the introduction of the microprocessor, powered wheelchairs have been able to accommodate the needs of people with more severe disabilities. Microprocessors permit some features of the control system to be tuned to the abilities of the driver. Products now in development will allow the wheelchair to adjust itself to the habits and abilities of the user. Wheelchairs will be able to help drivers avoid obstacles or negotiate environments. Electric-powered wheelchairs will acquire greater capabilities. Stand-up wheelchairs that function as the primary wheelchair are rapidly improving. Wheelchairs that raise, lower, and provide standing support are on the horizon. Stair-climbing wheelchairs that are functional for daily use as an individual's primary wheelchair are being designed all over the world.

Microcontrollers are used to tune the powered wheelchair system to the user's individual needs. Many wheelchair controllers permit adjusting maximum speed, yaw velocity and acceleration, acceleration and deceleration rate, input filter parameters, and input device deadzone. A number of methods have been used to vary controller parameters. An external control unit can be used to interface with the wheelchair controller and, through a series of switches or key strokes, the wheelchair controller parameters are tuned. Another approach is to use the user interface (e.g., joystick, sip-&-puff device, ultrasonic control device) to tune the wheelchair controller. This is accomplished by selecting the program mode, usually done by using a switch. Then a series of "menus" is used to tune each parameter of interest.

Microcontrollers improve control not only by permitting repeatable tuning and control of certain system parameters, but also by allowing implementation of dynamic control algorithms. The most common control variable is speed. A typical speed control algorithm uses tracking, or contour, control to have the wheelchair automatically follow the desired speed profile set by the user, by varying the input device, regardless of terrain or slope. Hence the wheelchair/rider system will move at the same speed up an incline as it will down an incline for the same user-desired speed.

Looking into the future, wheelchair users will benefit from better products. Some companies are developing and even introducing innovations in service. The long-distance diagnosis of wheelchair problems by on-board modems and other technologies will become available. People will be able to plug their wheelchair into a telephone and have the dealer or manufacturer download maintenance and driving records. This information will be used to provide maintenance and plan repairs. Repairs will be made faster and more efficiently, with less inconvenience to the consumer. In the future, wheelchair manufacturers and dealers will work more closely to provide better service. Models are already being employed where service personnel come to the consumer. In some cases, dealers provide loaner wheelchairs similar to the consumer's personal wheelchair.

Reforms in the payments for durable medical equipment, including wheelchairs, will require more flexible payment plans. It is likely that manufacturers will need to introduce financing programs similar to those offered by automobile manufacturers. People with disabilities are a growing segment of the consumer market, and are gradually becoming more affluent. This market trend will help consumers obtain those features that are not covered by insurance. Dealers and manufacturers will need to provide clinicians and consumers with guidance to assemble a financing package, including funding from multiple sources (e.g., private insurance, government programs, personal finances). Powered wheelchairs are the most exciting area for future technological development, for personal freedom, and as a business proposition.

## References and Further Reading

Amori R. D. (1992) Vocomotion—An intelligent voice-control system for powered wheelchairs. *Proceedings RESNA International '92*, 421–423.

Aylor J. H., Thieme A., Johnson B. W. (1992) A battery state-of-charge indicator. *IEEE Transaction on Industrial Electronics*, 39, 5, 398–409.

Aylor J. H., Byun H., Kauzlarich J. J. (1991) A user survey on backup power for powered wheelchairs. *Proceedings RESNA 14th Annual Conference*, Kansas City, MO, 234–236.

Aylor J. H., Johnson B. (1981) *Proceedings RESNA 4th Annual Conference*, Washington DC, 87–90.

Bailey D. M., DeFelice T. (1991) Evaluating movement for switch use in an adult with severe physical and cognitive impairments. *American Journal of Occupational Therapy*, 45(1):76–79.

Baldwin J. D., Thacker J. G. (1991) Structural reliability assessment techniques applied to tubular wheelchair frames. *Proceedings RESNA 14th Annual Conference,* Kansas City, MO, 237–239.

Baumgartner E. T., Yoder J. D. (1994) An automatically-guided powered wheelchair for the severely disabled. *Proceedings 17th Annual RESNA Conference,* Nashville, TN, 350–352.

Bell D. A., Levine S. P., Koren Y., Jaros L. A., Borenstein J. (1993) Shared control of the NavChair obstacle-avoiding wheelchair. *Proceedings RESNA 16th Annual Conference,* Las Vegas, NV, 370–372.

Bell D.A., Levine S.P., Koren Y., Jaros L.A., Borenstein J. (1994) Design criteria for obstacle avoidance in a shared-control system. *Proceedings 17th Annual RESNA Conference,* Nashville, TN, 581–583.

Bennett L. (1987) Powered wheelchair bucking. *Journal of Rehabilitation Research and Development,* 24, 2, 81–86.

Bourhis G., Pino P. (1993) Man/machine cooperation for the piloting of an intelligent electric wheelchair. *Proceedings Second European Conference on the Advancement of Rehabilitation,* 13.1.

Brooks L. (1994) Use of devices for mobility by the elderly. *Wisconsin Medical Journal,* January.

Brown K. E., Inigo R. M., Johnson B. W. (1987) An adaptable optimal controller for electric wheelchairs. *Journal of Rehabilitation Research and Development,* 24, 2, 87–98.

Brubaker C. E., (1988) Survey of powered wheelchair problems and features. *Proceedings of Wheelchair IV,* Washington DC, RESNA Press, 68–75.

Carlson C. W. (1995) Understanding EMI. *Team Rehab Report,* January, 32–33.

Chase J., Bailey D. M. (1990) Evaluating potential for powered mobility. *American Journal of Occupational Therapy,* 44(12):1125–1129.

Choy T. T. C., Koo J. T. K. (1992) An electric wheelchair with special features. *Proceedings RESNA International '92,* Toronto, Canada, 310–312.

Cooper R. A. (1994) Observability and controllability of scooters. *Proc IEEE-EMBS 16th International Conference,* 16(1):488–489.

Craig I., Nisbet P. (1993) The smart wheelchair: An augmentative mobility "toolkit." *Proceedings Second European Conference on the Advancement of Rehabilitation,* 13.1.

Department of Veterans Affairs. (1990) Choosing a wheelchair system. *Journal of Rehabilitation Research and Development—Clinical Supplement No. 2,* March.

Dunham J., Roberson G., Inigo R. M. (1993) A direct current to three-phase invertor for electric wheelchair propulsion. *Proceedings RESNA 16th Annual Conference,* Las Vegas, NV, 373–375.

*Electromagnetic Compatibility for Industrial Process Measurement and Control Equipment.* (1984) IEC 801-3.

*Electromagnetic Compatibility Requirements for Powered Wheelchairs and Motorized Scooters.* (1994) ANSI/RESNA Draft Standard, version 1.5, November.

Fisher W. E., Garrett R. E., Seeger B. (1988) Testing of gel-electrolyte batteries for wheelchairs. *Journal of Rehabilitation Research and Development,* 25, 2, 27–32.

Fiss J., Markmeller B., Luebben A. J., Collins R. A. (1993) More patterns in power mobility repairs. *Proceedings RESNA 16th Annual Conference,* Las Vegas, NV, 376–378.

Ford M. R., Kauzlarich J. J., Thacker J. G. (1992) Powered wheelchair gearbox lubrication. *Proceedings RESNA International '92,* Toronto, Canada, 316–318.

Ford M. R., Thacker J. G., Kauzlarich J. J. (1991) Improved wheelchair gearbox efficiency. *Proceedings RESNA 14th Annual Conference,* Kansas City, MO., 146–147.

Grant D. A., Gowar J. (1989). *Power MOSFETS theory and applications.* New York, NY: John Wiley & Sons.

Gregson P. H., Kirby R. H. (1992) Development of a 'smart' powered wheelchair: A progress report. *Proceedings RESNA International '92*, 424–425.

Guerette P., Caves K., Nakai R., Sumi E., McNeal D., Hoffer M. (1994) Determining the appropriateness of integrated control of assistive devices. *Rehabilitation Research and Development Progress Reports 1992–1993*, 408–409.

Hendriks J. L., Rosen M. J., Berube N. L. J., Aisen M. L.(1991) A second-generation joystick for people disabled by tremor. *Proceedings RESNA 14th Annual Conference*, Kansas City, MO., 248–250.

Hoyer H., Hoelper R. (1994) Intelligent omnidirectional wheelchair with a flexible configurable functionality. *Proceedings 17th Annul RESNA Conference*, Nashville, TN, 353–355.

Inigo R. M., Shafik K. T., Park C. W. (1990) An improved AC-DC converter for electric wheelchair propulsion. *Proceedings RESNA 14th Annual Conference*, Kansas City, MO., 148–150.

Jaffe D. L. (1981) Smart wheelchair. *Proceedings RESNA 4th Annual Conference*, Washington DC, 91–93.

Jamieson J. R., Nowack P. F. Model-based reasoning for industrial control and diagnosis. *Control Engineering*, 39(7):120–128.

Jaros L. A., Bell D. A., Levine S. P., Borenstein J., Koren Y. (1993) NAVCHAIR: Design of an assistive navigation system for wheelchairs. *Proceedings 16th Annual RESNA Conference*, Las Vegas, NV, 379–381.

Johnson B. W., Aylor J. H. (1981) Modelling of wheelchair dynamics for the design of a microcomputer-based controller. *Proceedings IEEE-IECI Annual Conference*, 70–75.

Junkman B. C., Aylor J. H., Kauzlarich J. J. (1988) Estimation of battery state-of-charge during charging using the charge recovery process. *Proceedings RESNA 11th Annual Conference*, 280–281.

Kamenetz H. (1969) *The Wheelchair Book: Mobility for the Disabled.* Springfield, IL: C. C. Thomas.

Kauzlarich J. J., Thacker J. G., Ford M. R. (1993) Electric wheelchair drive train efficiency. *Proceedings RESNA 16th Annual Conference*, Las Vegas, NV, 310–312.

Kauzlarich J. J., Dwyer M. A. (1982) Test of nickel-zinc battery for wheelchairs. *Proceedings RESNA 5th Annual Conference*, 110.

Kauzlarich J. J., Ulrich V., Bresler M., Bruning T. (1983) Wheelchair batteries: Driving cycles and testing. *Journal of Rehabilitation Research and Development*, 20(1):31–43.

Korba L., Park G., Farley R., Durie N., Roy O. Z. (1990) Development of a wheelchair controller: Conversion to a microcontroller. *Proceedings*, Washington, DC: RESNA Press, 199–200.

LaPlante, M. (1991) The demographics of disability. *Milbank Quarterly*, 69 Suppl 1–2:55–77

Lavanchy C. (1992) Comparative evaluation of major brands of lead-acid batteries. *Proceedings RESNA International Conference*, Toronto, Canada, 541–543.

Lefkowicz A. T., Wierwille W.W. (1992) Validation of a PC-based perspective-view wheelchair simulator. *Proceedings RESNA International '92*, 415–417.

Lipskin R. (1970) An evaluation program for powered wheelchair control systems. *Bulletin of Prosthetics Research*, 121–129.

Martin D. L., Aylor J. H. (1993) Improving wheelchair efficiency through intelligent diagnostics. *Proceedings RESNA 16th Annual Conference*, Las Vegas, NV, 367–369.

McNeil J. M., Americans with Disabilities: 1991–92. *Data From the Survey of Income and Program Participation*, P70–33.

Mohamadi M. C, Aylor J. H., Schwab A. J. (1992) A fault-tolerant optical joystick control integrated circuit for a powered wheelchair. *Proceedings RESNA International '92*, Toronto, Canada, 307–309.

National Center for Health Statistics (1992). Public Use Data Documentation, National Health Interview Survey of Assistive Devices, 1990. NCHS, Hyattsville, MD.

Nisbet P. D., Craig I. (1994) Mobility and mobility training for severely disabled children: Results of the "Smart" wheelchair project. *Proceedings 17th Annual RESNA Conference*, Nashville, TN, 41–343.

Orpwood R. (1993) A powered mobility aid for pre-school children with cerebral palsy. *Proceedings Second European Conference on the Advancement of Rehabilitation*, 9.1.

Pence R., Inigo C., Inigo R. M., (1991) A new method for electric wheelchair propulsion. *Proceedings RESNA 14th Annual Conference*, Kansas City, MO., 151–153.

Philipson L., Heckathorne C. W. (1981) The use of a microprocessor as a versatile controller for a powered wheelchair. *Proceedings RESNA 4th Annual Conference*, Washington DC, 84–86.

Pickles B., Topping A. (1994) Community care for Canadian seniors: An exercise in educational planning. *Disability and Rehabilitation*, 16(3):181–189.

Powell F., Inigo R. M. (1992) Pressure sensitive joystick and controller for front wheel steering wheelchairs. *Proceedings RESNA International '92*, Toronto, Canada, 304–306.

Powell F., Inigo R. M. (1992) Microprocessor-based D.C. brushless motor controller for wheelchair propulsion. *Proceedings RESNA International '92*, Toronto, Canada, 313–315.

Prevalence of Disabilities and Associated Health Conditions—United States, 1991–1992. *The On-line Journal of Current Clinical Trials*. 4, 164 950105 MMWR 43(40), Oct. 14, 1994.

Ramamurthi K., Agogino A. M. (1993) Real-time expert system for fault-tolerant supervisory control. *ASME Journal of Dynamic Systems, Measurement, and Control*, 115:219–225.

Riley P. O., Rosen M. J. (1987) Evaluating manual control devices for those with tremor disability. *Journal of Rehabilitation Research and Development*, 24, 2, 99–110.

Schauer J., Kelso D. P., Vanderheiden G. C. (1990) Development of a serial auxiliary control interface for powered wheelchairs. *Proceedings RESNA 13th Annual Conference*, Washington, DC, 191–192.

Schlemer M. R., Johnson D., Granic J. (1993) Powered wheelchair mobility simulator. *Proceedings RESNA 16th Annual Conference*, Las Vegas, NV, 357–359.

Scooters (1991) *Product Comparison and Evaluation*. REquest, Rehabilitation Engineering Center, National Rehabilitation Hospital.

Scott C. M., Prior R. E. (1978) Mobility engineering for the severely handicapped. *Bulletin of Prosthetics Research*, 10(30), 248–255.

Shung J. B., Tomizuka M., Auslander D. M., Stout G. (1983) Feedback control and simulation of a wheelchair. *ASME Journal of Dynamics Systems, Measurement and Control*, 105, 96–100.

Shung J. B., Stout G., Tomizuka M., Auslander D. M. (1983) Dynamic modeling of a wheelchair on a slope. *ASME Journal of Dynamics Systems, Measurement and Control*, 105, 101–106.

Silberberg, J. L. (1993) Performance degradation of electronic medical devices due to electromagnetic interference. *Compliance Engineering*, 25–39, Fall.

Sonn U., Grimby, G., (1994) Assistive devices in an elderly population studied at 70–76 years of age. *Disability and Rehabilitation*, 16, 2, 85–93.

Stefanov D. H. (1994) Powered wheelchair controller with dynamic stability checking. *Rehabilitation Research and Development Progress Reports 1992–1993*, 410–411.

Stout G. (1979) Some aspects of high performance indoor/outdoor wheelchairs. *Bulletin of Prosthetics Research*, 10(32), 330–332.

Teft D., Furumasu J., Guerette P. (1992) Cognitive predictors of successful powered wheelchair control in very young children. *Proceedings RESNA International '92*, 412–414.

Thacker J. (1978) Wheelchair dynamics. *University of Virginia REC Annual Report*, 41–44.

Ulrich V., Bresier M., Kauzlarich J. J. (1980) Wheelchair battery testing. *Proceedings RESNA 3rd Annual Conference*, 132–133.

van Woerden J. A. (1993) M3S: A general purpose interface for the rehabilitation environment. *Proceedings Second European Conference Advancement Rehabilitation Technology*, Stockholm, Sweden, 22.1.

Wakaumi H., Nakamura K., Matsumura T. (1992) Development of an automated wheelchair guided by a magnetic ferrite marker lane. *Journal of Rehabilitation Research and Development*, 29, 1, 27–34.

Whitmeyer J. J. (1993) A modification of joystick assemblies to limit the excursion and force applied by the user. *Proceedings RESNA 16th Annual Conference*, Las Vegas, NV, 360–361.

Widman L. M., Cooper R. A., Robertson R. N., Ster J. F., Grey T, (1993) Evaluation of an isometric joystick for power wheelchair control, *Proceedings 16th Annual RESNA Conference*, Las Vegas, NV, 364–366.

Wilson A. B., Jr., (1992) *Wheelchairs: A Prescription Guide, 2nd ed.* New York, NY, Demos.

Winkler F. W., Zuber D. (1991) Development of an analog controller interface to relate steered front wheels to powered rear wheels. *Proceedings RESNA 14th Annual Conference*, Kansas City, MO., 140–142.

Witters D., Weigle R. (1993) FDA/CDRH proposed EMC addition to ANSI/RESNA WC/14. US Food and Drug Administration, June 13.

Witters D. M., Ruggera P.S. Electromagnetic compatibility (EMC) of powered wheelchairs and scooters. *Proceedings 16th IEEE-EMBS International Conference*, Baltimore, MD, 16, 2, 894–895.

# CHAPTER

# 9

# Specialized Wheelchairs

*Chapter Goals*

☑ To know how to set up and adjust specialized wheelchairs
☑ To know state-of-the-art research and product development
☑ To understand person-to-device interface and access

## 9.1 Reclining Wheelchairs

Reclining wheelchairs allow the user to change sitting posture through the use of a simple interface, e.g., switch (see Figure 9.1). Some common reclining wheelchairs are shown in Figure 9.2. Changing seating posture can extend the amount of time a person can safely remain seated without damaging tissue or becoming fatigued. Determining the optimal range of seating postures is difficult and is best approached by clinical teams. Reclining wheelchairs assist in performing pressure relief. Changing seating position redistributes pressure on weightbearing surfaces, alters the load on postural musculature, and changes circulation. Changing position can also facilitate respiration. Elevating the legs while lowering the torso can improve venous return and decrease fluid pooling in the lower extremities

If the joints of the wheelchair do not follow the anatomical paths of the user, shear forces will result. Reclining systems that attempt to follow anatomical joint

**FIGURE 9.1** Schematic for reclining wheelchair seat. Arrows indicate the displacement between the user's back and the wheelchair backrest. Unless the back slides or the wheelchair's pivots follow the body's anatomical joint centers, shear forces will result.

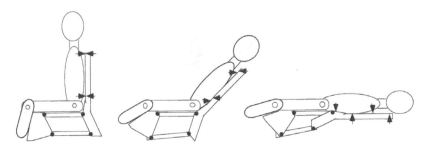

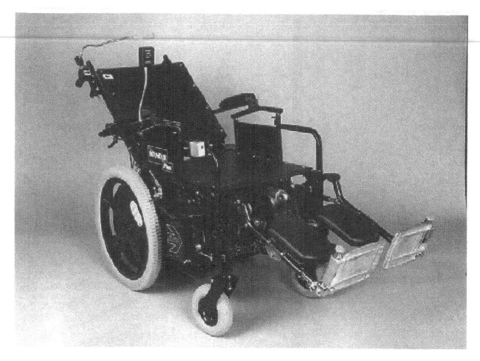

A

**FIGURE 9.2**　Adult reclining seat wheelchairs. Both of these wheelchairs include powered elevating legrests and powered reclining backrest. (Photographs courtesy of (a) 21st Century Scientific, and (b) Wheelchairs of Kansas)

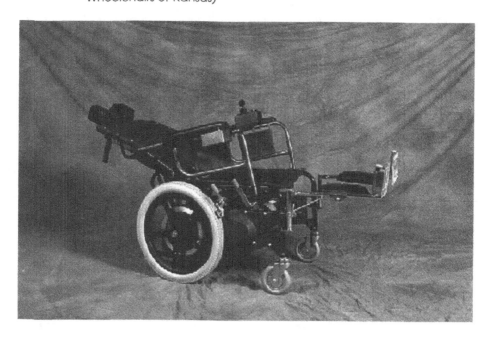

B

centers are called low-shear. These forces can be minimized by allowing the seat and backrest to freely translate while rotating about a hinge joint located near the user's hip; these systems are called zero-shear. Without an anti-shear mechanism up to 11 centimeters of displacement can take place between the person's back and the wheelchair's backrest. Displacement may also take place at the knee if the axis of rotation of the anatomical knee and wheelchair do not coincide. This does not usually present a problem because of the low mass of the lower limbs, which move in response to the wheelchair. The length of the legrests presents a greater potential problem. If the legrests are too short, then high forces can be placed on the bottom of the feet in the reclined position. Therefore, legrest length should be carefully adjusted and verified throughout the range of motion.

## 9.2 Tilt-in-Space Wheelchairs

Tilt-in-space systems are often characterized by the location of their pivot mechanisms (Figure 9.3). When the location is near the backrest, the chair is said to have a rear-pivot system. When tilting, the rear-pivot system raises the user's knees above his/her whole body center of gravity. The pivot point can also be placed under the front edge of the seat base, in which case the chair is said to have a forward-pivot system. With forward-pivot systems the user's buttocks are lowered to effect tilting. A counterbalance effect, which reduces the forces required to adjust position, can be obtained by placing the pivot near the center of the seat (i.e., center-pivot system). Springs and dampeners can be used to provide a suspended seating system. The springs and dampeners can be adjusted to create a floating-pivot system. Floating-pivot systems can provide a wide variety of tilt angles. Tilt-in-space systems must be stabilized in their resting positions. Three common methods are used to maintain seating position with tilt-in-space systems: mechanical locking pin, cable lock, and adjustable gas springs. Tilt-in-space wheelchairs with a cable lock are shown in Figure 9.4. All of these locks have been proven effective. There are some difficulties with tilt-in-space wheelchairs. The wheelchairs are heavier

**FIGURE 9.3**  Schematic for tilt-in-space mechanism. The user remains in the same position but orientation changes. This allows pressure to be redistributed.

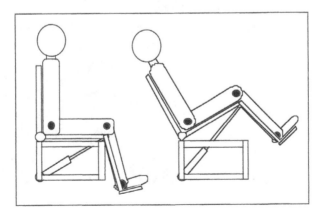

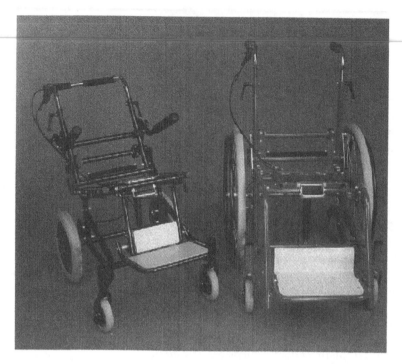

A

**FIGURE 9.4**   Photograph of tilt-in-space wheelchairs with upholstery removed (a). Both wheelchairs use cable locking mechanisms. (b) A tilt-in-space wheelchair (Photographs courtesy of (a) Otto Bock Orthopaedic Industry, Inc., and (b) Permobil, Sweden)

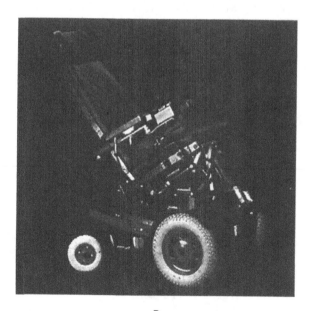

B

than standard wheelchairs, are less stable, and can require greater turning diameter when reclined.

A potential problem with tilt-in-space and reclining seating systems is that the body may not remain in a stable position after transitioning through several seating orientations. Sliding or stretching during reclining or tilting can cause undesirable shear forces, excite spasticity, and bunch clothing.

## 9.3 Variable Seat Height Wheelchairs

Many activities can be promoted by using a variable seat height wheelchair. Lowering seat height can make it simpler to get under tables and desks. Picking up objects from the floor can also be assisted by an adjustable seat height. Access to the floor is an important feature for promoting the cognitive and social development of children. Children often play, explore the environment, and interact with other children at ground level. Children who use wheelchairs can benefit from being able to access the ground. Some wheelchairs provide powered floor access for children (see Figure 9.5). Adults who use wheelchairs may also desire the ability to lower the wheelchair seat to the floor. This can allow parents who are wheelchair users to play with their children, or people to garden. As the person is lowered to the floor by the wheelchair, stability is influenced. Some wheelchairs move the batteries as they lower the person in order to maintain the balance of the wheelchair and rider. Some seat-lowering mechanisms alter the legrest angle in order to get closer to the ground. It is important to assure that the rider has a suitable range of motion to use this feature safely.

The ability to raise or lower the seat can also provide several advantages (Figure 9.6). The mechanism for raising or lowering the seat may be manual or

**FIGURE 9.5** Electric-powered wheelchair with the ability to lower the rider to near floor level (Photograph courtesy of Permobil, Sweden).

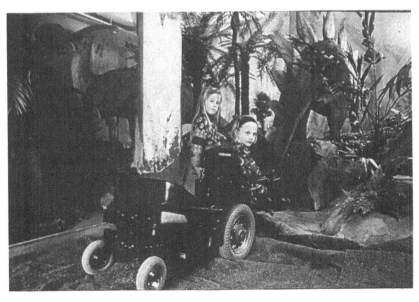

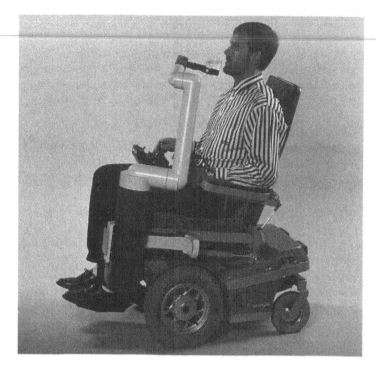

A

**FIGURE 9.6** Electric-powered wheelchair with a lowering/elevating seat. The seat is in the lowest position. A robotic arm has been mounted to the wheelchair to aid in manipulating objects (a). A woman using an elevating wheelchair seat to apply cosmetics (b). (Photographs courtesy of Permobil, Sweden)

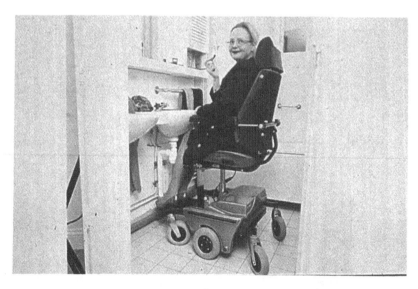

B

electrically powered. Lowering the seat makes access to desks and tables easier. When retrieving items from the floor or placing them in low cabinets, a lower seat height can be beneficial. Lowering the seat height tends to make the wheelchair more stable. Therefore, lowering the seat height can be helpful when maneuvering the wheelchair on steep ramps or slopes. The added stability of being able to lower the seat height can be of considerable benefit on slide slopes. Raising the seat height also offers several benefits. Items on high shelves or in high cabinets can be obtained by using an elevating seat. Elevating the seat height is also helpful for viewing people at eye level. Tasks such as cooking and washing can also be simplified with an elevating seat height. Many powered wheelchair controllers cause the speed of the wheelchair to decrease as the seat height is raised. This is because increasing seat height tends to decrease the stability of the wheelchair. Most wheelchair manufacturers do not recommend elevating the seat on a slope or uneven terrain.

## 9.4 Stand-up Wheelchairs

Stand-up wheelchairs are not a new phenomena, but they are gaining in popularity. As early as the 1950s people were developing stand-up wheelchairs. Early models were heavy and large, which limited their success. More recently stand-up wheelchairs have become lightweight and transportable (see Figure 9.7). Stand-up wheelchairs offer a variety of advantages over standard wheelchairs. They provide easy access to cabinets, shelves, counters, sinks, and many windows. Many activities around the home are made easier by using a stand-up wheelchair. Cooking, washing dishes, and ironing clothes are simple from a stand-up wheelchair and do not require significant home modifications. In the workplace, stand-up wheelchairs help to make presentations at "white board," to access copiers, and to interact with colleagues. The ability to perform some occupations is greatly enhanced by using a stand-up wheelchair. Machine operators or machinists can perform normal job functions with minimal modifications to the worksite using a stand-up wheelchair. Physicians and surgeons can examine patients and perform procedures safely and effectively using stand-up wheelchairs.

Greater integration of people with disabilities into society has created new avenues for specialized technologies. Stand-up wheelchair manufacturers have benefitted from the increased desire of people with disabilities to be active at home, school, and work, and in the community. In many cases stand-up wheelchairs allow people to perform activities without significant architectural modifications. This has tremendous potential for overcoming both physical and social barriers that have prevented wheelchair users from gaining greater access to employment, education, and community services. For example, a schoolteacher could use a stand-up wheelchair to conduct physics experiments at a standard laboratory bench without the need to completely remodel the entire classroom. This should not be interpreted to mean that society does not have an obligation to eliminate architectural and social barriers. However, specialized technology provides greater flexibility when making individual accommodations.

Stand-up wheelchairs are more complex than most manual or electric-powered wheelchairs. Several decisions must be made prior to selecting and fitting a stand-up wheelchair. The rehabilitation team must work with the individual to

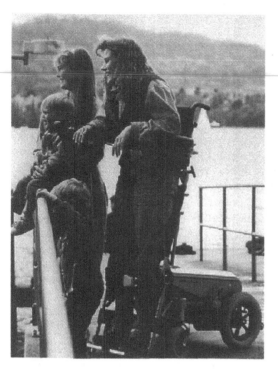
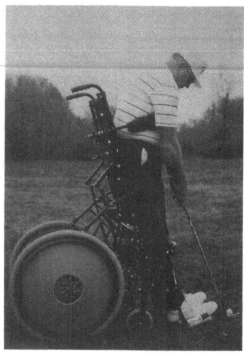

**A**

**B**

**FIGURE 9.7** Stand-up wheelchairs can assist with a variety of activities. A lightweight electric-powered stand-up wheelchair is shown in (a). Manually lifting and manually propelled stand-up wheelchairs are being used to play golf in (b). A father is playing with his children in (c) using a manually propelled stand-up wheelchair with power lifting mechanism. (Photographs courtesy of (a) Levo Incorporated, (b) LDC Corporation of America, and (c) Levo Incorporated)

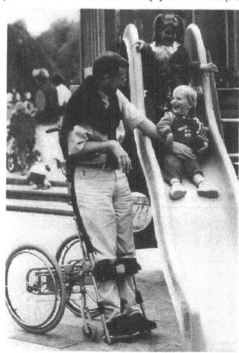

**C**

determine if the stand-up wheelchair should have an electric-powered base or whether it should be manually propelled. Stand-up features are integrated into some power wheelchairs with minimal trade-offs (i.e., no additional weight or size). Manually powered stand-up wheelchairs are heavier than lightweight manual wheelchairs. Currently the weight of manually propelled stand-up wheelchairs is between 30 and 60 pounds (13.6 to 27.3 kilograms). Some of the weight can be attributed to the lifting mechanism. All electric-powered wheelchairs with a stand-up feature use a separate electric drive system for the stand-up mechanism. Manually powered stand-up wheelchairs may use a manual lifting mechanism or an electric-powered lifting mechanism.

Greater strength is required to operate a manual lifting mechanism. For this reason, most stand-up wheelchairs use devices that reduce the effort required to manually move to a standing position. This has been accomplished using springs (e.g., coil or gas-filled) to help act against the force of gravity. Other stand-up wheelchairs use a cam mechanism that provides the person more leverage when just lifting from the sitting position and less as he/she nears the upright position. Effectively, the amount of force required to transition from sitting to standing alters with position to help the person overcome gravity. Screw-jack type mechanisms have also been employed to assist with lifting. A screw-jack type mechanism is often heavier and more complex than the other mechanisms, but it allows the person to hold position anywhere between sitting and standing. Moreover, screw-jack mechanisms require less force to operate. All of the lifting mechanisms have their strengths and weaknesses.

When selecting a stand-up wheelchair the activities for which the wheelchair will be used must be considered. For example, will the wheelchair need to be transported and if so does it fold or disassemble? Will the stand-up wheelchair be used outdoors or on uneven terrain? The manufacturer can provide folded dimensions, overall dimensions, and static stability angles. For manually powered stand-up wheelchairs, the manufacturer can provide dynamic stability results. It is important to ensure that the stand-up wheelchair is in compliance with American National Standards Institute (ANSI) and Rehabilitation Engineering and Assistive Technology Society of North America (RESNA) standards.

The fitting of a stand-up wheelchair is very important. Most clinicians are familiar with the requirements for obtaining proper static seating posture in a wheelchair. Few are familiar with dynamic seating posture. While using a stand-up wheelchair the posture of the individual changes dramatically. Therefore, it is necessary to align the pivot mechanism for the knees with the center of joint rotation for the individual's knees (see Figure 9.8). Misalignment can place stress on the knee and tibia, which may lead to a fracture or joint laxity. Rotation at the hip is also an important consideration. Improper selection of seat depth and legrest length can cause the individual's torso to be unstable in the standing position, can place excess force on the knees and lower limbs, and can induce shear forces along the seat and backrest. Shear forces in the seat and backrest can lead to the development of decubitus ulcers. Fortunately, the guidelines for selecting seat depth, seat width, and backrest height used for traditional sit-down wheelchairs appear to be appropriate for most stand-up wheelchairs. Some individuals can benefit from the additional stability provided by a lap belt and chest support. These supports must be adjusted with the individual in the wheelchair while going through the complete range of motion provided by the wheelchair.

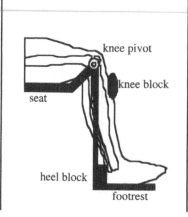

**FIGURE 9.8**    Stand-up wheelchair knee pivot must be aligned with the natural knee joint center to reduce forces that may cause bone fractures or tendon laxity.

All individuals considering a stand-up wheelchair should be examined by a physiatrist knowledgeable in assistive technology. Individuals with severe osteoporosis may be at risk for injury when using a stand-up wheelchair. The physiatrist must also determine whether the individual has sufficient range of motion to safely transition from sitting to standing. Standing alters the hemodynamics of the individual. Some people may require a training regimen prior to being able to operate a stand-up wheelchair independently.

The cost of a typical lightweight manual wheelchair ranges from about $1,000 to $2,000, depending on the quality and features. A manual stand-up wheelchair is likely to cost between $4,000 and $6,000. Typically, an active duty electric-powered wheelchair will cost $3,000 to $8,000; if stand-up features are added, cost increases to $7,000 to $14,000. The additional cost must be justified in terms of better health and greater activity level. Health, activity level, and satisfaction are major contributors to quality of life. Stand-up wheelchairs may be purchased by third-party payers for several reasons. Stand-up wheelchairs may be necessary or may be the most cost-effective means of returning to employment. For example, a lathe operator could return to work with minimal accommodation by using a stand-up wheelchair. In such cases, the stand-up wheelchair may be purchased through a vocational rehabilitation agency or by the employer. A private or government insurance company may purchase a stand-up wheelchair in lieu of costly home modifications to a kitchen. There are some medical indications for using stand-up wheelchairs. People who regularly use stand-up wheelchairs may be at lower risk for osteoporosis, have improved blood flow, and less spasticity. Stand-up wheelchairs may also provide psychological benefits such as improved peer interaction.

It is important to realize that many wheelchair users have access to greater financial resources than previously. Through moderate success in employment and education, some wheelchair users have the means to purchase stand-up wheelchairs. In such cases, the individual must decide whether the potential benefits justify the expense.

## 9.5 Mobile Standing Frames

There are some products that provide mobility solely in the standing position (see Figure 9.9). This class of mobility device is considered a mobile standing frame. Products have been developed for both adults and children. The children's products are by far more popular. They are designed for use on near-level surfaces with

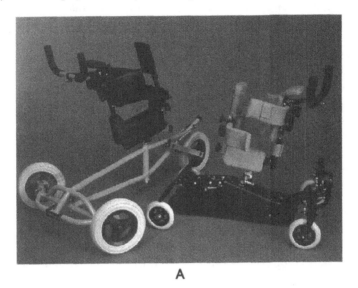

A

**FIGURE 9.9**  Photographs of various mobile standing frames designed for use by children with lower extremity impairments (Photographs courtesy of (a) Ottobock Orthopaedic Industry, Inc., and (b) & (c) Mulholland)

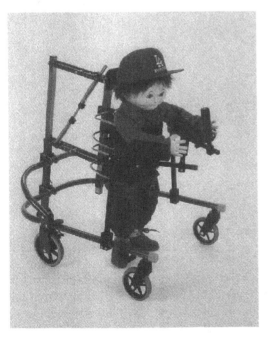

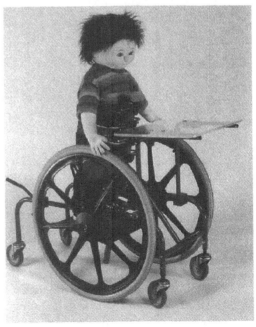

B                                                     C

few transitions (i.e., changes from tile to carpet, door thresholds). Mobile standing frames serve a valuable function. Many activities in which children participate are intended to be done standing. A mobile standing frame allows children with disabilities to participate in these types of activities equally with their peers. This helps in their social development. Passive standing may also assist with the physical development of children with disabilities. Mobile standing frames are also often more maneuverable than a wheelchair. This makes the mobile standing frame more suitable for some activities in busy classrooms. Standing also provides a different perspective on the surroundings from sitting in a wheelchair. This may be beneficial for the development of children with disabilities.

Adults may also benefit from mobile standing frames. Although they perform functions similar to stand-up wheelchairs, they are more suitable for some applications. For example, most stand-up wheelchairs are immobile in the standing position. Therefore, the person must transition from standing to sitting to change position. Mobile standing frames provide mobility in the standing position. A standing frame may be more suitable for a machine operator who needs to move around the workstation to change tools and parts. Typically, these tasks are performed in a small area with a level concrete floor. A mobile standing frame may also be better suited than a stand-up wheelchair for working in a small kitchen. Mobile standing frames are used by some teachers to write on the chalkboard or conduct demonstrations at a laboratory bench.

Assessment for use of a mobile standing frame is similar to that for a standing wheelchair. The individual must be able to tolerate standing and must not have severe osteoporosis. A very important consideration when evaluating a mobile standing frame is whether the person can safely and reliably enter and exit. Many mobile standing frames require an assistant to help the rider, or the rider must be strong enough and flexible enough to enter/exit the mobile standing frame. Some training and practice are required to be able to use a mobile standing frame safely and effectively.

## 9.6 Stair Climbing

Significant progress has been made toward increasing architectural accessibility. More buildings provide wheelchair access and facilitate greater mobility within the community. Public transportation has become easier to use as well. Many trains and buses include lifts, ramps, or level platforms. Air travel has also been simplified. Airlines provide onboard wheelchairs and other devices to allow wheelchair users to access an aircraft seat. Despite the many improvements in accessibility, barriers to wheelchair users remain.

Stairs are an obstacle that continue to face wheelchair users. It is unlikely that stairs will be removed from our communities at any time in the near future. Stairs are of historical and architectural importance. Some wheelchair designers and manufacturers have introduced products to address stair climbing. Stair-climbing wheelchairs can be classified as multi-purpose or single-purpose. A multi-purpose stair-climbing wheelchair is intended to be used for general wheelchair driving (i.e., for common activities of daily living). Single-purpose stair-climbing wheelchairs are intended for use on stairs and for very short distances (e.g., on stair landings).

Stair-climbing wheelchairs can be grouped into three broad categories: assistant operated, jointly operated, and independently operated. Assistant operated stair-climbing wheelchairs are used on landings and stairs (see Figure 9.10). These devices can only be operated by an assistant. The most common configuration is for the assistant to operate the wheelchair from behind the occupant. The controls are often placed on a handle attached to the backrest. While ascending or descending stairs, the assistant always remains on the upstairs side of the wheelchair. While operating the wheelchair under normal circumstances, the assistant must not be required to provide more than 10 kilograms (22 pounds) of force to control operation and maintain balance. Under emergency circumstances, the assistant may be required to exert greater force in order to ensure the safety of the wheelchair rider. By remaining on the upstairs side of the wheelchair, the assistant can decide when releasing control of the wheelchair is an appropriate action with minimal risk of injury from the falling wheelchair. Most stair-climbing wheelchairs incorporate safety systems.

Jointly operated stair-climbing wheelchairs are operated by the rider and an assistant. The basis for joint operation is that less training is required of the assistant. Ideally, an assistant could be a passer-by willing to receive a few minutes of instruction from the wheelchair rider. A common scenario is for the wheel-

**FIGURE 9.10** Photograph of assistant operated stair-climbing wheelchair (Photograph courtesy of Scalamobil, Norway)

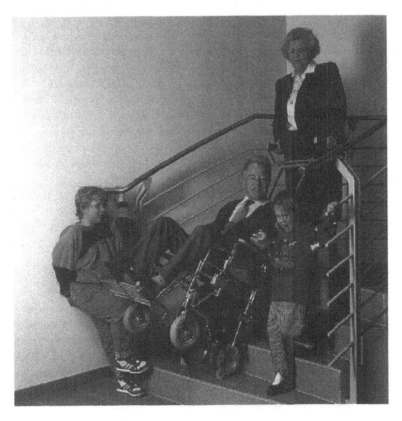

chair rider to drive to the stairs and initiate the transition to stair mode. The wheelchair rider then transfers control to the assistant, who in turn operates the wheelchair on stairs. Jointly operated stair-climbing wheelchairs may use two sets of controls or a single control on a tether for use at both rider and assistant operating positions.

Independently operated stair-climbing wheelchairs, as the name implies, do not require an assistant to traverse stairs. Typically, the driver can operate the stair-climbing wheelchair much like a standard power wheelchair and then change modes for stair traversing. Stair traversing may be accomplished by initiating a program that allows the wheelchair controller to assume operation on stairs, or the driver can retain control and maneuver the wheelchair upstairs.

Stair-climbing wheelchairs are overwhelmingly electric-powered. Some manually propelled stair-climbing wheelchairs have been developed. The low speed and inefficiency of manually propelled stair-climbing wheelchairs have inhibited their ability to obtain profitable market penetration. Electric power provides a viable solution to the power problem and accomplishes stair climbing for people with a wide variety of impairments. Climbing stairs requires a substantial amount of energy and hence reduces the range of the wheelchair. For example, a stair-climbing wheelchair may be able to travel 15 kilometers down a flat road or climb 100 stairs. Of course, the driver can participate in a combination of these activities. The amount of time that the wheelchair can be driven without recharging depends on the tasks it is used to perform.

In some cases, the stair-climbing device can be an add-on unit to a manual wheelchair. This has been accomplished by designing mechanisms for fastening a stair-climbing device to a manual wheelchair. Such devices can be transported to the stairs or attached to a manual wheelchair when stairs are encountered. Devices are also available where the manual wheelchair rolls onto it and is locked in place. These devices are typically located near stairs and used by multiple people.

Several types of mechanisms are used to accomplish the engineering of stair climbing. The most common means are to use tracks or wheel clusters. Tracks are essentially belts with protrusions that provide traction on the stairs. Tracks can be used to accommodate a wide variety of stairs, including spiral stairs. Tracks are inefficient on flat surfaces when compared to wheels. Therefore, tracks are mostly used only for stair climbing. Wheel clusters can provide effective stair climbing and efficient community driving. Clusters cannot climb the range of stairs that can be climbed by a track (see Figure 9.11). Clusters use a combination of either three or two wheels (see Figure 9.12). The wheels rotate around their own axes and rotate around a cluster axis. Driving is accomplished by the rotating wheels, whereas rotation about the cluster axis is used for traversing stairs.

## 9.6.1 Stair-Traversing Device Standards

The International Standards Organization (ISO) has developed test methods and performance levels for stair-traversing devices. The stair-traversing device standard incorporates methods for evaluating static stability, stair stability, static strength, impact strength, fatigue strength, energy consumption, and evaluation of controls. The ISO standard is helpful for determining the performance and level of safety of a stair-climbing wheelchair. Many of the methods are similar to those used for electric-powered wheelchairs.

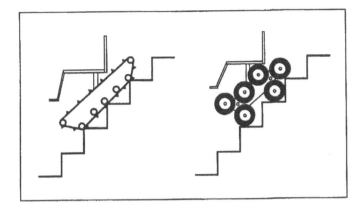

**FIGURE 9.11** Illustration of track (left) and cluster (right) type stair-climbing wheelchairs. The track covers a wide area over the stairs and uses the nose of the stairs. The distance between the wheels on a cluster and the rise/run of the stairs must be similar in order to climb stairs.

The ISO standard is intended to assist manufacturers in producing safe and high-quality products, clinicians to compare and select products, and riders to use reliable and effective stair-climbing wheelchairs. It is particularly important for stair-climbing wheelchairs to meet standards to ensure their safety and effectiveness.

### 9.6.2 Selecting a Stair-Climbing Wheelchair

Stair-climbing wheelchairs can be very complex. They are arguably the most complex form of wheelchair. When the stair-traversing device supports a manual wheelchair, the wheelchair must be securely attached. The stair-traversing device and

**FIGURE 9.12** Illustration of two- and three-wheeled clusters used for stair climbing. The clusters can rotate about a common axis and about each wheel's hub (see inset). The combination of rotation about the common axis and the wheel axes provides the stair-climbing ability.

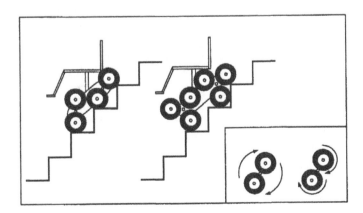

wheelchair must be compatible to ensure safe operation. Also, the stair-traversing device must include safety systems. Seat belts and in some cases shoulder harnesses must be positioned to provide support during normal and emergency operation. Standard postural support and control hardware may not be adequate.

Positioning of the controls required to operate the stair-climbing wheelchair is an important consideration. Stair-climbing wheelchairs go through dramatic changes in orientation. The forces of gravity applied through the body change and will alter posture. This may influence the ability to operate the access devices. Clinicians, including rehabilitation engineers, need to consider the effects of changes in body orientation that occur during stair traversing when selecting and placing access devices (i.e., operating controls). The position of an assistant must also be included.

Seating is also an important consideration when selecting a stair-climbing wheelchair. Most stair-climbing devices change the user's seating position to maintain stability and achieve sufficient foot clearance to traverse steps. This requires assessment of a user's range of passive motion, and active range of motion against gravity. Some stair-climbing wheelchairs use legrest elevation, hip and knee flexion, seat tilt, and backrest recline to obtain sufficient stability and clearance for safe stair traversing. Clinicians and riders must carefully review the operation of the stair-climbing wheelchair with reference to the user's abilities.

The cognitive abilities of the user must be considered when determining the suitability of a stair-climbing wheelchair to meet a user's needs. The ability to make rational and wise decisions is required to safely operate a stair-climbing wheelchair. Stair-climbing devices can require complex decision making and, if used improperly, they can lead to harm. The type of stair-climbing wheelchair will depend on the rider's ability to make appropriate choices.

## References and Further Reading

Agrawal V. P., Chandra R. (1979) Optimization of a chair mechanism for partially disabled people for sitting-standing and sitting-lying motions. *Medical and Biological Engineering and Computing,*17, 671–682.

Andersson G. B. J., Oertengren R. (1974) Lumbar disc pressure and myoelectric back muscle activity during sitting. III. Studies on a wheelchair. *Scandinavian Journal of Rehabilitation Medicine*, 3, 122–127.

Andersson G. B. J., Murphy R. W., Oertengren R., Nachemson A. L. (1979) The influence of backrest inclination and lumbar support on the lumbar lordosis in sitting. *Spine*, 4, 52–58.

Babbs C. F., Bourland J. D., Graber G. P., Jones J. T., Schoenlein W. E. (1990) A pressure-sensitive mat for measuring contact pressure distributions for patients lying on hospital beds. *Biomedical Instrumentation Technology*, 24, 363–370.

Bergen A. F., Presperin J., Tallman T. (1990) *Positioning for Function: Wheelchairs and Other Assistive Technologies.* Valhalla, NY, Valhalla Rehabilitation Publications.

Cook A. M., Hussey S. M. (1995) *Assistive Technologies: Principles and Practices.* St. Louis, MO, Mosby.

Cooper R. A., McGee H., Apreleva M., Albright S. J., Van Sickle D. P., Wong E., Boninger M. L. (1995) Static stability testing of stand-up wheelchairs. *Proceedings RESNA '95 Annual Conference*, Vancouver, BC, Canada.

Cooper R. A. (1991) A comparison of pulmonary functions of wheelchair racers in their racing and standard chairs. *Proceedings 14th Annual RESNA Conference*, Kansas City, MO, 245–247.

Dempster W. (1955) *Space Requirements of the Seated Operator*. WADC Technical Report 55–159, Wright-Patterson Air Force Base, OH.

Ferguson-Pell M. W. (1980) Design criteria for the measurement of pressure at body/support interfaces. *Engineering in Medicine*, 9, 209–214.

Flippo K. F., Inge K. J., Barcus J. M. (1995) *Assistive Technology: A Resource for School, Work, and Community*. Baltimore, MD, Paul H. Brookes Company.

Galvin J. C., Scherer M. J. (1996) *Evaluating, Selecting, and Using Appropriate Assistive Technology*. Gaithersburg, MD, Aspen Publishers.

Gilsdorf P., Patterson R., Fisher S., Appel N. (1990) Sitting forces and wheelchair mechanics. *Journal of Rehabilitation Research and Development*, 27, 3, 239–246.

Goosens R. H. M., Snijders C.J. (1995) Design criteria for the reduction of shear forces in beds and seats. *Journal of Biomechanics*, 28, 2, 225–230.

Grady J. H., Kuipers I. (1993) Modular systems in wheelchairs: Purpose in relation to function. *Proceedings Second European Conference on Advancement of Rehabilitation Technology*, Stockholm, Sweden, 33.1.

Grieco A. (1986) Sitting posture: An old problem and a new one. *Ergonomics*, 29, 345–362.

Hunt J. T. (1993) Standing tall. *Team Rehab Report*, 4, 6, 17–20.

ISO Working Group 9. (1994) *Stand-up wheelchair draft standard*. WG 09–01, April.

Jacobs K., Bettencourt (1995) *Ergonomics for Therapists*. Newton, MA, Butterworth-Heinemann.

Katz R. T., Rymer W. Z. (1989) Spastic hypertonia: Mechanisms and measurement. *Archives of Physical Medicine and Rehabilitation*, 70, 2, 144–155.

Keegan J. J. (1953) Alterations of the lumbar spine related to posture and seating. *Journal of Bone and Joint Surgery*, 35–A, 589.

Laenger C. J., Lee J. H. (1991) Small improvements in seating hardware. *Proceedings RESNA 14th Annual Conference*, Kansas City, MO, 353–355.

Seelen H. A. M. (1993) Dynamic sitting posture and impaired postural control in seated spinal cord injured people. *Proceedings Second European Conference on Advancement of Rehabilitation Technology*, Stockholm, Sweden, 33.2.

Sengupta D., Sherwood A. M., McDermott M. (1974) Comparative evaluation of control surfaces for disabled patients. *27th ACEMB*, Philadelphia, PA, 356.

Shapcott N., Bar K. (1990) Seating simulation as an aid to assessment. *Proceedings RESNA 13th Annual Conference*, Washington, DC, 111–114.

Shaw C. G. (1993) Seat cushion comparison for nursing home wheelchair users. *Journal of Assistive Technology*, 5, 2, 92–105.

Shields R. K., Cook T. M. (1988) Effect of seat angle and lumbar support on seated buttock pressure. *Journal of the American Physical Therapy Association*, 68, 1682–1686.

Thacker J. G., Sprigle S. H., Morris B. O. (1994) *Understanding the Technology When Selecting Wheelchairs*. Arlington, VA, RESNA Press.

Trefler E., Hobson D. A., Taylor S. J., Monohan L. C., Shaw C. G. (1993) *Seating and Mobility for Persons with Physical Disabilities*. Tucson, AZ, Therapy Skill Builders.

van Eijk D., Bulsink D. (1993) Design of a series of positioning systems for handicapped children. *Proceedings Second European Conference on Advancement of Rehabilitation Technology*, Stockholm, Sweden, 9.2.

Warren C. G. (1982) Reducing back displacement in the powered reclining wheelchair. *Archives of Physical Medicine and Rehabilitation*, 63, 447–449.

Warren C. G. (1990) Powered mobility and its implications. *Journal of Rehabilitation Research and Development*, Clinical Supplement No. 2, 74–85.

Webster J. G., Ed. (1991) *Prevention of Pressure Sores: Engineering and Clinical Aspects.* Philadelphia, PA, Adam Hilger.

Winter D. A. (1990) *Biomechanics and Motor Control of Human Movement.* New York, NY, John Wiley & Sons.

Woo A. (1992) Standing options. *Team Rehab Report*, 3, 8, 39–44.

Zollars J. A., Axelson P. (1993) The back support shaping system: An alternative for persons using wheelchairs with sling back upholstery. *Proceedings RESNA 16th Annual Conference*, Las Vegas, NV, 274–276.

# CHAPTER 10

# Sports and Recreational Wheelchairs

## Chapter Goals

☑ To know basic setup and adjustment of sports and recreational wheelchairs
☑ To understand person-to-device interface and access

## 10.1 Introduction

Wheelchair sports and recreation have changed the way in which people with disabilities perceive themselves and the way in which they are perceived by society as a whole. The concept that someone in a wheelchair can be athletic and compete at high levels of sport has helped to remove the stigma of being sick that was long associated with a physical impairment. Wheelchair sports continue to be an important tool for social changes as well as individual rehabilitation. There is a growing trend toward integrated activities where people with and without physical impairments can participate in sports and recreational activities side by side. People with disabilities participate in nearly every recreational activity that exists. Some activities require specialized adaptations, whereas others use the same equipment. Recreation is an important aspect of peoples' lives. Good recreational habits can lead to a fuller and healthier life. People participate in a variety of recreational activities, from gardening to sky-diving. Recreational activities change over the life span as well. It is important for people with disabilities to learn healthy recreational activities during rehabilitation.

Shortly after World War II, Sir Ludwig Guttmann and his colleagues originated wheelchair sports as a rehabilitation tool at Stoke Mandeville Hospital in England. This developed out of the need to provide exercise and recreational outlets for the large number of young people recently injured in the war. News of Dr. Guttmann's success with the rehabilitation of his patients through the use of sports soon spread through Europe and to the United States. In 1948, he organized "Games" for British veterans with disabilities. In 1952, the Games developed into the first international wheelchair sporting competition for people with physical disabilities, with participants from the Netherlands, the Federal Republic of Germany, Sweden, Norway, and Israel. During this event, the International Stoke Mandeville Games Federation (ISMGF) was formed to govern and develop wheelchair sporting competitions. The ISMGF established ties to the International Olympic

Committee (IOC), thus expanding the scope of wheelchair sports. As the international sports movement for people with disabilities grew into international multi-disability events, the ISMGF was expanded to include all wheelchair sporting events. After the reorganization, the ISMGF was renamed the International Stoke Mandeville Wheelchair Sports Federation (ISMWSF). The first international games for the disabled were held with the Olympic Games in 1960 in Rome, Italy. The name "Paralympics" was coined during the 1964 Tokyo games and, as such, subsequently held every four years.

## 10.2 Racing Wheelchairs

In the early years of wheelchair racing, participants used bulky standard (depot-type) wheelchairs and did not compete in events with distances over 200 meters (see Figure 10.1). In the 1970s, athletes started to modify their wheelchairs for specific sports and began to take an interest in road racing. In 1975, a young man with paraplegia became the first person to compete in the Boston Athletic Association Marathon in a wheelchair. This opened the door for many future road racers, prompting Dr. Caibre McCann, a leading physician for the International Stoke Mandeville Games Federation (ISMGF), to say: "Running is natural, but propelling

**FIGURE 10.1**    Photograph of early depot-style racing wheelchair prior to specialization (Photograph courtesy of Rory Cooper)

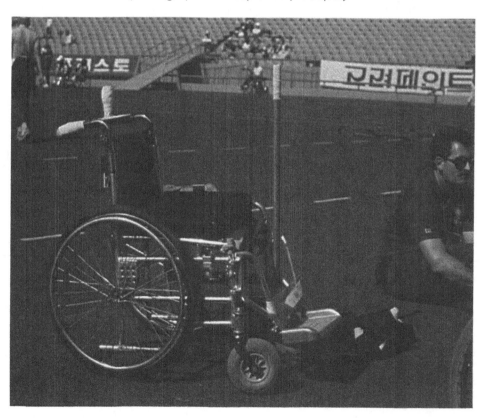

yourself in a wheelchair is an unnatural phenomenon. People never realize what a wheelchair athlete is capable of. This is a breakthrough in man's limits." Within a few years, several recognized U.S. road races initiated wheelchair divisions, and more people with disabilities began to train for these races than had ever been anticipated. In 1976, the ISMGF started to coordinate with other international sports organizations to launch a unified international sports movement for people with disabilities. Racing wheelchairs began to evolve as special-purpose pieces of equipment easily distinguishable from everyday wheelchairs. Distances on the track were extended to include races up to 1500 meters, and during this time the mile record was dropped to below five minutes.

The early 1980s saw the development of more sophisticated racing wheelchairs and training techniques. By 1985, most racing wheelchairs no longer had any components in common with everyday wheelchairs (which had also improved dramatically), and George Murray became the first wheelchair racer to break the four-minute mile. In the years that followed, wheelchair racing continued to progress with improved equipment, training, and nutrition; consequently, world records were continually being broken. Wheelchair racing began the path toward recognition as a legitimate Olympic sport in 1984 when the men's 1500 meter and the women's 800 meter wheelchair races were included as demonstration events in the Olympic Games held in Los Angeles. Wheelchair racing continued to be an exhibition event at the 1988, 1992, and 1996 Olympiads. Athletes and organizers continue to work for further integration of wheelchair sports into the Olympic movement. The general wheelchair user has also benefited from the advances brought about in wheelchair design by racing. The light weight and superior maneuverability of the sports wheelchair, once only used by athletes, has become the wheelchair of choice for many wheelchair users. The ultralight wheelchair has created an entire industry.

It is important that a racing chair fit the user properly. Racing chairs are similar to shoes in that a poorly fitted chair can be uncomfortable and awkward. A racing chair should fit as closely as possible without causing discomfort or pressure sores. Most manufacturers ask for a number of anatomical measurements when a chair is ordered. The most common measurements requested are hip width, chest width, upper-leg length, arm length, trunk length, height, and weight. It is important for the manufacturer to know of the athlete's special needs, such as asymmetry or limited range of motion. Disability etiology and racing ability are important to consider to properly fit a racing chair to its rider for maximum performance with least risk of injury.

Wheelchair racing, like any other sport, has rules to define competition. The purpose of wheelchair racing is to cover a predesignated course in a minimum amount of time and to finish ahead of the other competitors in the process. There are rules governing the conduct of the competitors and design of the equipment. These rules have been developed to make competition fair and equitable. The rules allow a wide variety of designs to be used and thus are not overly prohibitive. The racing wheelchair must be designed to meet the specifications of the rules and yet assist the racer in completing the course as rapidly as possible in a safe manner. Racing wheelchairs must be propelled by arm power only, and steered by hands and arms only. This leaves the uncompensated front wheel assembly susceptible to downhill turning moments due to road crown and caster flutter. These factors affect the energy required to propel the racing chair and thus the efficiency. Crown compensators and (on four-wheeled chairs) tie-rod linkages with Ackerman steering geometry effectively minimize the effects of crown and caster flutter. Racing chairs are steered by using a lever attached to the front fork(s) or trailing arm(s). The only reduction in steering is in the length of the lever.

Racing wheelchairs are propelled by hitting the pushrims as rapidly and with as much force as can be sustained for the distance required. Pushrims used on racing chairs are smaller than those used on chairs used for mobility. Pushrims are tubular rings of aluminum attached to the rear spokes. The attachment is made via threaded stand-offs with two spacers sandwiched around a spoke and clamped to the stand-off via a small bolt. A pushrim will have several attachments to the wheel. Pushrims may be coated to achieve higher friction between it and the athlete's gloves (a tire or a high-density foam coating are most common).

There are a variety of different designs for racing wheelchairs; however, most have some common characteristics. Racing wheelchair frames are constructed of aluminum (6061T6), chromolly steel (4130 or 4140), or titanium. Racing wheelchairs may be equipped with three or four wheels. In the infancy of wheelchair racing, most racing wheelchairs were designed with four wheels. However, most wheelchairs today use three wheels because of changes in rules and design innovations.

Athletes sit near rear axle height. Four-wheeled wheelchairs commonly employ a rectangular main frame with a cross-member immediately fore and aft of the seat (see Figure 10.2). Three-wheeled wheelchairs are similarly constructed using a triangular (as viewed from above) main frame (see Figure 10.3). The rear wheels are mounted rigidly to the frame by a threaded insert welded either

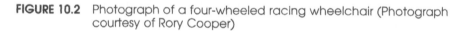

**FIGURE 10.2**   Photograph of a four-wheeled racing wheelchair (Photograph courtesy of Rory Cooper)

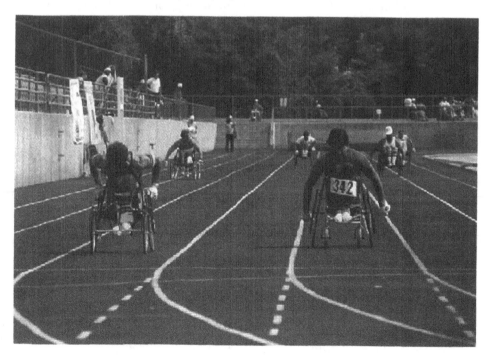

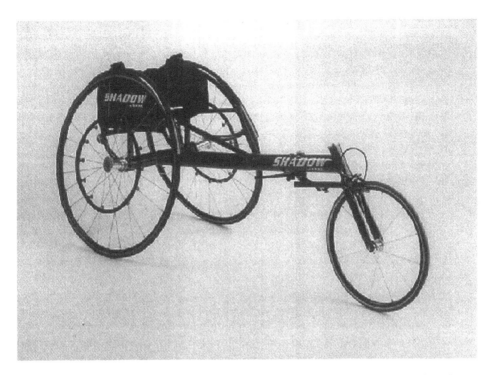

**FIGURE 10.3** Photograph of a three-wheeled racing wheelchair with a leading bicycle-type fork (Photograph courtesy of Quickie, a division of Sunrise Medical)

through the side frame tubes or into a cross-member. The rear wheel inserts are aligned such that there is no toe in/out and between 2 and 15 degrees of wheel camber. This helps to make the chair more stable and allows the athlete to reach the bottom of the pushrims without hitting the top of the wheels or pushrim. Toe in/out causes problems for wheelchair racers as it can cause a significant increase in rolling resistance if not aligned properly. Toe in/out may change with use, so some manufacturers incorporate an alignment mechanism into the frame. Three methods are commonly used: a cross-member is affixed to one side of the side frame via a bolt and spacers are used to lengthen or shorten the cross-member, hence aligning the rear wheels; a similar method employs a "turn-buckle" mechanism that can be expanded or contracted to align the rear wheels; another method uses an angled cross-member with the rear axle insert pressed into it, rotating the cross-member to align the rear wheels.

The seat cage is welded on top of the main frame, and serves the purpose of supporting the athlete. The seat cage should fit snugly around the athlete. Some elite racers use racing wheelchairs that incorporate seat and leg support as an integral unit. Elite athletes usually prefer a tighter-fitting seat cage than do novice athletes because they are more accustomed to pushing a racing wheelchair. The seat and leg support should hold the athlete solidly, so that his or her energy can be focused on propelling the wheelchair, and not on maintaining balance. A seat cage also offers the athlete greater control over the racing chair than does a conventional seat and provides some protection in the event of an upset. Seat cages have side panels to provide support and to prevent the athlete from rubbing against the wheels. Well-designed side panels follow the curvature of the wheel and allow the athlete a large range of motion fore and aft. Most seat upholstery is made of nylon or cotton canvas slung from the seat cage. Some racing chairs use plastic or fiberglass seats. Athletes typically use low-profile foam or air flotation cushions.

Racing wheelchair frames are designed to be stiff and lightweight. The typical racing wheelchair frame weighs less than five pounds, excluding the wheels. The frame and seat cage are made to fit each individual, for different disability etiologies and levels. The location of the rear axles with respect to the seat cage are dependent on experience and disability etiology. Experienced athletes with paraplegia prefer between 15 and 25 centimeters from the seat back to the rear axle inserts. Experienced athletes with quadriplegia prefer between 5 and 20 centimeters from the seat back to the rear axle inserts. More stable configurations are recommended for novice athletes. The seat cage upholstery adjustment and rear axle position must be such that the athlete can position his/her shoulders over the front edge of the pushrims and be able to reach the bottom of the pushrims with both arms.

Many athletes use three-wheeled racing wheelchairs. Advances in steering geometry and front wheel assemblies have contributed to improvements in race performance and safety. Front wheel assemblies are designed to follow the path selected by the athlete without requiring corrections from the pushrims. Two methods are commonly used to attach the front wheels to racing wheelchairs: trailing arm or fork. Trailing arm racing chairs have the front wheel(s) mounted on a cantilever axle. The frame is swept down to axle height, minimizing the moment arm of the ground reaction forces with respect to the front housing. This design also makes the front tires easily accessible in the event of a puncture. On four-wheeled trailing arm racing chairs the front wheels are mounted in line with the rear wheels, yielding the maximum allowable width and the most stable configuration. Three-wheeled racing chairs often use a leading fork, similar to those used on bicycles; this minimizes frame length for a given wheelbase, helps to improve high-speed handling, and makes the frame lightweight (see Figure 10.4).

Lightweight wheels have been designed and are commonly available for wheelchair racing. Racing wheelchair rear hubs have cantilever threaded axles (7/16 and 1/2 inch thread sizes are most common). The hub shells are made of aluminum alloy and are either standard or high flange. Spoke patterns are from 24 to 36 spokes per wheel. Tri-spoke composite wheels are also used on some racing chairs. Many athletes use Mylar wheel covers on their rear wheels. Front hubs are either fork mount or cantilever (5/16 or 7/16 axle). Front hubs are made for 10 to 20 spokes. Some athletes use composite disk wheels on their racing chairs. Front and rear wheels use aluminum alloy rims (18-millimeter wide). Rear wheels are typically 60 to 70 centimeters, whereas front wheels are typically 35 to 50 centimeters in diameter. Athletes use both clincher and sew-up tires. Clincher tires are usually used with latex tubes. Rear tires may weigh as little as 150 grams, while front tires may weigh as little as 75 grams. Racing wheels are radially spoked to reduce weight.

Many racing wheelchairs have features that aid in the athlete's performance or safety. Some of these features are a cycle computer that aids in pacing and training; a water bottle for fluid replacement; and caliper brakes (a safety feature to help control the tremendous speeds attainable on some downhill sections). Many races require brakes, and they make training safer. Athletes and clinicians must ensure that brakes can be reached from a comfortable position. The brake levers must be long enough and at the proper angle so that sufficient leverage can

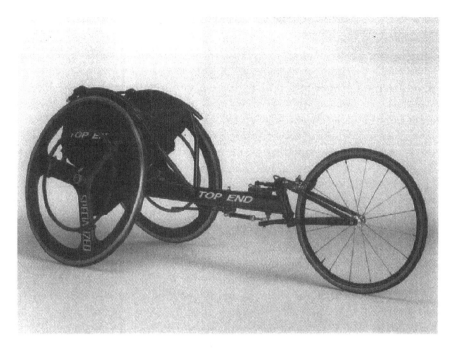

**FIGURE 10.4**   Photograph of a three-wheeled racing wheelchair with a low-profile leading edge fork (Photograph courtesy of Top End, a division of Invacare Corporation)

be applied to stop the racing chair. People with quadriplegia should be particularly critical. Most road and track races require helmets. Helmets have improved the safety of wheelchair racing, and all athletes should purchase a helmet when they purchase their racing wheelchair. The helmet must meet national safety standards and fit the athlete snugly. Many helmets provide some adjustment. It is also important that the helmet provide good airflow over the head. The head is a primary area for cooling the body of many wheelchair athletes. Aerodynamic helmets can enhance speed over no-helmet operation.

Racing wheelchairs come equipped with steering levers and compensators. These items make racing safer and more fun. However, all people are not alike. When ordering a racing wheelchair customers and manufacturers must ensure that compensators and steering levers are easily reached and operated by the athlete. The levers must be of sufficient length and in a position where the athletes effectively apply the necessary force and movement to operate these controls. Many compensator mechanisms come with stiff springs to ensure that the wheelchair tracks straight. To steer the wheelchair, adequate strength must be used to overpower the compensator. Softer springs or a longer steering lever can be requested to reduce the force required to steer the racing chair.

## 10.2.1 Positioning in a Racing Wheelchair

Racing wheelchairs are very user-specific, and athletes vary greatly in their abilities. Thus, it is difficult if not impossible to design a racing wheelchair effective for every athlete. This is one of the primary reasons that many racing wheelchairs are handcrafted for each individual based on his or her specific needs. The seat of the racing wheelchair should fit tightly to the body. Getting in a racing wheelchair should be like slipping on a glove. Many new athletes make the mistake of getting a loose-fitting wheelchair. Top athletes can only fit into their racers when wearing racing/training tights. To push properly the athlete has to sit properly. If the athlete is flexible enough and feels comfortable leaning on his/her knees, then the kneeling position is probably going to be fastest. If this is uncomfortable, after some trial period, or if the athlete has very good trunk control, then a more upright posture is best. When seated in the chair and kneeling or lying on the knees, the athlete should be able to touch the ground with both hands and be able to reach all the way around both pushrims. The center of each shoulder should line up with the front of each pushrim in the fully down position. The athlete should move the arms simulating stroking and test how difficult it is to breathe. Breathing must be synchronized with stroking, but if it seems difficult to breathe, the knees should be raised.

The wheelchair racing stroke can be divided into two primary phases: propulsion and recovery. Propulsion is when the arms are applying force, and recovery is when they are off the pushrims getting ready for the next stroke. In order to push a racing wheelchair effectively, the upper body must rapidly apply a large force to the pushrims. Theoretically, the greatest velocity can be achieved by applying a large force over a long time period. However, it is difficult for an athlete to effectively apply a large force during the entire propulsion phase. The use of larger muscles and more of the upper body can assist in developing greater force over the propulsion cycle. The result is a larger force value and longer time of application, which creates a larger change in the athlete's and wheelchair's momentum. However, the price for this higher mechanical of energy is a higher metabolic energy cost (i.e., the amount of energy used by the body).

A racing wheelchair stroke can be divided into five phases (Figure 10.5). The five phases are defined as follows: (1) pushrim contact (a); (2) pushing through to

**FIGURE 10.5**  Schematic illustrating the phases of an efficient racing wheelchair stroke

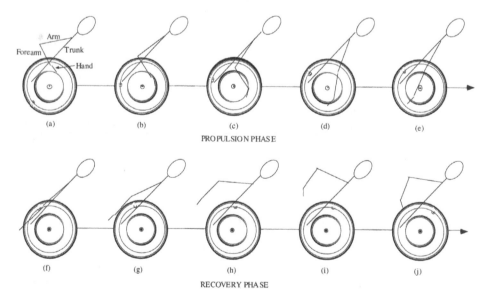

the bottom of the pushrims (b–d); (3) push-off or follow through (e); (4) elbow drive to the top (f–h); and (5) drive forward and downward (i–j). During the entire stroke the head should remain in line with the trunk. Head movement should be kept to a minimum. Elbow height before the drive forward and downward is critical to generating propulsion force. Maximal elbow height requires strength and flexibility. Optimal force transference from the body to the pushrim requires properly fitted and designed gloves, and a non-slip pushrim coating. The hand should be in line with the forearm at contact (i.e., wrist in the neutral position) to transfer maximum energy. The athlete must push continuously from contact through to the bottom of the pushrims. If the propulsion phase is done properly, the hand will push off the pushrim with a flick. Then the momentum of the arms carries the elbows upward until the elbows are lifted to their peak. When the elbows are at their peaks, the athlete should contract chest, shoulder, and arm muscles to punch the pushrims.

Some personal preferences should be considered when specifying a racing wheelchair. Athletes with paraplegia, quadriplegia, or amputated limbs have different preferences, and each person has his/her own abilities and anatomical structure. There are three basic seats to consider: kneeling bucket, kneeling cage, and upright cage. The kneeling position is very aerodynamic and has allowed some athletes to make tremendous improvements in their performance. Many athletes with paraplegia or quadriplegia use the kneeling position quite effectively. Athletes inexperienced with the kneeling position should use a kneeling cage. This affords them the option of sitting upright or kneeling and permits some adjustment of body position. Experienced athletes prefer a kneeling bucket because of the reduced weight and improved aerodynamics. Upright cage seats work well for athletes with lower limb amputations and for athletes with low levels of paraplegia. These athletes have the trunk control to adjust their body positions while racing. Athletes with contractures should order a cage seat unless they have substantial experience. Athletes are held in their racing chairs with straps and webbing. Additional padding or extra width can be requested to reduce the risk of developing pressure sores for people who are prone to skin breakdown. Although many competitors do not use a seat cushion in their racing chairs, the danger of skin breakdown makes use of a cushion advisable.

It is important that a racing wheelchair fit the user like a glove. A poorly fitting racing chair can be uncomfortable and awkward. A racing chair should fit as close as possible without causing discomfort or pressure sores. Most manufacturers ask for a number of anatomical measurements when a racing chair is ordered. The common measurements are hip width, chest width, upper-leg length, arm length, trunk length, height, and weight (see Table 10.1).

Manufacturers must be made aware of an athlete's special needs, such as asymmetry or limited range of motion (e.g., contractures). The manufacturer should be informed of any pelvic or spinal curvatures (e.g., lordosis, kyphosis), and whether the athlete is prone to fractures or skin breakdown. Type of disability and racing ability also are important factors that should be considered when specifying a racing wheelchair. A properly fitting racing wheelchair translates into maximum performance with minimum risk of injury. Wheelchair racing is an important part of the rehabilitation of many people with disabilities and is indeed a significant activity in the daily lives of many people. Exercise is an important modality in the well-being of all people, including those with mobility impairments, and exercise should be encouraged and methods developed.

**TABLE 10.1    Critical body measurements for design and selection of a racing wheelchair**

---

- *Hip width measurements*

    This is the distance between hip joints (greater trochanters). To measure this distance, the hands should be used to distinguish where each hip joint is located, and the distance between the hands should be measured.

- *Chest width measurements*

    When exercising, muscles fill with blood and expand. Consequently, this measurement should be taken with the chest expanded. In order for the top of the seat to be comfortable but snug, the chest measurement should be made after taking a deep breath and while flexing the chest and upper body muscles. The measurement is made across the back between the underarms.

- *Upper-leg length*

    This measurement is taken from the hip joint (greater trochanter) to the inside of the knee (i.e., popliteal area). If amputated above the knee, the residual limb length should be used.

- *Arm length*

    This measurement is taken from the underarm to the cleft between the thumb and index finger. Arm length is used to recommend the correct rear wheel and pushrim sizes.

- *Trunk length*

    This measurement is taken from the hip joints (greater trochanters) to the underarms.

---

## 10.3 Field Event Chairs

People with disabilities enjoy participating in field events as part of athletic competitions, such as club, shot put, discus, and javelin. The club is an event for people who are most severely involved (e.g., a person with C4–C5 quadriplegia). As the section title implies, field event chairs are not required to have wheels. Prior to the 1989 international athletics season, field event chairs needed to have wheels. At that time most field athletes used old depot-type wheelchairs that were as heavy as possible. This was because the weight of the wheelchair helped to make it stiffer and less likely to move while throwing an implement (e.g., shot put, discus, javelin). The rules describing the throwing chair were changed in order to modernize and revitalize the sport. This has led to some interesting new features.

Field event chairs are designed to provide a rigid base of support (see Figure 10.6). The chair is strapped to the ground within a 1.5-meter throwing circle. Straps are attached to the chair and to steel stakes pounded into the ground. The thrower has the option of requesting that the stakes be moved. However, in many competitions the stakes are in a fixed location to expedite setup. Throwing chairs include a means of leveling the seat. This helps the thrower to obtain the proper angle at release (e.g., 40–50 degrees). The seat of a throwing wheelchair usually

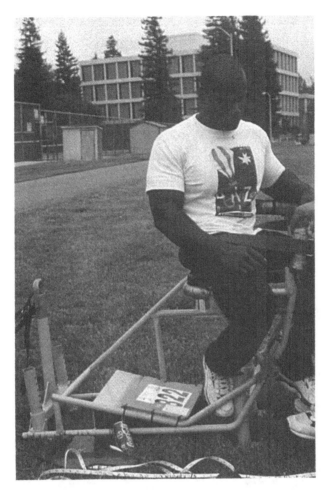

**FIGURE 10.6** Photograph of a field event chair designed for shot put, discus, and javelin throwing (Photograph courtesy of Rory Cooper)

has less than one centimeter of padding. This is because throwers desire the maximum sitting height, and the cushion is counted in the seat height. Throwers are not in the chair for very long. Hence, risk of pressure sores is not great. Throwers should be cautious during extended training sessions.

The feet are supported by a large footplate. The footplate is designed to allow the feet to move as the thrower changes body position. The frame of the throwing chair and straps may be used to restrict the movement of the feet. In order for a throw to be legal, no part of the body may extend outside the throwing area until the judge signals. Rails are used to guide the motion of the upper body through the throwing sequence. The shape of the rails is customized to the size and abilities of the user. Those with lower impairments and high skills use the least restrictive rails to guide the trunk, whereas the rails are more restrictive (providing greater support) for people who are more severely impaired or less skilled. The rails are padded to protect the thrower's body from the impact received while moving through the throwing motion.

The thrower and coach must be able to move the throwing chair into the throwing circle and secure it within a three- to five-minute period during major competitions. This has resulted in quick-release wheels being added to the throwing frame for transport. This has also led to simple attachment points and leveling mechanisms.

## 10.4 Off-Road Wheelchairs and All-Terrain Vehicles

Some people who use wheelchairs enjoy being outdoors. The desire to participate in sports and recreation similar to mountain biking has encouraged the development of specialized wheelchairs and off-road vehicles. Some wheelers, preferring not to wait for all trails to become accessible, have decided to acquire access to mountain bike trails by developing new vehicles or modifying existing equipment. Adaptive off-road vehicles open up trails that would be impassable in a conventional wheelchair. There are several versions of adaptive off-road vehicles.

The off-road wheelchair looks similar to a four-wheeled racing wheelchair from a distance, with large front wheels and a lot of rear wheel camber (see Figure 10.7). These chairs use wide knobby tires for added traction and resistance to puncture. Dual pushrims (two per rear wheel) may be used to help find the proper gear. Handlebars and four-wheel brakes help to control the chair on steep rough descents. The center of gravity is moved more forward of the rear wheels than in other chairs to provide additional stability. The steering geometry must also be designed to accommodate high speeds over rough terrain. The frame and wheels have to be made to withstand much higher forces than racing or conventional wheelchairs. The extra equipment and strength required of off-road wheelchairs makes them heavier (around 40 pounds for manual chairs). Mountain bike and

**FIGURE 10.7**   Photograph of an off-road wheelchair with suspension and disc brakes designed for downhill racing (Photograph courtesy of Peter Axelson and Beneficial Designs, Inc.)

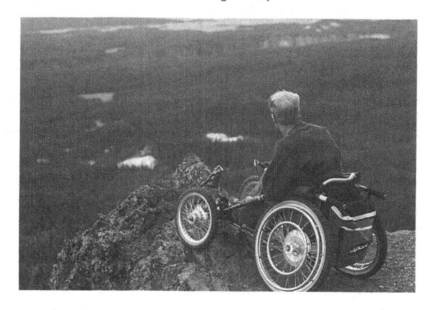

hiking trails tend to be steeper than paved roads or pathways. Off-road wheelchairs must be able to climb steep hills. This is accomplished by lowering the seat, moving the center of gravity forward, and lengthening the wheelbase. Two pushrim sizes make it easier to push on both hills and flat ground. Off-road wheelchair riding can be much more enjoyable with friends on mountain bikes. The friends can help pull the wheelchair with tow ropes attached to their mountain bikes. This can make going up long grades possible. In some areas tow ropes or ski lifts are used to help off-road wheelchair riders and mountain bikers to ascend to the top of a mountain. Once at the top, the expert off-road wheelchair rider can descend at speeds exceeding 50 kilometers per hour (30 miles per hour). Some downhill mountain bike races include off-road wheelchair divisions.

Conventional steering from the pushrims is insufficient for off-road use. The larger front wheels of an off-road wheelchair are steered using handlebars. The front wheels are connected via tie-rod linkage, and a spring compensator is used to center the front wheels when they are not being turned by the rider. Dynamic braking is required on off-road wheelchairs. The brakes are typically located on the handlebars to allow simultaneous braking and directional control. Conventional wheelchairs use wheel locks that restrict motion only when the wheelchair is stationary.

Some wheelchairs are designed more for utility use in rural environments. These wheelchairs look similar to ultralight wheelchairs, but they use larger casters and rear wheels (see Figure 10.8). This allows the rider to traverse rough terrain or to push over grass and unfinished surfaces easier. Utility type wheelchairs provide mobility in areas where a typical wheelchair is ineffective or very difficult to use.

Powered off-road vehicles are also available (Ontario Drive & Gear Limited, New Hamburg, Ontario, Canada; Recreatives Industries, Inc., Buffalo, New York). Several off-road amphibious vehicles can be totally hand-controlled. These vehi-

**FIGURE 10.8** Photograph of an off-road wheelchair designed for rural use (Photograph courtesy of Jim McCluskey, VA Pittsburgh Health Care System)

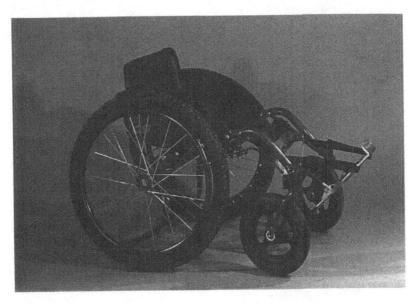

cles incorporate roll protection guards, a seat belt harness, and an on-board fire extinguisher. A swing arm and crane may be incorporated for some users. Many of these vehicles use six or more wheel drive and a vacuum-formed high-density poly-ethylene body. Two hand-held levers are used to turn and activate the brakes. The vehicles commonly use twist-grip throttles. These vehicles may climb hills as steep as 45 degrees. Vehicles use either internal combustion engines or electric motors. Off-road vehicles that use internal combustion engines are limited in certain areas, e.g., many national and state parks prohibit their use.

## 10.5 Beach Wheelchairs

Going to the beach is a popular pastime for many people. However, most wheelchairs are incapable of being driven any significant distance on a sandy beach. Wheelchairs tend to sink into the sand and become immobile. Short distances may be traveled by lowering the tire pressure. Specialized wheelchairs are available for use on sandy beaches. Most can be used in the water as well. Beach wheelchairs can serve as both a personal mobility device and a lounge chair (see Figure 10.9). Other beach wheelchairs require an assistant (see Figure 10.10). In order to drive effectively over soft sandy beaches, beach wheelchairs use wide tires and casters. The increased width reduces the amount of penetration into the sand made by the tires and casters. It is also common to use only a few pounds per square inch tire pressure. This helps to spread the weight of the person and the wheelchair over a wider area.

Beach wheelchairs do not require complex fitting. Most beach wheelchairs are designed to be stored near the beach and used by people as necessary. Some hotels and resorts rent or provide beach wheelchairs to their guests as a service.

**FIGURE 10.9** Photograph of a beach wheelchair (Photograph courtesy of Sean Shimada, University of Pittsburgh)

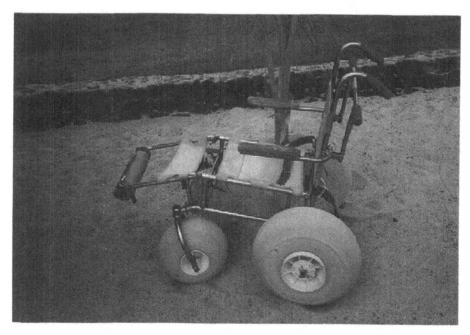

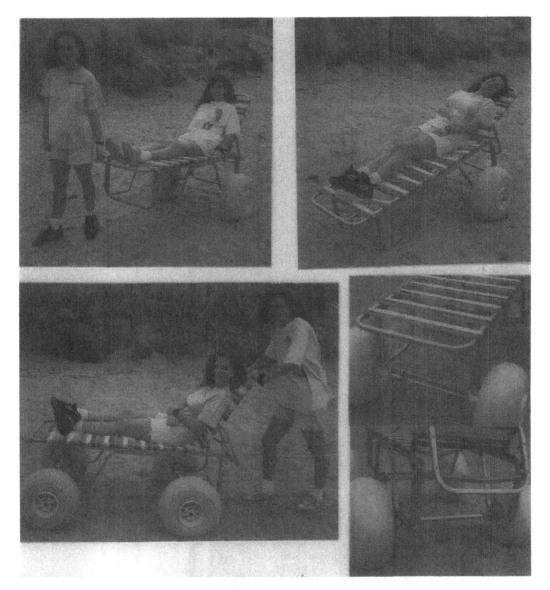

**FIGURE 10.10**   Photograph of a beach wheelchair that can be pulled by an assistant to provide access to sandy areas or water (Photographs courtesy of Roleez Wheel System)

Since most beach wheelchairs are one-size-fits-all and need to be propelled by an assistant, there is often no need for specialized fitting.

## 10.6 Court Sports Wheelchairs

Court sports wheelchairs are similar to ultralight wheelchairs designed for daily use, but they have some distinguishing features that make them more effective for use in specific sports. Court sports wheelchairs are often distinguishable by the extreme camber in their rear wheels and the small "roller blade"–type front casters. Court sports wheelchairs use rigid frames. The specific features of specialized court sports wheelchairs are described in the following sections.

### 10.6.1 Basketball Wheelchairs

Many of the current features of lightweight wheelchairs can be attributed to wheelchair basketball and wheelchair racing. Basketball wheelchairs must be lightweight to allow players to accelerate and brake rapidly in order to execute basketball plays. Although basketball is a noncontact sport, some incidental contact is inevitable. For this reason, players use spoke guards to cover the spokes of the rear wheels. Exposed spokes can be broken during a game or spoke parts of an opponent's chair can be lodged into spokes and disrupt a play. Spoke guards are made of high-impact plastic. Added benefits include making it easier to pick the ball up from the floor and providing space to identify a player's team affiliation.

Basketball wheelchairs are required to have forward anti-tip rollers or forward skids. Both anti-tip rollers and skids are designed to reduce the risk of forward falls and to minimize damage to the basketball court. Anti-tip rollers and skids are commonly mounted to the footrests. Some players use rear anti-tip casters. These help prevent backwards falls. This is especially important for people with higher levels of impairment. Rear anti-tip casters can make it more difficult to accelerate the wheelchair from contacting the ground as a player pushes. Basketball wheelchairs use four wheels: two large wheels in the rear used to push the wheelchair and two casters in the front for steering (see Figure 10.11). The front

**FIGURE 10.11**  Photograph of a four-wheeled basketball wheelchair (Photograph courtesy of Quickie, a division of Sunrise Medical)

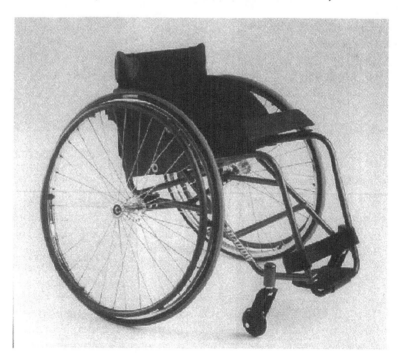

casters are nearly always 5-centimeter (2-inch) diameter polyurethane casters with precision roller bearings. The rear wheels are commonly 61 centimeters (24 inches) or 66 centimeters (26 inches) in diameter. High-pressure tires with no or very low profile tread are used on the rear wheels. High-pressure (120 psi to 200 psi) tires make it easier to push the wheelchair and make the wheelchair faster on the basketball court.

Camber is an important feature of basketball wheelchairs. Camber helps to make the wheelchair more responsive while turning. Camber also has the benefit of protecting the player's hands when two wheelchairs impact from the sides. The camber forces the wheels of two independent wheelchairs to hit at the bottom while leaving a gap at the top to protect the hands of each player.

Basketball wheelchairs typically have a near-level seat angle of about five degrees sloped toward the backrest. This is because the rules of basketball limit the maximum height of any portion of the seat. Therefore, athletes usually try to make their seat height as high as possible. Guards are a notable exception where a lower seat height and greater seat angle make the chair faster and more maneuverable for ball handling. Basketball wheelchairs often include loops for strapping. Strapping can be used to position a player to improve performance. Positioning has been used so effectively by some players that it has changed their functional classification.

### 10.6.2 Tennis Wheelchairs

In tennis there is no contact between opposing players, and in doubles partners must work as a team. Tennis is also a very fast sport despite the two-bounce rule applied for wheelchair players. The wheelchair player must be able to cover the entire court. Many players focus on the baseline and move forward as necessary to make a shot. Winning play requires quickness, speed, maneuverability, and agility. For these reasons, tennis wheelchairs have evolved to include several specialized features (see Figure 10.12). Tennis wheelchairs use three wheels. The rear wheels

**FIGURE 10.12**  Photograph of a tennis wheelchair with three wheels (Photograph courtesy of Quickie, a division of Sunrise Medical)

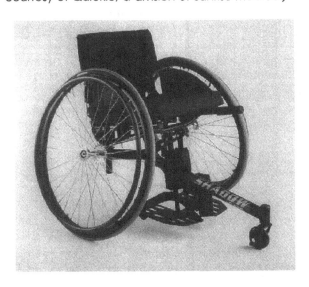

are typically 61 centimeters (24 inches) or 66 centimeters (26 inches) in diameter. They use high-pressure tires (120 psi to 200 psi) to lower rolling resistance on the court and increase speed. A single 5-centimeter (2-inch) diameter front caster is used. This allows the wheelchair to be light, making it more maneuverable and allowing it to accelerate faster. Camber is added to the rear wheels to increase lateral stability while reaching to the side with the racquet to make a shot, and to make the chair turn faster. Front or rear anti-tip casters are not commonly used on tennis wheelchairs.

The seating systems on tennis wheelchairs are also specialized for performance. Tennis players introduced the concept of radical seat angle. A steep seat angle or pitch helps to keep the player against the back of the seat. This gives the player greater control over the wheelchair and provides many people greater balance. The knees are abducted in a tennis wheelchair and feet are placed on the footrest behind the player's knees. By bringing the body close together, the inertia of the rider and wheelchair combined becomes lower. It is similar to a figure skater bringing her arms in to make her spin faster. By lowering the inertia, the player and wheelchair become more maneuverable. This helps the player to respond to shots by rapidly changing direction. Tennis wheelchairs commonly use a rigid footrest so that the feet remain in place and do not touch the ground while moving around. Most players strap their feet to the footrests. Handles are also incorporated into the front of the seats of tennis wheelchairs. The handles are used to help the player balance while leaning forward or to the side to hit the ball. The handles also help to keep the knees in place while playing.

### 10.6.3 Quad Rugby Wheelchairs

Quad rugby is a sport developed out of the desire of people with quadriplegia who have the ability to propel a manual wheelchair but who are not competitive at basketball to play a team sport. The rules of basketball favor people who are not as severely involved. Many of the top wheelchair basketball players do not use a wheelchair as their primary source of mobility. Therefore, people with low-level quadriplegia effectively had no team sport opportunities prior to quad rugby. Quad rugby is a combination of team handball and rugby. Contact is permitted and teams must carry the ball across their goal line to score. The ball may be passed or carried. There is tremendous interest in quad rugby.

The growth of quad rugby has brought about the development of specialized wheelchairs for quad rugby (see Figure 10.13). Quad rugby wheelchairs use four wheels. The rear wheels are typically 61 centimeters (24 inches) in diameter. The front casters are 5 centimeters (2 inches) in diameter with precision roller bearings. The rear wheels are radically cambered to around 15 degrees. This helps to protect the player from side impacts and glancing blows, and makes the chair turn faster. Four wheels are used to make the wheelchair more stable while maneuvering and during an impact with another wheelchair. The two front casters are less likely to penetrate the guards on a quad rugby chair that are used to protect the feet and legs. Guards wrap around the bottom of the wheelchair across the entire front of the chair from one rear wheel to another. The guards have the additional feature of making it more difficult to hook the wheelchair. If a wheelchair can be hooked, the player can be stopped and players from the opposing team can gain advantage.

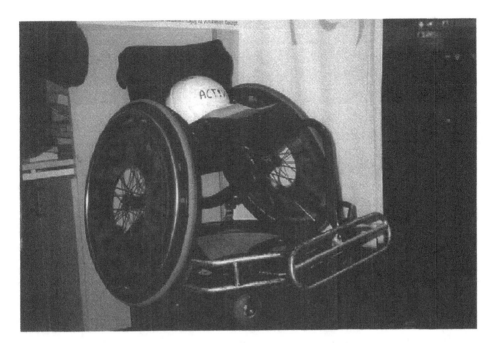

**FIGURE 10.13** Photograph of a wheelchair designed for playing quad rugby (Photograph courtesy of Rory Cooper)

Similar to tennis wheelchairs, quad rugby wheelchairs use a radical seat angle up to 20 degrees. This helps the player to maintain balance and maneuver more effectively. The knees are also abducted and the feet are behind the knees. In quad rugby players must be very quick and maneuverable. A stable seating position with the legs held close provides the user greater control over the wheelchair. Because the rules for quad rugby restrict team members to wheelchair users who are more physically impaired, the rules also require front and rear anti-tip casters. The anti-tip casters have the effect of providing the players some protection from forward and rearward falls, but they also help to protect the court during impacts. Quad rugby chairs are a hybrid of basketball and tennis wheelchairs.

## 10.7 Lever-Drive Wheelchairs

In order to obtain higher efficiency than is possible with a pushrim-propelled wheelchair, without making an entirely new vehicle, some designers have turned to the lever-drive wheelchair. Lever-drive wheelchairs are used in some regions as a primary source of mobility, most commonly in China and other countries in the Far East. Lever-drive wheelchairs provide effective mobility over open spaces or unfinished terrain (e.g., dirt roadways). In some countries where bicycle paths are prevalent, lever-drive wheelchairs are used as a secondary device to the wheelchair. In such cases, the lever-drive wheelchair serves much the same purpose as a bicycle. The lever-drive wheelchair is used to travel longer distances (e.g., five kilometers) from home to town and still be able to maneuver through a department store when arriving at one's destination.

Lever-drive wheelchairs are used as recreational devices by some people. Companies make adapters to wheelchair wheels that can be mounted onto many wheelchairs in order to convert them to lever drives. This allows a person to propel the wheelchair more rapidly and to use it more like a single-speed bicycle. There are no sanctioned competitions for lever-drive wheelchairs.

## 10.8 Arm-Crank Vehicles

People with mobility impairments want alternatives when choosing recreational activities. Some people are interested in physically demanding sports such as marathons or triathlons. Other people prefer touring. Alternatives to racing wheelchairs that offer the increased efficiency of levers and gears are attractive to some people. Alternatives to wheelchair locomotion have been in development for a number of years. The commercial availability of arm-crank recreational equipment was delayed because of lack of awareness among people with mobility impairments of the equipment's existence; the ineligibility of this type of product for purchase by insurance carriers; the high risk associated with production of low-volume adaptive recreation equipment, since liability insurance is difficult to obtain at a reasonable price; and the complexity of home-building an arm-powered vehicle. Presently there are only a few restrictions on arm-powered vehicles for use in competitions. The vehicle can use no motors or external energy sources and may have no structures that serve the sole purpose of reducing air/wind resistance.

Hand cycles are the bicycles of people with mobility impairments (see Figure 10.14). The present generation of hand cycles is geared much like mountain bikes with 15 to 21 gears. The wide range of gears gives riders the ability to select the

**FIGURE 10.14**   Photograph of a two-wheeled hand cycle. The low-speed casters have been retracted for cruising (Photograph courtesy of the Veterans Affairs Rehabilitation Research & Development Center, Palo Alto, California)

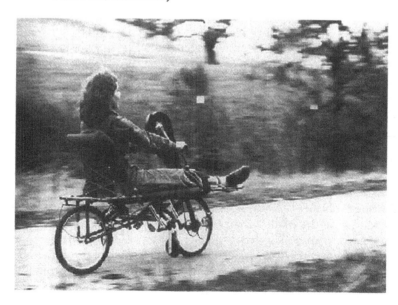

most efficient gear for the grade of the roadway. Whether going downhill or uphill, the rider searches for the optimal gear ratio. The goal is to keep pedal turnover high and effort low. A cadence of between 80 and 100 revolutions per minute minimizes energy consumption and risk of musculoskeletal injury. Before a person rides independently several factors must be considered. Where will most of the riding be done (beach, neighborhood, country, city)? What kind of riding will be done (recreational, racing, touring)? Is the hand cycle appropriate based on the abilities of the rider (disability etiology, physical function)? When the pedal(s) are fully extended (hands on the pedals, back against the backrest), are the elbows slightly bent?

The motivation for designing arm-powered vehicles is to create a vehicle that efficiently converts the user's energy to motion while maintaining control over the vehicle over normal-surface streets. Ideally, arm-powered vehicles would be designed to be transported in a passenger automobile without requiring disassembly. Standard bicycle components should be used whenever possible. Arm-powered vehicle frames are typically constructed from steel alloy (SAE 4130) tubing. Commonly, tubing ends are milled for best fit and stronger joints. Frames may be either brass welded (simple and inexpensive) or inert gas welded.

A limitation of most arm-powered vehicles is the balance of the pilot with the mobility impairment. Accustomed to using a wheelchair for mobility, many people have unlearned their ability to balance. The loss of some kinesthesia and neuromuscular control of the trunk and lower limbs makes balancing a bicycle more difficult. A bucket type seat as used on a racing wheelchair is effective in ameliorating these challenges for some people. Care should be taken when placing the rider's legs, as some positions may require placing the crank center farther away from the rider so that the cranks clear the lower legs. This may result in suboptimal center position and make steering more difficult at the front end of the crank cycle. Some bicycles position the rider low enough to the ground that the rider may place a hand on the ground when starting or stopping. Some people may prefer fully retractable side wheels. Arm-powered bicycles are turned by a combination of leaning and turning the crank arms about the steering axis. Using side wheels may limit the amount the rider can lean the bicycle. When side wheels are used they must be designed not to interfere with normal lean steering. Height of the center of gravity, the balance of the user, and the vehicle's steering geometry interact. These factors must be considered when designing arm-powered vehicles to make them safe and effective.

With many arm-powered vehicles the steering and drive train are interconnected. One of the primary design considerations of arm-powered vehicles is: how does one power the vehicle and maintain directional control? Some designs have decoupled the steering from the drive train with moderate success by using the tilt (from side-to-side) of the seat for steering (Figure 10.15). These vehicles have a large turning radius for their size. Arm-powered bicycles require finer steering control to maintain balance, so direct arm steering is used.

Crank arms may be positioned adjacent or opposed. Using the cranks opposed provides for greater mechanical efficiency. However, dampening must be used to minimize the moment about the head-set created by the opposed crank arms. This moment may cause the front wheel(s) to turn from one side to the other as the rider cranks the vehicle, which results in the rider and vehicle moving side-to-side when uncompensated. The undesired turning moment can be mini-

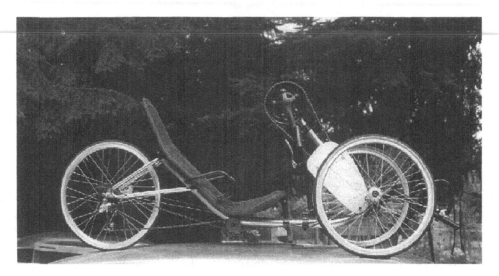

**FIGURE 10.15**   Recumbent three-wheeled arm cycle with lean steering
(Photograph courtesy of Varna Cycles)

mized with a friction dampener (nylon bushings in the head-set) or a viscous dampener. Steering a bicycle is different from steering a tricycle; the former is accomplished primarily by leaning with the front wheels turned opposite to the desired direction to initiate the turn. A tricycle, in contrast, relies on turning the front wheels in the direction of the turn without leaning (Figure 10.16).

It is important to have a wide range of gear ratios available in arm-powered vehicles, since the power output of the arms can be quite limited and fine increments are required to achieve optimal pedaling rates. A chain guard must be used

**FIGURE 10.16**   Photograph of a three-wheeled hand cycle with steering
accomplished by turning the crank from side to side
(Photograph courtesy of Varna Cycles)

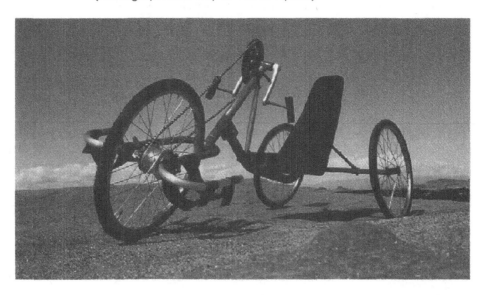

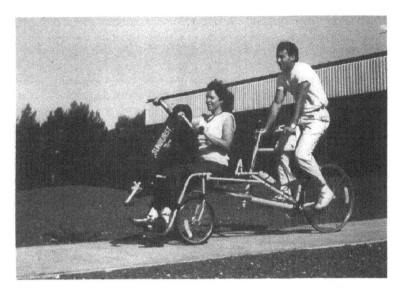

**FIGURE 10.17** Photograph of a tandem arm-crank and foot-pedal bicycle (Photograph courtesy of the Veterans Affairs Rehabilitation Research & Development Center, Palo Alto, California)

to help keep fingers out of the sprockets and to protect the rider in the event of an accident. Easily reachable, indexing type shift levers should be used.

Braking may be accomplished via standard bicycle brakes. Levers must be positioned so that they can be grasped with one hand. Typically, the rider will steer with one hand while braking with the other. Some arm-powered vehicles use a cam-activated brake, which is engaged by reversing the crank direction. This simplifies braking, but prohibits back pedaling for balance at low speeds and when attempting to maximize one's leverage on inclines.

An arm-powered vehicle does not have to be separate from the wheelchair. Add-on units have been designed to convert a wheelchair into an arm-crank vehicle. Some of these devices incorporate quick-release mechanisms used to attach a self-contained front-wheel gear-crank system. Another approach is to attach cranks to each of the rear drive wheels. This type of device may be quick-release as well. Quick-release add-on units are useful for people who desire a device that allows them to use their wheelchair as an arm-crank vehicle without transferring. When desired the user may remove the add-on unit and use the wheelchair normally. Add-on units are often easier to transport in an automobile. Usually performance is traded off for convenience with add-on units. However, add-on units are often less expensive and quite functional for recreational riders.

Power output of human-powered vehicles may be enhanced by using a tandem, where a leg crank is used by an ambulatory rider and an arm crank is used by the other rider (Figure 10.17). Tandems may be two- or three-wheeled. The combined power output of the arm-leg powered tandem is greater than the power output of the arm-powered vehicle alone. The ambulatory rider may sit either in front of or in back of the other rider. When the ambulatory rider sits in the rear he/she can sit higher and see over the other rider, providing both a clear view. When the ambulatory rider sits forward, a carriage can be used to allow the wheelchair rider to roll into the carriage and crank from the wheelchair. Steering is often performed by the ambulatory rider so that the cranking is decoupled from the steering. Shifting may also be done by the ambulatory rider so that pedaling does not have to be interrupted to change gears. The drive train of tandems is most efficient when each rider can pedal at his/her own pace and coast independently.

## References and Further Reading

Asato K. T., Cooper R. A., Baldini F. D., Robertson R. N. (1992) Training practices of athletes who participated in the National Wheelchair Athletic Association Training Camps. *Adapted Physical Activity Quarterly*, 9, 3, 249–260.

Beck K. (1992) Evergreen folding camper. *Paraplegia News*, 46, 7, 31–32.

Charles D., James K. B., Stein R. B. (1988) Rehabilitation of musicians with upper limb amputations. *Journal of Rehabilitation Research and Development*, 25, 3, 25–32.

Cooper R. A., Bedi J., Horvath S. M., Drechsler-Parks D., Williams R. (1992) Maximal exercise responses of paraplegic wheelchair road racers. *Paraplegia*, 30.

Cooper R. A. (1992) Contributions of selected anthropometric and metabolic parameters to 10K performance—A preliminary study. *Journal of Rehabilitation Research and Development*, 29, 3, 29–34.

Cooper R. A. (1989) Racing wheelchair crown compensation. *Journal of Rehabilitation Research and Development*, 26, 1, 25–32.

Cooper R. A. (1989) Racing wheelchair rear wheel alignment. *Journal of Rehabilitation Research and Development*, 26, 1, 47–50.

Cooper R. A. (1992) The contribution of selected anthropometric and physiological variables to 10K performance of wheelchair racers: A preliminary study. *Journal of Rehabilitation Research and Development*, 29, 3, 29–34.

Cooper R. A. (1989) An international track wheelchair with a center of gravity directional controller. *Journal of Rehabilitation Research and Development*, 26, 2, 63–70.

Cooper R. A. (1990) Wheelchair racing sports science: A review. *Journal of Rehabilitation Research and Development*, 27, 3, 295–312.

Cooper R. A. (1992) Racing wheelchair roll stability while turning: A simple model. *Journal of Rehabilitation Research and Development*, 29, 2, 23–30.

Coutts K. D. (1991) Dynamic characteristics of a sport wheelchair. *Journal of Rehabilitation Research and Development*, 28, 3, 45–50.

Engel P., Seeliger K. (1986) Technological and physiological characteristics of a newly developed hand-lever drive system for wheelchairs. *Journal of Rehabilitation Research and Development*, 23, 4, 37–40.

Galvin J. C., Scherer M. J. (1996) *Evaluating, selecting, and using appropriate assistive technology*. Gaithersburg, MD, Aspen Publishers.

Golbranson F. L., Wirta R. W. (1982) *Wheelchair III: Report of a workshop on specially adapted wheelchairs and sports wheelchairs*. RESNA Press, September.

Howell G. H., Brown D. R., Bloswick D. S., Bean J., Gooch J. L. (1993) Design of a device to exercise hip extensor muscles in children with cerebral palsy. *Journal of Assistive Technology*, 5, 2, 119–129.

Loverock P. (1989) The athlete of the future. *Los Angeles Times Magazine*, March, 12.

MacLeish M. S., Cooper R. A., Harralson J., Ster J. S. (1993) Design of a composite monocoque frame racing wheelchair. *Journal of Rehabilitation Research and Development*, 30, 3.

Maarlewski-Probert B. (1992) The RV industry is meeting the challenge. *Paraplegia News*, 46, 8, 21–23.

Rick Hansen Centre. (1988) Proceedings from a national symposium on wheelchair track and roadracing, Department of Physical Education and Sport Studies, University of Alberta.

Wade J. (1993) A league of its own. *REHAB Management*, 6, 5, 44–51.

# CHAPTER 11

# Selection
# of Seat Cushions

*Chapter Goals*

☑ To know criteria for cushion selection

☑ To know state-of-the-art research and product development

☑ To understand person-to-cushion interface

## 11.1 Stresses in Seated Tissue

When an individual sits on a cushion, a number of events take place. The interaction between the cushion and body tissue determines the user's comfort, function, and clinical safety. Distribution of stresses within the seating tissue affects the safety and effectiveness of the cushion. Wheelchair cushions are designed to provide pressure distribution for safe long-term seated posture, postural support, protection from vibration, and protection from shock. Poor distribution of stresses can lead to skin breakdown through a number of means. Normal stress is defined as force divided by the area over which it is applied (see equation (11.1)). High stresses can occur with large forces or with small areas.

$$\sigma_{Normal} = \frac{F}{A} \qquad (11.1)$$

The tissue either compresses or stretches in response to normal stress (see Figure 11.1). Localized stresses are a consequence of sitting.

Only when the body is suspended are the internal stresses minimized. Therefore, the stress must be distributed over the tissue based on the tissue's ability to withstand stress. Normal stresses act perpendicular to the skin, whereas shear stresses act parallel to the skin (see Figure 11.2). Sitting causes both normal and shear forces to exist within the seating tissue. Shear stress is applied force divided by the cross-sectional area (see equation (11.2)).

$$\sigma_{Shear} = \frac{F}{A_c} \qquad (11.2)$$

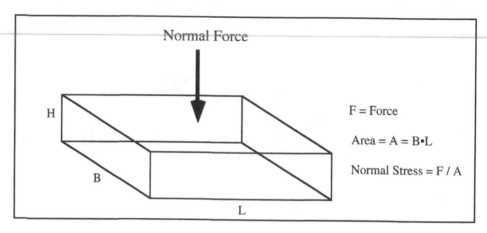

**FIGURE 11.1**    Normal forces, commonly known as pressure, cause materials to compress in response to compression forces and expand in response to tension forces.

Normal stress over bony prominences can cause a decrease in blood flow, or ischemia, which causes a lack of oxygen, anoxia, and nutrients. Anoxia and lack of nutrients promote tissue death, or necrosis. When normal stresses are applied capillaries are pinched off, or occluded, when the external pressure exceeds the internal tissue pressure. Capillary blood pressure is in the range of 32 mmHg as measured in the fingernail beds of healthy subjects, but can be as low as 12 mmHg. Friction and shear can cause skins abrasions. Shear also causes strain within the body tissue and can cause capillary occlusion. When shear is present, tolerance for normal stresses is reduced.

## 11.2 Seating Interface Response

Occlusion of blood flow, or tissue ischemia, is considered to be the primary factor in the formation of pressure sores. Cushions are often used to provide a stable base of support while seated and increase the time a wheelchair user can sit without risk of

**FIGURE 11.2**    Shear stresses act orthogonal to normal stresses and cause little change in tissue thickness.

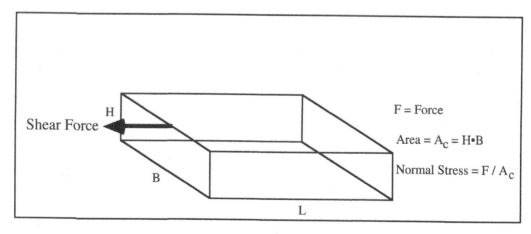

soft tissue injury. Pressure sores are of greatest concern, but several other changes occur within the seated tissue. Lymph flow is altered in seated tissue and there are changes in local tissue metabolism. There may also be localized edema within the seated tissue. All of these factors affect seated tissue integrity and viability.

External factors may also influence the health of seated tissue. Most professionals are aware that pressure contributes to the development of decubitus ulcers. However, pressure is only a single extrinsic factor. While seated, much of an individual's body weight must be supported by the seating interface. Individual anatomy, posture, contouring, and the cushion material influence how the body force is directed through the seated tissue. The magnitude of the force applied to the body tissue influences the tissue response. The sum of the forces over the entire seating surface must equal the magnitude of the applied force. However, the forces within specific segments of the seated tissue may vary significantly. Forces are vector quantities. The direction of the forces within the body tissue also influences the response of the tissue. The duration of the applied force also affects the underlying body tissue. Living tissue demonstrates a remarkable ability to adapt to stress. Adaptation is related to the magnitude, direction, and duration of the forces applied to tissue. The response of body tissue to the seating surface material and contour have led to two theories of seating interfaces. The response of the body to seating surface material and contour is illustrated in Figure 11.3. The shape of the free-

**FIGURE 11.3**    The internal pressure on the body's seated tissue and the deformation of the seated tissue are influenced by the compliance of the cushion and the degree of contouring. Compliance and contouring help to redistribute the forces applied by the cushion to the body.

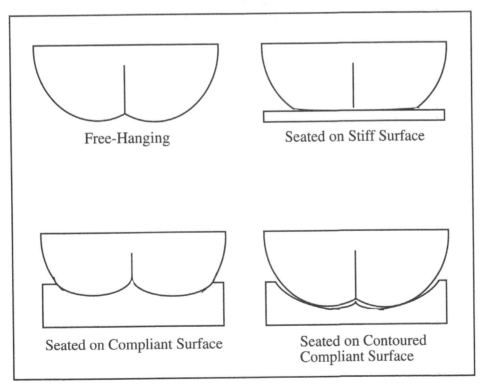

Free-Hanging

Seated on Stiff Surface

Seated on Compliant Surface

Seated on Contoured
Compliant Surface

hanging buttocks is most closely approximated with soft seating surfaces or deep contouring.

Pressure, shape, and deformation are interrelated. This has spawned two theories related to seating interfaces. For the sake of convenience, one theory will be called the interface pressure theory and the other the shape preservation theory. The interface pressure theory is based on a combination of clinical experience and pressure mapping measurements. Its origin can be traced back to prosthetic socket fitting. The interface pressure theory relies on the concept that there is a mapping between pressures measured at the interface and internal pressures. Moreover, the interface pressure theory implies that some seated tissue is more pressure-tolerant than other tissue in the region of the seated interface. Some people also propose that the pressure gradient cannot exceed a certain threshold for each individual. The gradient is used to represent the differences between pressures in a region. The gradient is proposed to be an indicator of shear forces within the seated tissue. There is considerable empiric evidence to support the interface pressure theory. Clinicians and wheelchair users often observe redness where pressure sores may develop. If pressure is removed by means of a cut-out or by sitting shorter periods of time, the redness typically recedes. This has led to the practice of measuring interface pressure using a mapping system, the goal being to reduce the peak pressure to under 150 mmHg and to prevent "large" gradients in pressure. Most of the current cushion technologies operate on the principle of lowering peak interface pressure and controlling the pressure gradient. The interface pressure theory is illustrated in Figure 11.4. External pressure applied by the cushion supporting gravity is reflected by a distribution of pressure within the body tissue at the seating surface. Several investigations have been conducted to relate external force applied by the cushion supporting a portion of the body's weight to internal pressure experienced by the body's tissue at the seating interface. Physical and computer models have been developed to estimate internal pressures. These models provide a qualitative presentation of how internal pressure may be distributed, and may lead to some insight into pressure sore development. Quantitative data have been difficult to obtain because of the complexity of body tissue and the inability to use pressure sensors internally.

The shape preservation theory takes a different perspective on how the body responds to external forces. Shape preservation relies on two basic assumptions: minimum occlusion of blood flow will occur when hydrostatic pressure is constant within the seating surface; and body tissue will experience minimal internal deformation when free-hanging shape is maintained. In simplest terms if the seating surface could be represented by a sack of water, then the cushion should be designed to preserve the unloaded shape of the sack. This would minimize the pressure within the sack and drive the pressure gradient to zero. Of course, body tissue is nonhomogeneous and may not respond like a sack of water. Shape preservation may still be effective if muscle, fat, and connective tissue respond to pressure similarly. Another assumption implicit in the shape preservation theory is that the tissue has an even distribution of capillaries and that the tissue is well capillarized. If capillaries are evenly distributed throughout the tissue, then constant hydrostatic pressure may reduce occlusion of blood flow by maintaining an even cross-sectional area of the capillaries. This is illustrated in Figure 11.5. If pressure is equal in every direction around a capillary, its area will be reduced radially, whereas if pressure is placed uniaxially the capillary may collapse. The amount of reduction in the capillary radius for hydrostatic loading is dependent on the com-

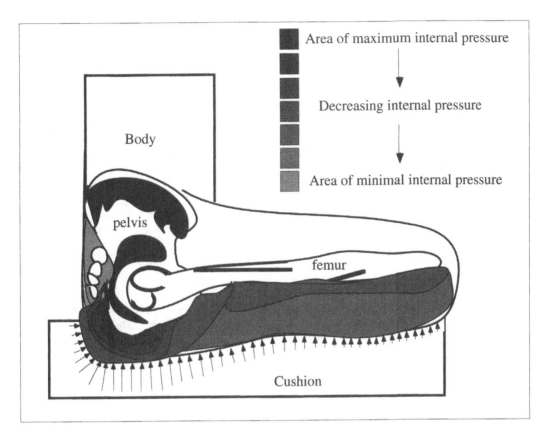

**FIGURE 11.4** External forces applied by the cushion to support the seated portion of the body weight often result in an uneven pressure distribution within the body. Altering the distribution and direction of the cushion forces may lead to more desirable internal pressures.

pressibility of the body tissue, the capillary wall, and blood. Water is typically considered to be an incompressible fluid. Supporters of the shape preservation theory argue that body tissue has compressibility properties near to those of water. Uniaxial loading does not trap the capillary or surrounding tissue, allowing it to deform in response to the load. This may cause the capillary wall to collapse and occlude blood flow.

Shape preservation of the seated buttocks may be obtained by treating the cushion more like an orthosis. If the body tissue within the seating surface is captured to remain within a semi-rigid container, shape can be preserved. The basic concept of a shape preservation cushion is presented in Figure 11.6. A potential problem with shape preservation is that it may interfere with movement for pressure relief, and that the optimal static seating posture may not coincide with the optimal dynamic seating posture required to propel a wheelchair. The optimal cushion based on the interface pressure theory is likely to be faced by similar problems. However, the shape preservation theory indicates that a semi-rigid shell is necessary to minimize occlusion, whereas the interface pressure theory may be able to reduce internal pressure by selecting the compliance of the seating surface. Time will tell whether these two theories can be unified and whether a single or multiple solutions to the problem of pressure relief will ultimately result from research in this area.

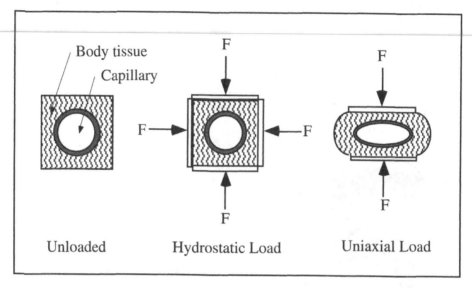

**FIGURE 11.5**  The capillary assumes its natural shape when unloaded and blood flows freely. Under hydrostatic pressure the capillary may reduce in size, causing an increase in capillary pressure. With uniaxial loading the capillary wall may collapse, causing occlusion of blood flow. The response of the capillary and the subsequent blood flow is dependent on the loading around the capillary wall.

## 11.3 Pressure Measurement Systems

Seating pressure is often associated with compression of body tissue, muscle, and fat. However, a large percentage of the body is fluid (about 98%), which is incompressible. Body fluid under pressure within tissue, fat, and muscle is in shear. For example, compressing a balloon filled with water against a hard table causes the

**FIGURE 11.6**  By using a rigid volume to constrain the body tissue under loading, near hydrostatic loading may be obtainable.

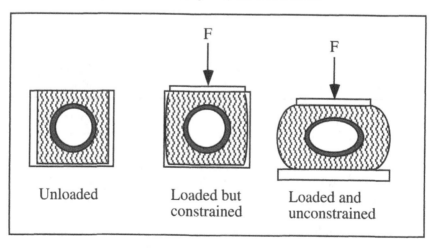

balloon to flatten. This is because the water moves parallel (shear) to the compression force. When a person sits on a flat surface, the fluid in the buttocks does not compress but moves parallel to the exerted force. The buttocks flatten at the center and extend outward at the sides. The shear pressure exerted on the tissue and the distortion of the buttocks are related. To minimize distortion of the buttocks and thus damage to the tissue, the resting shape of the buttocks has to be maintained. Several approaches have been investigated for the optimal pressure distribution in wheelchair seating.

Static seating pressure measurements have long been applied in the field of rehabilitation. There are two major types of pressure monitors: simple single-point pressure static pressure monitors, and pressure mapping systems. Systems are currently available that can measure from 64 to 2000 data points in a single second. In order to have a repeatable sensor orientation, many systems attach their sensors to a flexible membrane. The stiffness of the membrane may affect the ability of the sensors to conform to the surface of the buttocks and thus to measure normal force on contoured surfaces. To effectively analyze pressure distribution on a seated surface, time variations in pressure changes must be measured.

Dynamic pressure measurement is required as people move over time and pressure varies as they move. Pressure must be measured over time for various activities, and the time-pressure profile could be used to develop appropriate cushion and seating systems. Seat interface pressure changes as a person pushes a wheelchair. Pressure may vary from 50 mmHg to 200 mmHg for a single point on the seat during the propulsion recovery phase. Pressure measurement systems should enable clinicians and designers to make informed decisions about the effectiveness of products.

### 11.3.1 Variables Produced by Seating Pressure Mapping Systems

Many seating pressure mapping systems measure force over a small sensor with a known area. Referring to Figure 11.7, the area (A) of a single sensor is given by equation (11.3),

$$A = a \bullet b \tag{11.3}$$

With a force sensor of fixed area, the pressure (p) is simply the force (F) divided by the area (A),

$$p = \frac{F}{A} \tag{11.4}$$

The pressure as defined in equation (11.4) is equivalent to the normal stress described by equation (11.1). Pressure sensing arrays typically use color or shading as options for displaying pressure. Current systems use a finite number of sensors with a fixed area and location. The map of the pressure, as shown in Figure 11.7, indicates where contouring or other forms of pressure relief may be warranted.

A simple variable used to evaluate and select cushions is the mean or average pressure. The mean pressure is determined for all sensors,

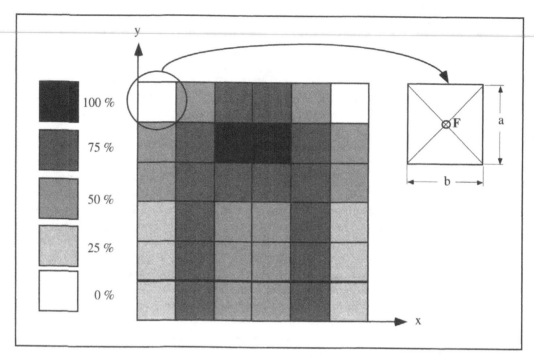

**FIGURE 11.7** Illustration of pressure and center of pressure calculation from an array of force sensors

$$P_{mean} = \frac{1}{N} \sum_{i=1}^{N} p_i = \frac{1}{N \cdot A} \sum_{i=1}^{N} F_i \qquad (11.5)$$

More information about the variability can be gained by calculating the median pressure. The median is determined by ranking all of the pressure values and then finding the midpoint. If the pressures are symmetrically or evenly distributed, the mean and the median will yield similar results. Comparison of the mean and the median indicates whether there are some high or low values that must be looked at more closely. Many people concern themselves with the maximum pressure recorded by the pressure map. This may be misleading. The sensors used on pressure-sensing maps are subject to a variety of sources of error, and use of a single value may lead to erroneous decisions. Peak values should be considered but should be viewed as pieces of information from a set. When comparing cushions, some people prefer to use a truncated mean. The truncated mean is calculated by discarding the minimum and maximum values and calculating the mean based on the remaining values.

The total contact area between the cushion and the buttocks is a useful value when evaluating cushions. A larger contact area helps to reduce the pressure required to be supported by a given region. If the contact area is large, it becomes simpler to lower the pressure in sensitive regions because the pressure over the entire surface will be lower. Every sensor has a fixed area over which it acts, so the contact area can be estimated by counting the number of sensors that register a force or pressure above the factory-determined minimum.

Symmetry and placing of the mapping system can be checked by using the center of pressure. The center of pressure has long been used in force platform analysis as a measure of how the foot places pressure on the ground. Seating map center of pressure is very similar. The center of pressure is the weighted sum of the forces acting over the pressure mapping system. The result is the location where an equivalent force could be applied to cause the same moments about the x and y axes of the pressure mapping system. The main reasons for using center of pressure for seating are to see if the person is moving the center of mass around while measurements are being taken, and to help ensure that the pressure mapping system is aligned in the same location when making multiple measurements. Center of pressure is taken by summing the moments about each axis and setting them equal to zero,

$$\sum_{i=1}^{N} M_x = 0 \qquad \sum_{i=1}^{N} M_y = 0 \tag{11.6}$$

We will first look at the sum of the moments about the y axis as defined in Figure 11.7,

$$Fx_{cop} = F_1x_1 + F_2x_2 + F_3x_3 + \cdots + F_Nx_N$$
$$Fx_{cop} = \sum_{i=1}^{N} F_ix_i \tag{11.7}$$

The pressure or force sensing array provides the force for each sensor ($F_i$), and one can measure the distance between each sensor ($x_i$). The total force seen by the array is equal to the sum of the forces seen by each of the sensors,

$$F = F_1 + F_2 + F_3 + \cdots + F_N$$
$$F = \sum_{i=1}^{N} F_i \tag{11.8}$$

Equations (11.7) and (11.8) provide the information needed to determine the center of pressure from the y axis,

$$x_{cop} = \frac{\sum_{i=1}^{N} F_ix_i}{\sum_{i=1}^{N} F_i} \tag{11.9}$$

The center of pressure from the x axis produces a similar result,

$$y_{cop} = \frac{\sum_{i=1}^{N} F_iy_i}{\sum_{i=1}^{N} F_i} \tag{11.10}$$

Movement of the x and y coordinates of the center of pressure ($x_{cop}$, $y_{cop}$) indicate that the person or the mat have shifted. Shifting may influence the interpretation of the pressure mapping results because many clinicians rely on anatomical landmarks to be located above specific sensors.

We will examine the center of pressure for the specific example given in Figure 11.7. In this example each sensor has x dimension b, and y dimension a. The force acting at each sensor ($F_i$) is located within the middle of the corresponding sensor (i.e., at b/2, a/2). For simplicity, we will assume that 100% is equal to 100 mmHg, and that the sensors are linear. Given this information, we are prepared to determine the center of pressure.

Let us determine (F), the total force applied to the force sensing array. There are 36 sensors in Figure 11.7, therefore (F) is sum of the forces from each of these sensors. Moving from left to right and bottom to top,

$$F = 25 + 75 + 50 + 50 + 75 + 25 + 25 + 75 + 50 + 50 + 75 + 25$$
$$+ 25 + 75 + 50 + 50 + 75 + 25 + 50 + 75 + 75 + 75 + 75 + 50$$
$$+ 50 + 75 + 100 + 100 + 75 + 50 + 0 + 50 + 75 + 75 + 50 + 0$$

$$F = 2000 \text{ mmHg} \tag{11.11}$$

Because the process is similar, we will only determine the center of pressure from the y axis. The moment needs to be determined next; this calculation relies on the position of each of the sensors.

$$
\begin{aligned}
Fx_{cop} = \tfrac{b}{2} \big[ &25 + 3(75) + 5(50) + 7(50) + 9(75) + 11(25) \\
+ &25 + 3(75) + 5(50) + 7(50) + 9(75) + 11(25) \\
+ &25 + 3(75) + 5(50) + 7(50) + 9(75) + 11(25) \\
+ &50 + 3(75) + 5(75) + 7(75) + 9(75) + 11(50) \\
+ &50 + 3(75) + 5(100) + 7(100) + 9(75) + 11(50) \\
+ &0 \ \ + 3(50) + 5(75) \ \ + 7(75) \ \ + 9(50) + 11(0) \big]
\end{aligned}
$$
$$Fx_{cop} = (b/2)12000 \tag{11.12}$$

The x coordinate of the center of pressure is determined by dividing the results of equation (11.12) by the result of equation (11.11),

$$x_{cop} = Fx_{cop} / F = 6000b / 2000 = 3b \tag{11.13}$$

A few checks can be used to determine whether the center of pressure location seems reasonable. If the pressure map appears symmetrical about a line, then one of the center of pressure coordinates should be close to the line of symmetry. The second check is that the center of pressure must lie within the dimensions of the pressure map.

The pressure gradient may also be an important measure when evaluating and selecting cushions. If the difference between two adjacent pressure sensors is large, then large shear forces may exist, which could lead to tissue damage. The gradient ($\Delta$) is taken as the difference between the pressures (p) divided by the distance (d) between the sensors,

$$\Delta_{i\text{-}j} = \frac{p_j - p_i}{d} \tag{11.14}$$

The gradient can be visualized by plotting the pressures recorded by each sensor as a mesh plot (i.e., a plot shows pressure as hills and valleys). Figure 11.8 shows the pressures presented in Figure 11.7 as a mesh plot. The differences

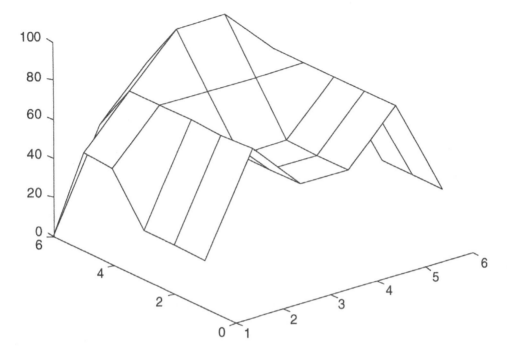

**FIGURE 11.8** A mesh plot of the pressures presented in Figure 11.7. The mesh plot illustrates the pressure gradients as steep slopes between adjacent sensor measurements

between adjacent pressures are illustrated by steep transitions. When selecting or evaluating a cushion, high-pressure gradients should be avoided.

### 11.3.2 Bladder Pressure Sensors

Bladder sensors readily conform to the curvature of human soft tissue, have good repeatability, and are inherently insensitive to shear forces and temperature changes. Ideally, the sensor would not induce any changes in the tissue or tissue-cushion interface. Seating pressure measurements typically range from 0 to 1500 mmHg. Some researchers have placed sensors over the ischial tuberosities or have taped sensors directly over the skin.

Switch-activated bladder pressure sensors rely on an interior switch to indicate pressure equilibrium. An air bladder is placed at the skin-cushion interface. The client is appropriately positioned, then the air bladder is inflated and the pressure in the bladder increases. The switch opens when the pressure in the air bladder equals that of the tissue. A pressure gage can be used to indicate pressure upon switch open. This process can also be reversed (i.e., deflate the bladder until the switch closes).

An array of bladder sensors can be made by using two sheets of airtight flexible material molded to form a set of pockets forming a grid of switch-activated pressure sensors. The pressure in each pocket can be measured to yield an estimate of the seating pressure distribution. However, the pad may act as an air flotation cushion, reducing the pressure gradient especially around high-pressure areas.

Bladder sensors can also be integrated with other pressure sensors to produce a pressure contour. The Oxford air bladder system consists of a $3 \times 4$ matrix of sensors. A microprocessor-controlled system inflates each of the bladder sensors individually. Each sensor is multiplexed to the microprocessor and a semiconductor pressure transducer. A vacuum pump holds each sensor deflated. The sensor of interest is activated and begins to inflate with a constant mass flow. When the pressure in the bladder exceeds that of the external tissue, it begins to inflate, producing a change in volume and reducing the rate at which internal pressure increases. The pressure is recorded at this inflection point, the bladder is deflated, and the process is repeated by the next sensor. A larger number of bladders are required to achieve a useful pressure contour.

Water can be used as an incompressible fluid to transmit seat interface pressure to a remote pressure transducer. Flexible, typically nonelastic bladders filled with water are connected to a diaphragm-type pressure transducer. When force is exerted on the active bladder, the pressure developed is transmitted via a capillary to the transducer, which produces a proportional voltage. Caution must be used to avoid overfilling the bladders and creating stresses on the walls of the bladder that will produce a nonlinear response. The height of bladder sensors may cause the person's weight to shift and cause measurement error.

### 11.3.3 Conductive Polymer Force-Sensing Resistors

Devices for measuring pressure can be useful in identifying localized areas of high pressure. However, the skin pressure is lower than the interior pressure around bony prominences, where most ulcers begin. Two recent innovations have developed that may dramatically improve cushion design and prescription. The first is the development of low-cost, low-profile dynamic force sensors that can be arranged in an array to yield a model of the pressure distribution on the surface of the buttocks. The second is the development of noninvasive techniques for measuring the distribution and geometry of tissue and to model tissue behavior under various loads (e.g., finite element analysis). The combination of a sensor array and a model of tissue behavior could lead to an understanding of how cushions need to be designed to prevent pressure sores.

Recently, conductive polymer sensors have become commercially available, which with some modification may be suitable for measuring cushion interface pressure. Conductive polymer resistive force sensors (Interlink) with some adaptations may make it suitable for measuring cushion interface pressure. Conductive polymer resistive force sensors are inexpensive, lightweight, and small. However, they are sensitive to how pressure is applied, and their response is nonlinear. In addition, they have been used in some applications without knowledge of how they operate. This may produce erroneous results. The development of a reasonably priced normal force-sensing mat or pressure-sensing pants may yield the external loading data required for finite element or other models of the internal distribution of pressure within the buttocks. This could lead to improvements in cushions and reductions in pressure sores. However, the properties and limitations of these sensors need to be understood before they are applied. The efficacy of the data is dependent on the quality of the sensor.

Conductive polymer resistive force sensors consist of three main parts: 1) a round piece of mylar coated with a circle of a conductive polymer ink, 2) a thin metallic ring with an inside diameter slightly larger than the diameter of the conductive polymer, and 3) another round piece of mylar with traces printed onto it in a pattern of interlocking fingers. The leads come from the piece of mylar with the fingers printed on it. Without any force on the sensor, the resistance is nearly infinite (the fingers do not touch and the air gap prevents conduction through the polymer ink). As pressure is applied the conductive polymer ink begins to touch the traces of the opposite mylar film and the resistance between the leads drops (the resistance of the polymer ink remains constant). As more pressure is applied the contact area increases and the resistance drops further. However, the contact area depends on where the pressure is applied; there is greater contact with fingers in some areas than there is in others. The range is typically between 12M ohms and 100 ohms. This range is large enough to be measured by very simple circuitry.

### 11.3.4 Capacitive Pressure Mats

Capacitive sensors can be made very sensitive, linear, and inexpensive. Typically, larger capacitance requires simpler circuitry, but implies larger physical size. Individual capacitive transducers do not show significant promise for seat interface pressure measurement. However, a mat of woven conductive strips may be a solution. A capacitor is a charge storage device that can be described by three physical parameters:

$$C = \frac{\varepsilon A}{d} \tag{11.15}$$

where $\varepsilon$ describes the dielectric material, $A$ is the effective plate area, and $d$ is the separation distance between the plates. Typically, capacitive transducers work on the principle of varying $A$ or $d$. A method of developing a useful capacitive transducer pressure-sensing mat was proposed by Babbs et al. (1990), who used two orthogonal arrays of ribbon-like conductor. The arrays are separated by low-hysteresis foam rubber. Current is sensed between a pair of conductors on either side of the foam with a 5-kHz voltage source. All unused conductors are grounded to avoid cross-talk while measurements are made. The foam compresses as force is applied, which brings the ribbon-like conductors closer together, increasing the capacitance.

## 11.4 Properties of Pressure Relief Cushions

There are two basic types of seating systems used with wheelchairs: linear systems and contoured systems. Linear seating systems are planar in that the seat and back surfaces are flat and only conform to the weight of the user. For many wheelchair users a simple linear seating system or a standard contour is very effective. Foam, gel, dry flotation (air) cushions, and honeycomb are the most common cushion materials.

### 11.4.1 Linear Foam Cushions

Various densities and types (polyurethane, urethane, T-foam, Sunmate) of foam are commonly used in linear seating systems (see Figure 11.9). Foam has been shown to offer the lowest maximum pressure over the seating surface when the

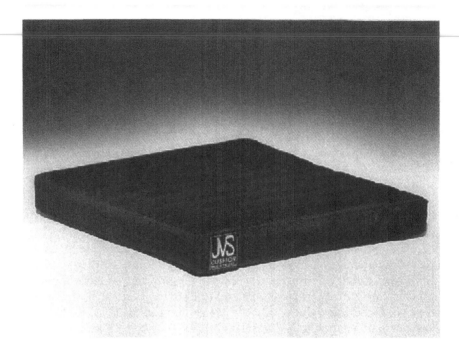

**FIGURE 11.9**   Photograph of a linear foam cushion (Photograph courtesy of JVS Cushion)

appropriate densities and contours are used. However, foam has a tendency to deteriorate at an undesirable rate. A very significant advantage of foam over other materials is that it is inexpensive. The raw material for a foam cushion costs only a few dollars. The added cost to make a cushion comes from the sculpting or contouring, which requires clinical skills in order to make foam work most effectively for pressure relief.

Standard polyurethane or urethane foams are made from plastic that has been processed to incorporate large numbers of air bubbles. These air bubbles within the foam cause a cross-link structure. When foam is loaded, it behaves like a spring for small forces and displacements. As greater load and displacement are applied, the cross-links begin to buckle and the foam begins to behave nonlinearly. If further load is applied, the cross-links fully buckle and the foam begins to behave like a compressible solid. This is shown graphically in Figure 11.10. Little is understood about how these properties are best manipulated to form a pressure relief cushion. For this reason people use foams of various densities and stiffnesses.

Density of foam relates to the amount of air that is trapped in the plastic matrix. Higher-density foams tend to be heavier because they contain more plastic. As density increases, stiffness also increases. However, stiffness and density are not the same properties. Stiffness refers to the slope of the force-displacement curve during the linear region (i.e., before the cross-links begin to buckle). Foam is also characterized as open-cell or closed-cell. Closed-cell foam is made such that it is less permeable to fluid.

Foam cushions can be made by contouring a single piece of foam or by combining foams of different stiffnesses. There are also specialty foams such as T-foam or Sunmate foam. These specialty foams are made to have gel-like properties while

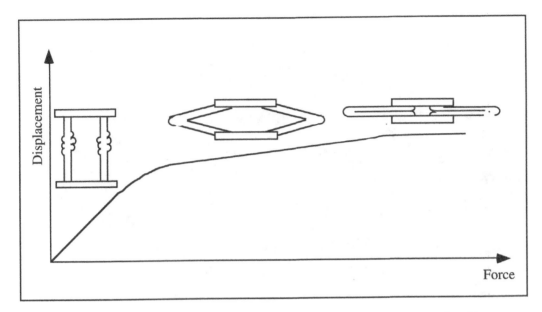

**FIGURE 11.10**  The cross-links of foam change the force/displacement relationship as force is increased. This nonlinear behavior of foam has not been fully exploited in cushion design.

maintaining some desirable properties of foam. T-foam and Sunmate foam have negligible linear regions. They compress like a standard foam, although slower. However, they have memory that retards them from returning to their resting shape. Hence, when a person sits on them, they tend to come to equilibrium with the sitting tissue. The foam then responds slowly to changes in position. T-foam or Sunmate foam can be used to give some additional stability to standard foam cushions. Foam is an excellent material for cushions, but it has low durability and rapidly loses its pressure-relieving properties with use. Most foam cushions need to be replaced annually.

### 11.4.2 Air Flotation Cushions

Air flotation cushions provide an excellent example of cushion design based on the interface pressure theory. If one were to sit on a balloon full of air, the pressure over the entire seating surface would be equal. This is due to the air in the bag shifting to conform to the seated surface to equalize the internal pressure. A balloon full of air does an excellent job of distributing the pressure over the seating area. However, the pressure would be distributed indiscriminately. In order to better control interface pressure, many air flotation cushions use multiple compartments, contouring, and baffling (Figure 11.11). Multiple compartments allow interface pressure to be regulated from one compartment to another. The pressure within a particular cell (balloon) will be constant. The pressure at the skin interface may be regulated by shaping the balloon. Balloon shape may lower pressure within the tissue by altering the way in which the body tissue deforms. Some cushions use foam in combination with air bladders to control the pressure within the cushion, and in turn the interface pressure (Figure 11.12). The combination

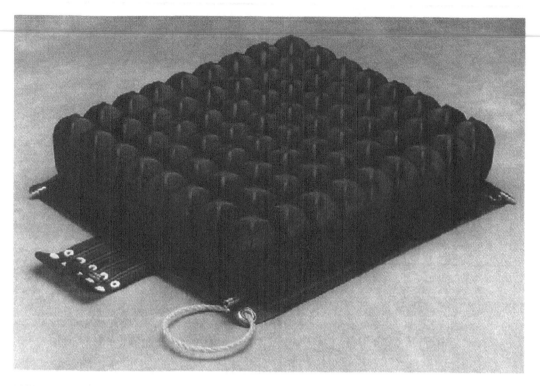

**FIGURE 11.11**   Photograph of a multi-cell air flotation cushion with flexible membrane
(Photograph courtesy of Roho Incorporated)

of foam and air flotation assumes that the compression of the foam within the bladder will regulate pressure to direct it away from low tolerant regions and toward regions of higher pressure tolerance.

A problem with air cushions is that they may lose their air and simultaneously their ability to provide pressure relief. Some air cushions require considerable maintenance. In some case, users should bring repair kits with them when traveling. Air cushions will also change their properties with changes in altitude. The most common instance is when flying on an airplane. The air pressure within the cushion can change considerably from take-off to cruising altitude.

### 11.4.3 Gel Flotation Cushions

Gel cushions use an electrolyte gel in a closed plastic or latex pocket. The gel conforms to the body and provides a nearly even pressure distribution. Gel is essentially a viscous fluid. Viscosity is used to define a fluid's resistance to flow. Because gel behaves like a fluid, it will work much like air to equalize pressure over the entire seating surface. This is because the gel will move to come to a constant pressure within its container. Baffles can be used to control the flow of the gel just as with air cushions. The pressure distribution can be altered by using a stiff base (e.g., plastic or foam) to provide some contouring (Figure 11.13). The high viscosity of the gel prevents it from moving rapidly within its container. This property allows the gel cushion to provide a more stable seating surface than an air

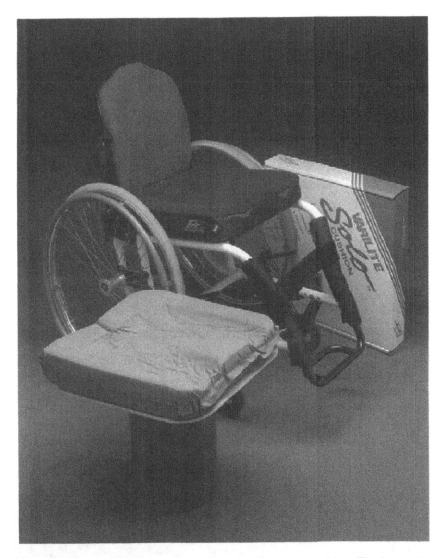

**FIGURE 11.12** Photograph of a foam-filled air flotation cushion (Photograph courtesy of Varilite Incorporated)

cushion. However, the high viscosity of a gel cushion also limits its shock-absorbing properties.

Gel cushions often suffer from excessive weight by many users, and their properties are subject to changes in temperature. Some types of gel may actually freeze during extremely cold weather, or if the cushion becomes cold the user's body may need to exert considerable energy to heat the cushion. The weight of gel cushions has been altered by some cushion manufacturers making lightweight gels (Figure 11.14). Lightweight gels may act more like whipped cream. Light weight is typically accompanied by lower viscosity. Lower viscosity provides greater shock-absorbing properties. Gel cushions do not change their properties significantly with changes in atmospheric pressure. Users of gel cushions must check with man-

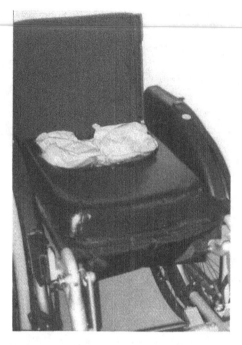

**FIGURE 11.13**  Photograph of a gel-based flotation cushion with a rigid foam base
(Photograph by Rory Cooper)

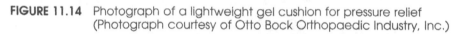

**FIGURE 11.14**  Photograph of a lightweight gel cushion for pressure relief
(Photograph courtesy of Otto Bock Orthopaedic Industry, Inc.)

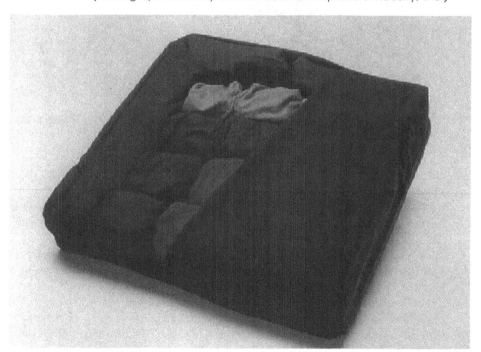

ufacturers about possible allergic reactions from contact with the gel. Gel cushions may develop leaks with time and use.

### 11.4.4 Honeycomb

Honeycomb materials are made to exploit linear properties of some polymers (types of plastics). When these polymers are molded into a honeycomb, they behave like a collection of springs (i.e., similar to the linear behavior of foam). Honeycomb cushion materials have an advantage over foam in that the manufacturer can carefully control the properties of the honeycomb material and the resulting cushion. Honeycomb cushions can be contoured like foam (Figure 11.15). However, honeycomb cushions are typically contoured by the manufacturer for some standard shapes. Honeycomb cushions can be made to greatly simplify cleaning, which makes them more attractive than foam in institutions that may have multiple people sharing a single cushion. Of course, air and gel flotation cushions can also be made easy to clean.

A drawback of honeycomb cushions is that they are considerably more expensive than foam, and they do not come in the wide variety of stiffnesses that foam does. Honeycomb materials may have a larger linear range than foam. There also are indications that honeycomb materials may be more durable than foam.

### 11.4.5 Seat Bases

Seat bases may be either rigid or a cloth sling. In either case the seat should be stiff and provide a stable base for the cushion and user. Sling seats (seat and backrests) are constructed of synthetic materials with high tensile strengths. Nylon, cotton canvas, Kevlar®, or similar materials are used to provide the struc-

**FIGURE 11.15** Photograph of a honeycomb polymer-based cushion (Photograph courtesy of Supracor Incorporated)

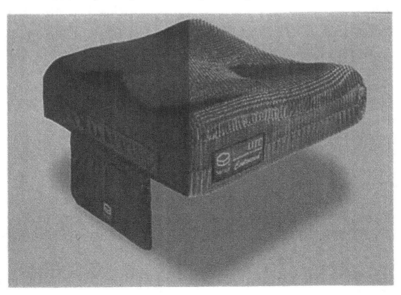

tural component of the seat or backrest sling. In many instances the structural material may be enclosed in a vinyl, naugahyde, or other water-resistant case, which acts as the interface to the user. Vinyl and naugahyde deform substantially under load and are not appropriate as structural seating materials. The exterior shell is often vacuum formed under heat to form a bond between the shell material and the structural material. Seats and backrests may be attached to the wheelchair frame in a variety of ways. One of the more common means is to sew a pocket into each lateral edge of the seat base and backrest upholstery. When attaching the base and backrest upholstery to the frame, a metal (steel or aluminum) slat is placed into the upholstery pocket. Screws are then inserted through the slat and into the frame. For backrests it is not uncommon to insert the backrest canes through the upholstery and to use grommets and oversized contoured washers to secure the backrest upholstery to the canes. A sufficient number of attachment points should be used to prevent the backrest upholstery from sliding down the canes in the event of a screw or grommet failure, or an upholstery tear. Other methods can be used to resist having the backrest upholstery slide down the canes in the event of component failure. The backrest upholstery can be sewn in a catenary so that equal tension is applied to the canes across the entire surface of the backrest, or a stiffening material (high-density foam) can be sewn into the upholstery. Seat base and backrest upholstery can also be attached using webbing or lacing.

Rigid seat bases and backrests have the advantage that their properties change little over time, so the cushion is always properly supported. However, a rigid seat base may weigh more, but as the application of composite materials becomes more widespread this should no longer be an issue. Aluminum, steel, fiberglass, Kevlar®, carbon fiber, and several plastics are used in making seat bases and backrests. Most wheelchairs are available in common sizes, so seat bases and backrests need to be made only for the sizes available. Rigid seat bases may incorporate some contouring to assist with proper seating positioning with hip supports, or they may be flat. Rigid or semi-rigid backrests may provide greater lumbar and lateral support than sling seats (Figure 11.16). Rigid seat bases and backrest supports form the foundation for many contoured seating systems, and they are becoming more popular.

## 11.4.6 Seating Positioning Equipment

Proper seating can be achieved for many people using standard seating and positioning equipment. The pelvis is often the foundation of the properly aligned seat. The structure, construction, and dimensions are critical in prescribing or designing a positioning pad or seating cushion. Seat cushions may have a squared edge, rolled edge, or beveled edge (Figure 11.17). Rolled or beveled edges are used to allow the knees to flex for people with contractures. The sagittal shapes of common seat cushions are shown in Figure 11.18.

Seat cushions commonly include a cut-out for the ischial tuberosities, an abductor pommel, and hip adductor contours (Figure 11.19). For people who require additional positioning or postural support, hip pads and/or hip belts can be used. For people with severe leg abduction or adduction, abductor or adductor pads can be attached to the seat pan. A cylinder of low-to-medium density polyurethane foam on a stainless steel or chromed mild steel pillar will pro-

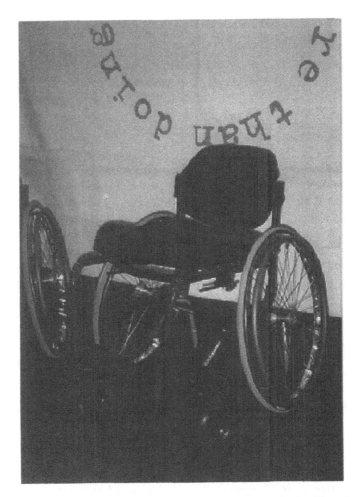

**FIGURE 11.16**  Photograph of an ultralight manual wheelchair with orthotic back support system (Photograph courtesy of Rory Cooper)

vide adequate support for even the most severe cases. Abductor or adductor pads can be prescribed or designed to be detachable or flip-down for easier transfers. Often a single cylinder is adequate; however, some people can benefit from two cylinders that can be independently adjusted laterally. A scissor board (i.e., a wedge of foam adhered to a semi-rigid material) with polyurethane foam can be used to reduce the risk of pressure sores at the knees when a narrow lateral separation is desired.

**FIGURE 11.17**  Cushion edge finish definitions

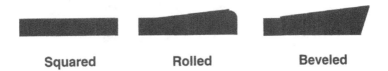

      **Squared**          **Rolled**          **Beveled**

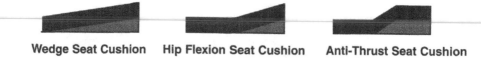

**Wedge Seat Cushion    Hip Flexion Seat Cushion    Anti-Thrust Seat Cushion**

**FIGURE 11.18**   Common seat cushion profiles

### 11.4.7 Custom-Contoured Cushions

Contour measurements can be made using vacuum forming or seating contour measurement systems. Typically such systems are used to create a contour representative of the client's seating profile. Vacuum forming methods are typically based on a flexible bag (e.g., latex, rubber) filled with styrofoam or foam rubber pellets. The bag is connected to a vacuum pump. The person to be molded is seated on the bead-bag and placed in approximately the desired position. Air is drawn from the bag, which becomes ever more rigid. While air is being drawn from the bag, the clinician and rehabilitation engineer/technician form the bead-bag around the client, pushing and pulling on the bag until the client is in the desired position. Air continues to be withdrawn from the bag until it becomes stiff, at which point the client can be removed from the chair. Vacuum forming systems are cost effective and relatively simple. Contour measurement systems are more effective when they mimic wheelchair seating (i.e., legrests are attached, armrests are used, backrest is at proper angle and of appropriate height). Once a male mold of the client's contour is completed, it must be transferred from the bead-bag to something that can be used to create a cushion. Many commercial contoured cushions are created using computer numerically controlled (CNC) foam milling machines. These machines use arrays to represent x, y, and z coordinates of the seating contour. Hence, some companies have developed mechanical or electromechanical panographs to convert the male mold to a graph or directly to a computer file. A panograph may simply consist of a set of bars with rounded tips that glide over the mold surface. The other ends of the shafts are connected to a pen or transducer. The sensors (fingers) of the panograph are indexed over the surface of the mold until a suitable representation has been created (Figure 11.20).

**FIGURE 11.19**   Illustration of cushion with hip adductor pads and pommel

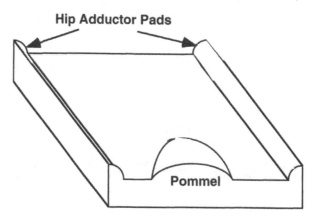

**Hip Adductor Pads**

**Pommel**

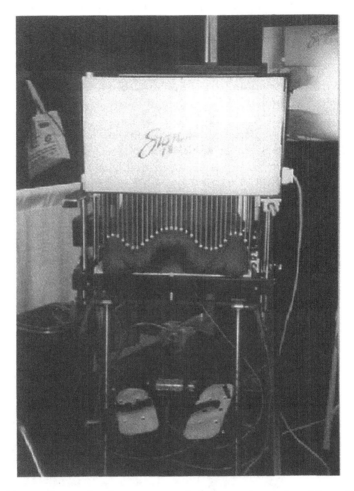

**FIGURE 11.20** Photograph of a panograph type contoured cushion digitizer (Photograph courtesy of Rory Cooper)

## 11.5 Computerized Shape Measurement

Systems have also been developed that directly measure the client's seating contour. This has been accomplished successfully in a number of ways. A simple method used to directly measure a client's seating contour is to punch an array of holes into a piece of foam. A plunger with a conforming head is placed through each hole in the foam. Each plunger is attached to its own stiff cable that runs through an incompressible flexible housing. On the other end of the cable there is either a pen or transducer to measure displacement. As the client sits on the sensor, the foam compresses and the plungers recess to create a portrait of the client's seating contour. If the foam is well characterized, the contour can be translated to an equivalent contour using a different foam with known density and compression properties. Each client must be seated properly and comfortably on the shape chair and shape sensor. Seat tilt angle, backrest angle, back height, footrest position, and armrest position must all be set properly to yield satisfactory results. Several sensors must be used to get an accurate contour profile; in some cases over 100 sensors are used to measure deflection.

More advanced systems have been developed that use linear variable displacement transformers (LVDT), linear potentiometers, or linear motors. Systems using LVDT's or potentiometers often use foam or coil springs to provide the necessary seating compliance. The preload force on coil springs can be set to simulate foams of different densities and compression properties. Coil springs behave linearly over a fairly large range, whereas foam does not. Linear motors offer greater flexibility than other seating pressure measurement systems, as linear motors can be operated to behave like springs or foam. Linear motors can also be operated in a closed loop, to apply or withdraw pressure at desired points or to alter the shape of the contour. Position and/or force transducers are required to create closed-loop contour measurement systems (see Figure 11.21). Direct-seating contour measurement systems are most appropriate for people who only require moderate seating and postural support. Such systems do not offer the same degree of postural support as bead-bag systems.

**FIGURE 11.21**    Photograph of a closed-loop computer-controlled machine for designing custom-contoured cushions (Photograph courtesy of Dr. David Brienza, University of Pittsburgh)

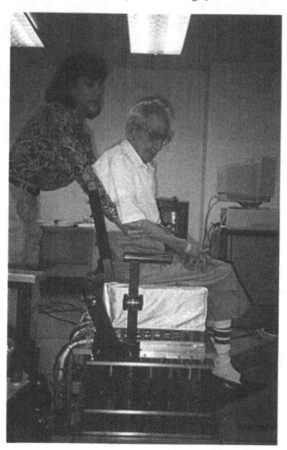

## References and Further Reading

Agrawal V. P., Chandra R. (1979) Optimisation of a chair mechanism for partially disabled people for sitting-standing and sitting-lying motions. *Medical and Biological Engineering and Computing*, 17, 671–682.

Andersson G. B. J., Oertengren R. (1974) Lumbar disc pressure and myoelectric back muscle activity during sitting. III. Studies on a wheelchair. *Scandinavian Journal of Rehabilitation Medicine*, 3, 122–127.

Andersson G. B. J., Murphy R. W., Oertengren R., Nachemson A. L. (1979) The influence of backrest inclination and lumbar support on the lumbar lordosis in sitting. *Spine*, 4, 52–58.

Axelson P. (1993) Wheelchair comparison. *Sports 'N Spokes*, 18, 6, 34–40.

Babbs C. F., Bourland J. D., Graber G. P., Jones J. T., Schoenlein W. E. (1990) A pressure sensitive mat for measuring contact pressure distributions for patients lying on hospital beds. *Biomedical Instrumentation Technology*, 24, 363–370.

Bennet L., Kavner D., Lee B. K., Trainor F. A. (1979) Shear versus pressure as causative factors in skin blood flow occlusion. *Archives of Physical Medicine and Rehabilitation*, 60, 309–314.

Brienza D. M., Chung K.-C., Brubaker C. E., Kwiatkowski R. J. (1993) Design of a computer-controlled seating surface for research applications. *IEEE Transactions on Rehabilitation Engineering*, 1, 1, 63–66.

Brienza D. M., Brubaker C. E., Inigo R. M. (1989) A fiber optic force sensor for automated seating design. *Proceedings 12th Annual RESNA Conference*, New Orleans, LA, 232–233.

Brienza D. M., Chung K. C., Inigo R. M. (1988) Design of a computer aided manufacturing system for custom contoured wheelchair cushions. *Proceedings International Conference of the American Association for Rehabilitation Therapy*, 312–313.

Brienza D. M., Gordon J., Thacker J. (1989) A comparison of force transducers suitable for an automatic body support contour system. *Proceedings 12th Annual RESNA Conference*, New Orleans, LA, 238–239.

Bush C. A. (1969) Study of pressures on skin under ischial tuberosities and thighs during sitting. *Archives of Physical Medicine*, 50, 207.

Chow W. W., Odell E. I. (1978) Deformations and stresses in soft body tissues of a sitting person. *Journal of Biomechanical Engineering*, 100, 79–87.

Chung K. C., DiNello A. M., McLaurin C. A. (1987) Comparative evaluation of pressure distribution on foams and contoured cushions. *Proceedings 10th Annual RESNA Conference*, 323–325.

Cooper R. A., Ward C., Ster J. F., (1992) Characterization and development of a resistive sensor for measuring cushion interface force. *Proceedings 15th Annual RESNA Conference*, Toronto, Canada, 627–629.

Cooper R. A., (1991) High tech wheelchairs gain the competitive edge. *IEEE Engineering in Medicine and Biology Magazine*, 10, 4, pp. 49–55.

Cooper R. A., (1991) A comparison of pulmonary functions of wheelchair racers in their racing and standard chairs. *Proceedings 14th Annual RESNA Conference*, Kansas City, MO, 245–247.

Dempster W., (1955) Space requirements of the seated operator. *WADC Technical Report*, Wright-Patterson Air Force Base, OH, 55–159.

Dinsdale S. (1974) Decubitus ulcers in swine: Role of pressure and friction in causation. *Archives of Physical Medicine and Rehabilitation*, 55, 147–152.

Ferguson-Pell M. W., Cardi M. D. (1993) Prototype development and comparative evaluation of wheelchair pressure mapping system. *Journal of Assistive Technology*, 5, 2, 78–91.

Ferguson-Pell M. W., Cardi M. (1992) Pressure mapping systems for seating and positioning applications: Technical and clinical performance. *Proceedings RESNA International '92*, Toronto, Ontario, Canada, 219–221.

Ferguson-Pell M., Cochran G. van B., Palmieri V. R., Brunski J. B. (1986) Development of a modular wheelchair cushion for spinal cord injured persons. *Journal of Rehabilitation Research and Development*, 23, 3, 63–76.

Ferguson-Pell M. (1990) Seat cushion selection. *Journal of Rehabilitation Research and Development*, clinical supplement, 2, 49–73.

Ferguson-Pell M. W. (1980) Design criteria for the measurement of pressure at body/support interfaces. *Engineering in Medicine*, 9, 209–214.

Garber S., Krouskop T. (1982) Body build and its relationship to pressure distribution in the seated wheelchair patient. *Archives of Physical Medicine and Rehabilitation*, 63, 17–20.

Garber S., Krouskop T., Carter R. (1978) System for clinically evaluating wheelchair pressure-relief cushions. *American Journal of Occupational Therapy*, 32, 565–570.

Gilsdorf P., Patterson R., Fisher S., Appel N. (1990) Sitting forces and wheelchair mechanics. *Journal of Rehabilitation Research and Development*, 27, 3, 239–246.

Gilsdorf P., Patterson R., Fisher S. (1991) Thirty-minute continuous sitting force measurements with different support surfaces in the spinal cord injured and able-bodied. *Journal of Rehabilitation Research and Development*, 28, 4, 33–38.

Goosens R. H. M., Snijders C. J., (1995) Design criteria for the reduction of shear forces in beds and seats. *Journal of Biomechanics*, 28, 2, 225–230.

Grieco A. (1986) Sitting posture: An old problem and a new one. *Ergonomics*, 29, 345–362.

Grady J. H., Kuipers I. (1993) Modular systems in wheelchairs: Purpose in relation to function. *Proceedings Second European Conference on Advancement of Rehabilitation Technology*, Stockholm, Sweden, 33.1.

Kadaba M., Ferguson-Pell M., Palmieri B. S., Cochran G. V. B. (1984) Ultrasound mapping of the buttock-cushion interface contour. *Archives of Physical Medicine and Rehabilitation*, 65, 467–469.

Katz R. T., Rymer W. Z. (1989) Spastic hypertonia: mechanisms and measurement. *Archives of Physical Medicine and Rehabilitation*, 70, 2, 144–155.

Keegan J. J. (1953) Alterations of the lumbar spine related to posture and seating. *Journal of Bone and Joint Surgery*, 35–A, 589.

Kwiatkowski R., Inigo R. (1992) The design of a computer aided seating system. *Proceedings RESNA International '92*, Toronto, Ontario, Canada, 216–218.

Kwiatkowski R. J., Inigo R. M. (1993) A strain gage force sensor for a computer aided seating system. *Proceedings RESNA 16th Annual Conference*, Las Vegas, NV, 292–294.

Laenger C. J., Lee J. H. (1991) Small improvements in seating hardware. *Proceedings RESNA 14th Annual Conference*, Kansas City, MO, 353–355.

Le K. M., Masden B. L., Barth P. W., Ksander G. A., Angell J. B., Vistnes L. M. (1984) An in-depth look at pressure sores using monolithic silicon pressure sensors. *Plastic and Reconstructive Surgery*, 754–756.

Levine S. P., Kett R. L., Ferguson-Pell M. (1990) Tissue shape and deformation versus pressure as a characterization of the seating interface. *Assistive Technology*, 2, 93–99.

Lim R., Sirett R., Conine T. A., Daechsel D. (1986) Clinical trial of foam cushions in the prevention of decubitus ulcers in elderly patients. *Journal of Rehabilitation Research and Development*, 25, 2, 19–26.

Mooney V., Einbund M., Rogers R., Stauffer E. (1971) Comparison of pressure distribution qualities in seat cushions. *Bulletin of Prosthetics Research*, 129–143.

Noble P. C., Goode B., Krouskop T. A., Crisp B. (1984) The influence of environmental aging upon the loadbearing properties of polyurethane foams. *Journal of Rehabilitation Research and Development*, 21, 2, 31–38.

Perr A., Lincoln A., McGovern T. (1992) Pressure distribution on contoured wheelchair cushions utilizing the electronic shape sensor. *Proceedings RESNA International '92*, Toronto, Ontario, Canada, 213–215.

Reddy N. P., Palmieri V., Cochran G. V. B. (1981) Subcutaneous interstitial fluid pressure during external loading. *American Physiological Society*, R327–329.

Sacks A. H. (1989) Theoretical prediction of a time-at-pressure curve for avoiding pressure sores. *Journal of Rehabilitation Research and Development*, 26, 3, 27–34.

Seelen H. A. M. (1993) Dynamic sitting posture and impaired postural control in seated spinal cord injured people. *Proceedings Second European Conference on Advancement of Rehabilitation Technology*, Stockholm, Sweden, 33.2.

Sengupta D., Sherwood A. M., McDermott M. (1974) Comparative evaluation of control surfaces for disabled patients. *27th ACEMB*, Philadelphia, PA, 356.

Shapcott N., Bar K. (1990) Seating simulation as an aid to assessment. *Proceedings RESNA 13th Annual Conference*, Washington, DC, 111–114.

Shapcott N., VanNote D., Kelly C., Bouge T., Lenker J. (1991) A vinyl vacuum forming for covering FIP systems. *Proceedings RESNA 14th Annual Conference*, Kansas City, MO, 367–369.

Shaw C. G. (1993) Seat cushion comparison for nursing home wheelchair users. *Journal of Assistive Technology*, 5, 2, 92–105.

Shaw G. (1985) Rigid pelvic restraint. *Proceedings RESNA 8th Annual Conference*, Memphis, TN, 409–411.

Shields R. K., Cook T. M. (1988) Effect of seat angle and lumbar support on seated buttock pressure. *Journal of the American Physical Therapy Association* 68, 1682–1686.

Sopsato B. A., Chung K.-C., McLaurin C. A. (1990) Prescribing customized contoured seat cushions by computer-aided shape sensing. *Proceedings RESNA 13th Annual Conference*, Washington, DC, 103–104.

Sprigle S., Schuch J. Z. (1993) Using seat contour measurements during seating evaluations of individuals with SCI. *Journal of Assistive Technology*, 5, 1, 24–35.

Sprigle S., Cron L. (1992) Development and evaluation of wheelchair cushion prototypes. *Proceedings RESNA International '92*, Toronto, Ontario, Canada, 519–521.

St-Geoges M., Valiquette C., Drouin G. (1989) Computer-aided design in wheelchair seating. *Journal of Rehabilitation Research and Development*, 26, 4, 23–30.

Sunita M. M., Sprigle S. H. (1993) Effects of undeformed contour and cushion stiffness at the buttocks-seat interface. *Proceedings RESNA 16th Annual Conference*, Las Vegas, NV, 286–288.

Tchang F. (1993) Guide to research results: seating materials and fabrication methods of 12 North American centers. *Proceedings RESNA 16th Annual Conference*, Las Vegas, NV, 268–270.

van Eijk D., Bulsink D. (1993) Design of a series of positioning systems for handicapped children. *Proceedings Second European Conference on Advancement of Rehabilitation Technology*, Stockholm, Sweden, 9.2.

Warren C. G. (1982) Reducing back displacement in the powered reclining wheelchair. *Archives of Physical Medicine and Rehabilitation*, 63, 447–449.

Warren C. G. (1990) Powered mobility and its implications. *Journal of Rehabilitation Research and Development*, clinical supplement no. 2, 74–85.

Winter D. A. (1990) *Biomechanics and Motor Control of Human Movement.* New York, NY, John Wiley & Sons.

Zollars J. A., Axelson P. (1993) The back support shaping system: an alternative for persons using wheelchairs with sling back upholstery. *Proceedings RESNA 16th Annual Conference,* Las Vegas, NV, 274–276.

# CHAPTER 12

# Seating Postural Support Systems

*Chapter Goals*

☑ To know basics of mounting and adjusting postural support systems
☑ To become familiar with research and product development
☑ To understand person-to-device interface and access

## 12.1 Introduction

All wheelchair users require some degree of postural support. The simplest form of postural support uses a linear sling back and a linear sling seat (Figure 12.1). For some people linear systems provide adequate support. Other people who are more severely impaired or at risk for developing postural deformities require greater postural support. Greater postural control can be obtained by using off-the-shelf products for most cases. In a few cases, custom-fabricated postural support systems are necessary. Postural control seating systems are commonly used with children to ensure proper postural development and to prevent skeletal deformities. Many adults require postural control systems for the same reasons. Some children and adults have postural anomalies that need to be accommodated to promote good health and maximize function. There are a wide variety of products used to promote good seating posture and functional seating for wheelchair users.

Postural support systems must often be integrated into a wheelchair that may or may not have been designed in concert with the seating system. Therefore, it is important to consult a seating specialist to ensure that the seating hardware is securely and properly attached to the wheelchair. All positioning straps and hardware must be securely attached to the wheelchair and seat base as well. A rehabilitation engineer should be consulted to prevent damaging the structural integrity of the wheelchair.

Pressure sores and skin breakdown are extremely important for many people who use postural support systems. People should check themselves or be checked routinely for redness. Bony prominences and sites where postural supports come in contact with the body are especially important. The trochanters, ischial tuberosities, and coccyx are all areas that require watching. If red or pink skin areas do not fade away within 30 minutes a physician should be consulted. People can help to prevent skin problems by eliminating wrinkles in areas that contact the

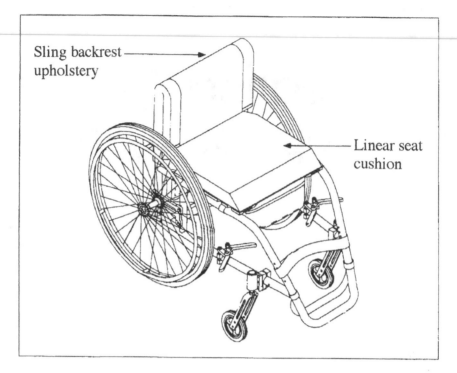

Sling backrest upholstery

Linear seat cushion

**FIGURE 12.1**   Ultralight wheelchair with linear seat cushion and sling backrest upholstery. This type of wheelchair is commonly used by active people.

wheelchair or postural support hardware. Tight clothing should be avoided. The skin should be checked frequently after making any changes to the wheelchair or seating system. Excessive moisture can promote skin breakdown. Therefore, clothing and diapers should be changed after becoming moist or soiled. With some care a properly adjusted and maintained postural support system can promote good health and maximal function.

Postural support systems can be customized to meet individual needs. Most systems are available with a variety of covers (e.g., vinyl, lucre, bare). Plastic, wood, or metal can be used to reinforce areas for additional support and control. Special mounting hardware can be provided by manufacturers upon request or developed by local rehabilitation engineers.

Postural supports and positioning hardware are primarily used by people with cerebral palsy, spina bifida, osteogenesis imperfecta, or advanced muscular dystrophy. However, people who have spinal cord injury, severe multiple sclerosis, arthrogryposis, arthritis, traumatic brain injury, stroke, lower limb amputations, or some severely impaired elderly persons can benefit from postural supports. More recently, postural control has gained greater attention among active wheelchair users as a means of improving comfort, increasing function, and preventing some of the debilitating effects associated with long-term wheelchair use. Proper positioning can help to improve pulmonary function. The ability to use the hands and arms to perform activities of daily living may be increased through positioning (see Figure 12.2). Positioning helps to orient the skeleton and the distribution of stresses within soft tissues. This can be used to help prevent or control pelvic and spinal deformities, and to prevent pressure sores.

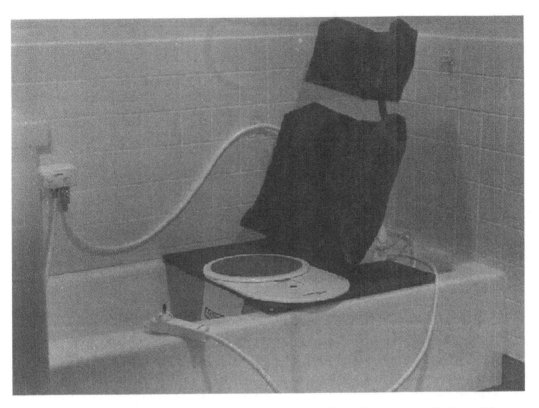

**FIGURE 12.2**  Contoured seating system used with a bathtub insert to facilitate bathing (Photograph courtesy of Clarke Health Care Products Inc.)

## 12.2 Leg and Feet Supports

Most wheelchair users require support for the feet and legs. Positioning of the feet and legs influences seating pressure, lower extremity joint angles, and seating posture. The traditional "rule of thumb" is to obtain a sitting posture ankle angle of 90 degrees, knee angle of 90 degrees, and a hip angle of 90 degrees. Recently, this thinking has been challenged for functional seating. Recall from earlier chapters that some wheelchairs are designed with much different seating angles than the traditional 90-90-90. This is because other seating angles may provide greater mobility or function during specific activities. For example, having the feet tucked under the seat (i.e., knee angle of less than 90 degrees) assists with playing wheelchair basketball by making the wheelchair more maneuverable and compact.

There are three basic types of legrests: rigid, swing-away, and elevating. Swing-away footrests are commonly used on cross-brace folding wheelchairs. They help to ease forward transfers by swinging to the side and being easily removed (see Figure 12.3). Typically, swing-away legrests are removed by undoing a latch, lifting the legrest upwards, and then rotating the legrest outwards. This shortens the wheelchair for stowage and frees the front area of the wheelchair. With the legrest removed, the area in front of the seat is open to simplify access to the seat. Having the area clear in front helps with forward and standing transfers. Swing-away legrests provide a fixed knee and ankle angle. The legrest angles are selected when ordering the wheelchair. Manufacturers provide a wide variety of legrest

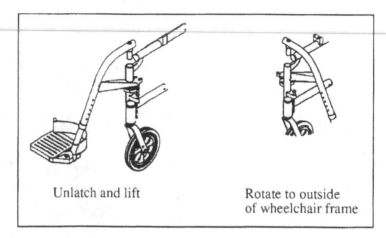

Unlatch and lift                    Rotate to outside
                                    of wheelchair frame

**FIGURE 12.3**   Swing-away legrest. The legrest is unlatched and lifted to move to
the side. This assists in transferring. Swing-away legrests can typically
be removed easily as well.

angles in order to accommodate individual anatomy, physiology, and preference.
However, a shallow legrest angle allows the legs to protrude farther in front of the
wheelchair. This will require more space to maneuver the wheelchair.

Elevating legrests are used to accommodate people who do not have the flexibility to use a standard angle on a swing-away legrest or for people who need to
change their sitting posture because of physiological conditions. Elevating legrests
are used to reduce edema and/or blood pooling in the lower extremities. Elevation
of the legrest can be manual or power operated. Manually operated elevating
legrests use a latch to set the legrest angle. The latch needs to be manually released
and the leg placed in the desired position. The latch is then returned to its locked
position. Power elevating legrests use small motors to lift and lower the legrests. A
calf pad is used with elevating legrests to help support the lower legs and foot over
the range of legrest angles through which the leg can be elevated (see Figure
12.4). For some people pressure relief can be improved or pain can be reduced by

**FIGURE 12.4**   Elevating legrest with calf pad

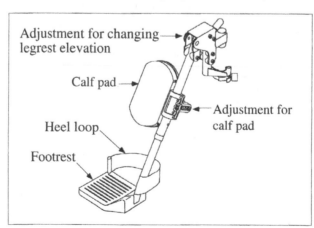

Adjustment for changing—
legrest elevation

Calf pad —

                                                —Adjustment for
Heel loop                                        calf pad

Footrest

elevating the legs. Elevating legrests allow sitting posture to be changed periodically.

There are several types of footrests. The most common categories are composite flip-up, tubular flip-up, and rigid. Examples from these categories are shown in Figure 12.5. Most wheelchairs come with several footrest options, and a variety of footrests can be used with each legrest type. Flip-up footrests help to provide access to the wheelchair seat. By flipping the footrests up, a person can place the feet in front of the seat to transfer or, if possible, to stand. Composite footrests are the most common type of foot support. A heel strap is used to maintain foot position while using the wheelchair. Tubular flip-up footrests are preferred by some active wheelchair users. They provide a more sporty appearance and can be more durable. Flip-up footrests are mounted to the legrest using a telescoping tube. The footrest length can be adjusted by selecting the appropriate adjustment hole or by loosening a pinch clamp and setting the legrest length prior to tightening. The legrest length should be set so that the person's feet sit firmly on the legrests.

Some wheelchair users prefer a rigid frame. Most wheelchairs used for sports have rigid frames. Rigid-framed wheelchairs can be provided with a wide selection of legrests and footrests. In order to get the stiffest and most responsive rigid-

**FIGURE 12.5** Common footrests used on wheelchairs. Upper footrests both flip up to simplify transfers. Rigid footrests are commonly used on rigid wheelchairs.

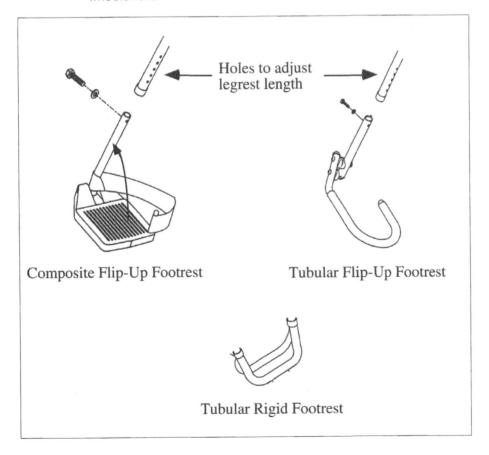

Holes to adjust legrest length

Composite Flip-Up Footrest

Tubular Flip-Up Footrest

Tubular Rigid Footrest

framed wheelchair, rigid footrests are used. A rigid footrest acts like part of the frame structure. Since rigid footrests remain fixed in place, the wheelchair user must adapt other transfer techniques. The side-to-side transfer is most commonly used. Highly skilled wheelchair users can learn forward transfer with rigid footrest wheelchairs. Many children's wheelchairs are available with rigid footrests. This is sometimes simply to accommodate growth. Forward anti-tip rollers can be placed on both rigid and swing-away footrests. Forward anti-tip rollers were originally designed for court sports. The rules for basketball and quad rugby require forward anti-tip rollers to reduce forward falls and damage to floors. Anti-tip rollers may help some wheelchair users in reducing forward falls. Care should be taken not to set the anti-tip casters too low so that they do not interfere with driving over common obstacles (e.g., door thresholds, sidewalk cracks). For the same reason it is important to properly set the legrest clearance. The legrests should be approximately 50 mm (2 inches) from the floor. This will help to clear common obstacles. For tall people the seat angle or seat height can be increased.

Some people can benefit from padded footrests or footstraps. These devices act to help position the feet for greater function and body control. When footrest positioning is important, the lower thigh area should be resting on the wheelchair seat. There should be no gap between the bottom of the thighs and the seating surface; otherwise the footrest may need to be lowered. A pressure map can be used to determine the proper pressure distribution on the seat.

## 12.3 Armrests

Wheelchair armrests are used for a multitude of activities. The primary purpose of armrests is to provide good resting posture for the arms. However, armrests provide a variety of other functions that assist the wheelchair user. Armrests assist with pressure relief for the buttocks and thighs. By placing their hands on each armrest, some wheelchair users can push up and elevate their buttocks and thighs from the seating surface. This helps to encourage blood flow and may reduce the risk of developing pressure sores. Armrests are also used to assist with transfers. The armrests are the easiest point on the wheelchair for some people to grasp while transferring. Using the armrest may also help to increase clearance height between the wheelchair seat and the individual's buttocks. Armrests are used to stabilize someone when reaching for objects from the floor or on places high within the person's reachable space. Armrests are also used to attach objects to control the wheelchair (e.g., a joystick on an electric-powered wheelchair) or to simplify some tasks (e.g., a cup holder).

Wheelchair armrests are available in a variety of styles. Some armrests are equipped with "skirt guards" that help to keep clothing and skin from rubbing against the tires of the wheelchair. Armrests can be used to help maintain sitting posture by positioning the person's hips in the wheelchair. Some armrests are no more than fenders that help to keep dirt and water from the tires off the wheelchair user. The most common armrest styles are fixed, flip-back, and removable. Fixed armrests are bolted or permanently attached to the wheelchair. This type of armrest is most common on low-end wheelchairs designed for temporary use within institutions (e.g., hospitals). Flip-back and removable armrests are available on many models of wheelchair. Flip-back armrests are hinged at the back near the intersection of the seat and backrest. Some flip-back armrests use a latch in the front to help secure them in place. Flip-back armrests move out of the way to assist with transfers and reaching to the side, but remain with the wheelchair so that the user does not need to find a place to put them or be concerned with their being misplaced. Removable armrests usually fit into two sockets. Commonly, the front socket contains a latch to lock the armrest in place. Removable armrests may be used to assist with transfers and sideways reaching. They also have the advantage of reducing the weight of the frame when removed. This may make stowage in an automobile or airplane easier. Some people prefer to use their wheelchairs without armrests at times.

Armrests are also classified by whether they are adjustable or set, the length of the arm pad, and whether they mount to the side or the back of the wheelchair. Adjustable armrests may be moved up and down, and forwards and backwards to position the arms in a comfortable and functional position. Up-and-down adjustment is commonly accomplished by using the bracket that attaches the arm pad to the lower (skirt guard) portion of the armrest (see Figure 12.6). Fore-and-aft motion is done by moving the armrest pad. Armrests with short armrest pads are called desk-length armrests; otherwise they are full-length armrests (see Figure 12.7). As the name implies, desk-length armrests allow the wheelchair user to sit closer to a table or desk without removing the armrests.

Side-mounted armrests tend to add to the overall width of the wheelchair, up to 25 millimeters (1 inch) in some cases. However, some people prefer a narrower wheelchair. To accommodate these customers, wheelchair manufacturers developed the wrap-around armrest. The wrap-around armrest attaches at the back of the wheelchair and comes forward above the wheel eliminating the need for the extra width (see Figure 12.8).

Armrest pads may simply be padding placed over a tube or they may range to a highly contoured pad for positioning the arm and hand. A contoured pad can provide greater control over an electric-powered wheelchair by providing accurate positioning of the arm and hand. Contouring can also provide greater support for

**FIGURE 12.6** Components of an adjustable height wheelchair armrest

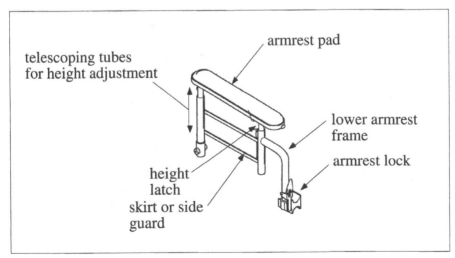

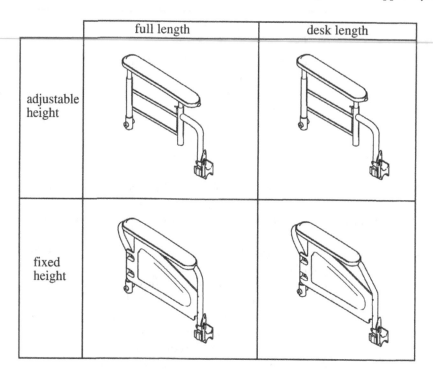

|  | full length | desk length |
|---|---|---|
| adjustable height |  |  |
| fixed height |  |  |

**FIGURE 12.7**   Common types of armrests used on wheelchairs

**FIGURE 12.8**   Ultralight manual wheelchair with wrap-around armrests

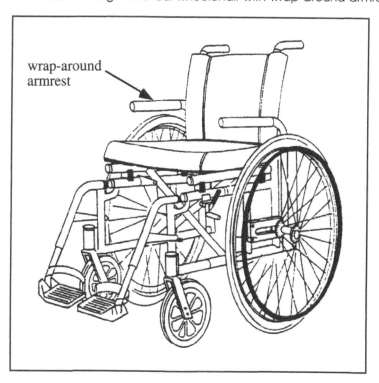

wrap-around armrest

the hand and arm. Many people do not require contouring, but its impact can be tremendous for people who may benefit from the additional support and positioning. Contoured armrests may be selected from standard shapes or at additional cost they can be custom made.

## 12.4 Pelvic Positioning

Proper positioning of the pelvis cannot be maintained without selecting the proper seat depth. There must be clearance between the front edge of the seat and the back of the person's knees. For children, about 25 millimeters (1 inch) is appropriate, whereas 50 millimeters (2 inches) is considered appropriate for adults. However, clinical judgment must be exercised in each case. In order to obtain proper seating posture, the clinician must determine the desired hip flexion angle. In some cases, the proper hip flexion angle must be determined in the wheelchair. On most wheelchairs, hip flexion angle is adjusted by pivoting the backrest. Some wheelchairs allow for the seat angle to be adjusted to set hip flexion angle.

Pelvic support and positioning can be achieved using a pelvic belt, lap belt, subasis bar, or antithrust cushion (see Figure 12.9). These devices can help to pre-

**FIGURE 12.9**  Methods for positioning the pelvis to maintain proper posture in a wheelchair

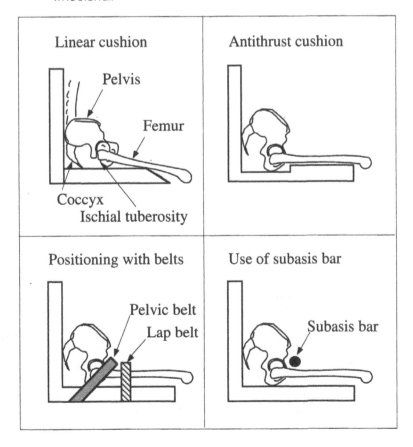

vent or correct a slouching posture with an unacceptable postural pelvic tilt. In some cases combinations of these devices must be used. Pelvic support for minor cases can be provided by using a seat belt and an antithrust seat cushion. The antithrust seat helps to maintain posture by positioning the ischial tuberosities. The pelvic belt or subasis bar must be positioned snugly (e.g., about two adult fingers should be able to fit between the belt and the abdomen). The pelvic belt or subasis bar should prevent the person from sliding forward on the seat even when the occupant wiggles or squirms. The pelvis should be maintained in a neutral position against the backrest. The latch on the pelvic belt must be selected to meet the physical and cognitive abilities of the user. The pelvic belt should not slip or become unlatched inadvertently. If attached to the wheelchair, the pelvic belt or subasis bar should be used whenever the person is sitting in the wheelchair. For some people the pelvic belt or subasis bar works in concert with thoracic supports. If the pelvic belt or subasis bar is not adjusted properly with the pelvis against the backrest, the child may slump in the seat such that the thoracic supports can bruise or abrade the underarms. In some cases choking may occur, which could lead to death. If an antithrust seat is used, the step in the seat must be positioned in front of the ischial tuberosities such that the proper pelvic angle is maintained.

In some cases an abduction pommel may be required (see Figure 12.10). A pommel promotes alignment of the heads of the femurs with the acetabulum. The abduction pommel is positioned between the wheelchair user's knees. An abduction pommel may be as simple as a wedge placed with the narrow end facing the groin. An abduction pommel can be mounted asymmetrically to counteract a strong adduction on one side. The pommel should be adjusted until the clinician is satisfied that the desired effect has been achieved. The abduction pommel must be sized to remain clear of the groin. Abduction pommels are not used to hold people within their wheelchair seats.

## 12.5 Back Supports

Backrests may also be contoured to provide additional support for those people who need it (Figure 12.11). Two common approaches used are a flat back base with additional supports or a back base with curved sides. The width and height of the back base should be determined based on the user's mode of mobility (e.g., manual, attendant-propelled, power) and postural support needs. For people who use manual wheelchairs the backrest should follow the individual's frontal contour and the height should not extend four (4) centimeters below the scapula. The height should be sufficient to provide comfortable support, and to provide a base to push against. Generally, the higher the degree of impairment, the taller the backrest must be to provide adequate support. Contour can be added to backrests via carved foam, foam in place, standard contours, or custom-molded/carved contours. People with significant loss of lateral stability may benefit from fixed or adjustable lateral trunk supports (see Figure 12.12). A depth of between 125 and 200 mm is sufficient for most people. The height and width depend on the individual's anatomy. When using lateral supports many backrest plates require reinforcement. Scoliosis support systems can provide additional support for proper positioning for greater comfort and better control over the wheelchair. Scoliosis supports should be prescribed or designed to be independently adjustable (i.e.,

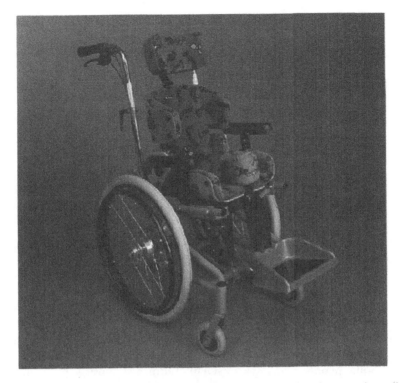

**FIGURE 12.10**  Children's tilt-in-space wheelchair with postural support seating system. This seat includes lateral hip supports, lateral chest supports, head rest, and abduction pommel (Photograph courtesy Otto Bock Orthopaedic Industry, Inc.)

**FIGURE 12.11**  Contoured backrest with rigid pan to provide postural support (Photograph courtesy of Metalcraft Industries )

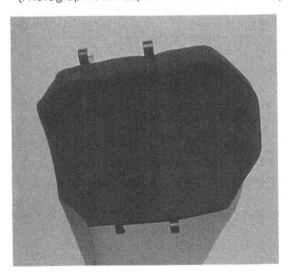

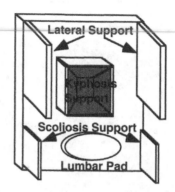

**FIGURE 12.12**  Illustration of backrest with postural support devices

inferior-superior, fore-aft, medial-lateral). Supports can be designed or prescribed to wrap around the trunk anteriorly, and may include a strap that wraps around the trunk for greatest support. Often the wrap-around scoliosis supports incorporate a quick-adjust mechanism (e.g., quick-release pin, knob head bolt) and a simply operated strap locking mechanism (e.g., Velcro, ring lock, or cam lock) to aid in transferring in and out of the wheelchair. Lateral and scoliosis supports require padding (i.e., typically 8 to 25 mm is sufficient depending on the applied force), and the person should be isolated from all fasteners.

Some people who use wheelchairs require kyphosis support devices. A backrest box is a means of providing appropriate seating for many people who require kyphosis support. Kyphosis backrest boxes are commonly made of a composite material (e.g., fiberglass, carbon fiber, Kevlar®). The kyphosis backrest box is filled with foam (i.e., typically a laminate of various types and densities of foams) that is cut out to match the placement of the kyphotic hump. This method relieves the hump so the person's back is positioned neutrally. Foam-in-place methods can be used instead of contouring the foam so that not only the kyphotic hump is accommodated, but the entire back as well.

People with extreme spasticity often have difficulty maintaining proper posture in their wheelchairs despite having adequate postural musculature. Side-wing controls or wrap-around backrests can be used to assist people with spasticity to maintain proper posture. Side-wings or wrap-around backrests are barriers added to the side of the wheelchair to confine the user within the backrest. Typically, a padded wall along the entire length of backrest of 100 to 150 mm high is effective.

A lumbar support can be added to the backrest of many wheelchairs for people who have difficulty maintaining the natural curvature of the spine (see Figure 12.13). Lumbar support is becoming widely used among wheelchair users. Lumbar support can improve balance with added comfort and mobility. A 75- to 100-mm thick piece of contoured foam the width of the back is placed in the lumbar area. Custom devices and systems can be designed for people with unusual postural support needs. A properly placed lumbar support can position the head squarely over the shoulders and improve pelvic alignment. For many wheelchair users a standard sling seat induces sacral seating. This can be corrected with a lumbar support. Spinal extension can be achieved with some people.

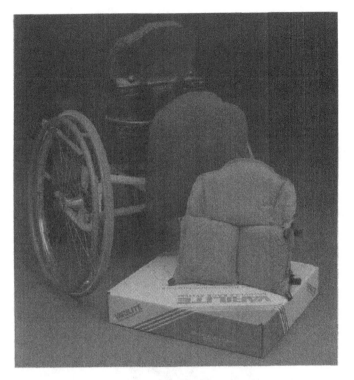

A

**FIGURE 12.13**   (a) Adult wheelchair with a lightweight molded rigid frame backrest with pneumatic cushioning and support. (b) Honeycomb
cushion and lumbar support designed to be lightweight and
adaptable to many different types of wheelchairs (Photographs
courtesy of (a) Cascade Designs Inc., and (b) Spuracor Inc.)

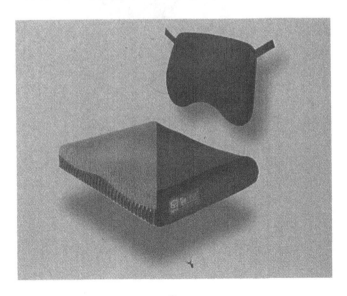

B

## 12.6 Chest Supports

Systems can be designed to provide chest and shoulder support to help people remain erect (see Figure 12.14). An H-strap system can often provide adequate postural support. With an H-strap system one strap wraps anteriorly around the chest under the arms while two straps originate in the center of the chest and go over the shoulders to keep the trunk erect. Portions of the straps in contact with the person must be padded. The padded portion is sometimes called a chest pad or H-pad. A D-ring, Velcro, or snap-buckle can be used to secure the H-strap system in place.

Shoulder straps or bars and thoracic vests (e.g., H-straps) must be adjusted snugly enough to maintain the person in the desired position safely and comfortably. The thoracic vest should be centered on the chest. The H-strap system must

**FIGURE 12.14**   Adjustable postural support and guidance system for children. This seating system includes pommel, hip lateral supports, thoracic lateral supports, and shoulder bars (Photograph courtesy of Mulholland)

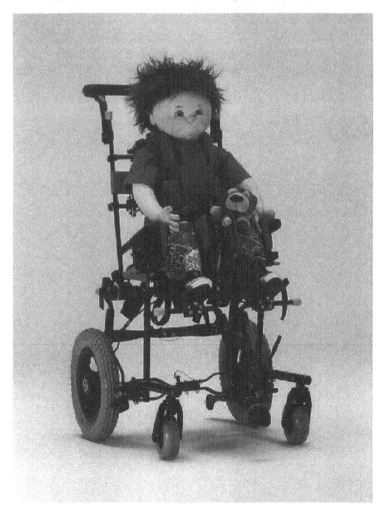

be secure across the chest, but not tight. An adult's fingers should be able to fit between the bottom of the vest or chest pad and the person's chest. The upper edge of the vest or chest pad must be at least 25 millimeters (1 inch) below the sternal notch. The upper edge of the vest or chest pad should under no circumstances rub against the person's neck. Chest supports must always be used in conjunction with pelvic supports. If a pelvic support is not used or improperly adjusted, the chest support may restrict or completely cut off breathing, which can lead to injury and even death.

Thoracic or lateral supports provide medial-lateral stability for people who do not have good trunk control (see Figure 12.15). Thoracic supports come in a variety of sizes and may be removable or swing-out. Lateral supports are made of metal brackets upholstered with foam padding. The metal provides the strength and stiffness required for providing medial-lateral stability. Because of the forces between the body and the pads, the support metal support brackets must be well-covered to prevent harming the wheelchair user. Swing-out and removable lateral supports should always be securely in place when the wheelchair is in use. Thoracic supports should be positioned snugly against the thorax without applying excessive pressure or causing discomfort. The tops of thoracic supports should be at mid-chest level (e.g., approximately the nipple line). Thoracic supports must not be placed at the underarms. Lateral supports may also be placed at the pelvis. This helps to control medial-lateral alignment of the spine. This is accomplished through the combination of a thoracic support, lateral thoracic supports, and

**FIGURE 12.15**  Adult-sized wheelchair with postural support seating system. This wheelchair includes an antithrust seat cushion, lateral thoracic supports, a winged headrest, and occipital supports. (Photograph courtesy of Metalcraft Industries)

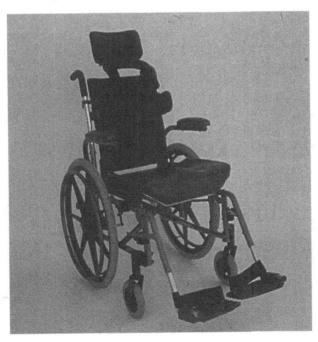

pelvic lateral supports. Through proper adjustment the pelvis and chest can be aligned to provide postural support and control.

Once all postural supports are in place and adjusted, the clinician should take a look at the person's overall body position. Ideally, the person will be centered in the seat. The buttocks will be firmly in the seat with the pelvis against the backrest. The hips should be level and the body weight distributed properly over the seating surface. This is best done using some type of pressure mapping system. The thighs and feet should be in anatomically neutral positions for seating. The lateral thoracic supports must not squeeze the chest area or compromise breathing. Caution should be taken to ensure proper adjustment of the chest and pelvic supports to prevent risk of choking or bruising. Shoulder straps and/or thoracic vests should pull the person's back against the wheelchair's backrest without applying undue pressure to restrict breathing or bruising (especially around the chest and neck).

## 12.7 Head Supports

In extreme circumstances people require head and neck supports (Figure 12.16). Head and neck supports often provide the necessary stability required to control a power wheelchair, environmental control unit, or communication device. Extensions are designed and added to the backrest structure to support the head and

**FIGURE 12.16**  (a) Adult-sized wheelchair with custom-contoured seating system with winged headrest and occipital supports. (b) Occipital head support. (Photographs courtesy of (a) Prairie Seating Corporation, and (b) Miller's)

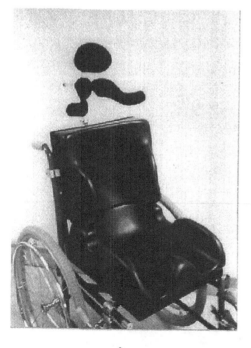

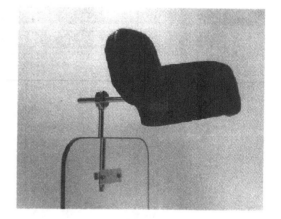

A                                                             B

neck. The degree of support required determines the type of head and neck support employed (see Figure 12.17). For people who require minimal head and neck support a simple flat headrest is sufficient. This type of headrest prevents the head from extending beyond the plane of the backrest, which is especially important if the seating system is tilted or reclined. To assist in transferring, a flip-down headrest can be used that can be moved out of the way without being detached from the backrest. Removable headrests can also be prescribed or designed. Curvature can be added to the headrest to keep the user's head within the confines of the headrest. A winged headrest includes foam wedges on either side of center to provide slight lateral head support. A vertical foam wedge on the headrest can help to keep the head upright rather than extended, and gives slight lateral support. A neck yoke, a U-shaped support, with foam padding can be used for lateral head support and to create neck flexion. Another means of providing moderate lateral support and neck flexion is to use an occipital headrest (i.e., a stiff U-shaped support padded with foam to fit the contour of the occipital region). Lateral head supports, padded arms extending on either side of the head, can be used to provide a high degree of support. For people with hydrocephalus a head sling can be used to relieve the head. A head sling is a padded shelf of molded material (e.g., plastic or composite) at the top of the backrest. Often the shelf is reinforced with a steel frame.

When assessing a person for a head support system, the clinician should be realistic in expectations. A good seating and head support system is unlikely to be a solution to all of a person's functional limitations. The clinician must work with

**FIGURE 12.17**  Wheelchair head and neck supports

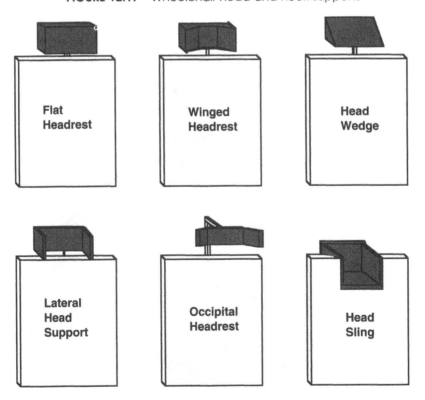

Flat Headrest

Winged Headrest

Head Wedge

Lateral Head Support

Occipital Headrest

Head Sling

the person to develop a plan for how the person will ultimately sit and function. Head control is difficult to evaluate and requires specialized knowledge. In many cases, evaluation kits and simulators are very helpful. A skilled clinician must determine the direction and the amount of force required to place the head in the desired position. Most systems attempt to bring the head to a neutral position. The clinician should be cautious to avoid placing excessive force while positioning the head. Many people who can benefit from head positioning systems can exert active muscle forces in addition to gravitational and passive connective tissue forces. After determining the amount of force and direction of force required, the desired support is duplicated by selecting head support hardware. Head supports should not apply pressure to the temporal area, the mastoid process, or the mandible. In most cases some functional tests with the head support hardware are required to verify improved function.

## 12.8 Custom Postural Support Hardware

Contoured seating systems are molded to fit the anatomy and anthropometry of the user (see Figure 12.18). Contoured seating systems may be made by hand-

**FIGURE 12.18** Custom-contoured seating system for a child requiring maximum support through a total contact seating system (Photograph courtesy of Danmar Products Inc.)

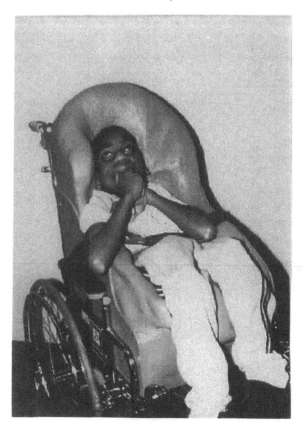

shaping foam and plywood, by using a bead-bag system to create a plaster mold or panograph of the seating contour, or by using foam-in-place techniques. The objective of contoured seating systems is to provide optimal postural support and control while minimizing pressure in sensitive areas. Custom-contoured cushions accommodate the natural shape of the person and minimize tissue distortion that may cause discomfort or pressure sores. Contoured cushions provide postural support and positioning. The user should settle comfortably into the cushion and be supported statically and dynamically. The cushion should also protect the user against sudden impacts, as when going off a curb.

Plywood and foam is perhaps the simplest and most time-consuming of the methods for developing contoured seating. However, plywood and foam requires a great deal of skill on the part of all involved (i.e., engineer, technician, clinician). Typically a piece of 6- to 12-mm interior plywood is cut to the shape of the seat base; in some instances a section is removed around the ischial tuberosities. A base of polyurethane, urethane, T-foam, or similar material is glued to the plywood base. The thickness of the foam base depends on the weight of the individual, the amount of fleshy tissue over the seating surface, and the health of the individual. Usually 50 to 150 mm of foam is used. Various densities of foam are used to provide support in some areas and pressure relief in others. Low-density foam is used around bony prominences that carry significant weight (e.g., ischial tuberosities, coccyx). The foam is contoured using carving tools, sand paper, and finally high-density foam for smoothing. The foam is shaped until the client and clinician are satisfied that adequate pressure relief and postural support have been achieved. This process is sometimes aided by having the client lie prone on the edge of a table with his/her legs hanging over the edge. A clinician can then lay up plaster of paris over the person's thighs, buttocks, and lower back to create a mold of the person's seated shape. The mold can then be used to create a positive or male mold of the person's seated shape, which can be used when contouring a seating system.

Foam-in-place is another method of directly developing a custom-contoured seating system. Foam-in-place requires a fair degree of technical and clinical ability to be successfully applied. A rubber, latex, plastic, or similar bag is filled with a liquid foam that when molded will form the contoured cushion. In some cases a 25- to 50-mm piece of foam is placed under or adhered to the bottom of the bag to provide a cushion base. A thin layer of foam (i.e., 8-mm thick medium-density foam) may be placed on top of the bag to provide a smooth finish. Usually the engineer or technician works from the side of the wheelchair, minimizing the mess and shaping the cushion with the clinician. The foam base is mixed with a catalyst and poured into the bag. Time is of the essence so it is best to make several dry runs with all parties involved. The client should wear thick clothing for protection from the 110–120 degree heat produced during the foam-curing process. The client is placed on the bag filled with liquid foam. The clinician and engineer/technician shape the foam to provide desired pressure relief and postural support. The client must be held in the desired position until the foam cures enough to maintain shape, at which time he/she can be carefully removed from the seat. When the foam is completely cured any excess material can be trimmed away. The bag is either separated from the foam and a vinyl cover vacuum-formed over the cushion, or if suitable the bag is cleaned and then glued to the foam with a permanent adhesive.

Another common method of creating a custom-contoured seating system is to use a vacuum bag approach. The person sits in a seating simulator with the body positioned as desired by the clinician and individual. The seating simulator includes latex bags filled with foam beads. Usually there is one bag for the back and another for the seat. The bags filled with beads are flexible and pliable when there is no vacuum. As air is pulled out of the bags, they become stiffer. At first they behave like clay and can be molded by the clinician to generate the desired postural support. As further vacuum is drawn from the bags, they become stiffer, eventually becoming nearly rigid. With the person out of the simulator a copy of the imprint can be made, by either making a plaster mold or using a digitizer. Plaster molds are seldom used because they are bulky and require too much space to store. Digitizers are cost effective and the stored shape can be easily edited and stored on a computer. Bead-seat cushions can be highly contoured to provide postural support and guidance (see Figure 12.19).

Shape-sensing technology and computer-assisted manufacturing can be used to produce custom-contoured cushions for precise seat and back support (see Figure 12.20). Custom carving may help to increase comfort and provide postural stability. Polyurethane foam is commonly used as the cushion material. The goal of custom contouring is to achieve maximum surface contact and containment of soft tissue over prominent areas. Maximum surface contact can be used to support

**FIGURE 12.19**   (a) Upholstered custom-contoured seating system made from digitizing a bead-bag seating simulator mounted to a lightweight wheelchair. (b) Foam custom-contoured seating system with water-repellent coating (Photographs courtesy of (a) Otto Bock Orthopaedic Industry, Inc., and (b) Danmar Products, Inc.)

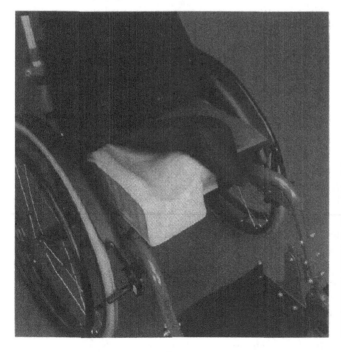

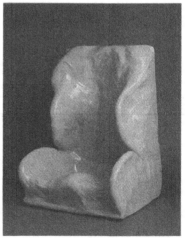

A                                                                    B

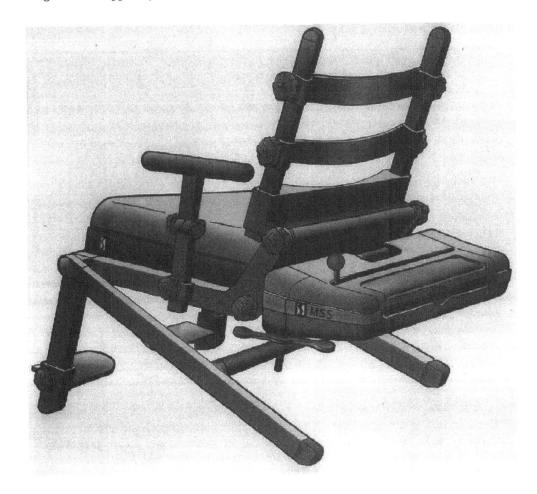

**FIGURE 12.20**  Direct seating contour measurement system used for custom carving seating systems (Photograph courtesy of PinDot, a Division of Invacare Corporation)

the trunk, pelvis, and lower extremities to provide some postural control. Surface contact and contouring help to create an antithrust effect. A major feature of shape-sensing technology and computer-assisted manufacturing is that complex orthopaedic complications can be recorded and accommodated. The person's information can be stored on a computer for immediate visualization, modification, and storage for future use. An efficient record can be kept of an individual's changes in posture over time or after interventions. This allows the clinician to develop an accurate quantitative and visual record of the person's seating history. Software is available for displaying cushion shapes, cushion cross sections, lateral views, and seating posture estimates. Shapes can be edited using contour shifting techniques and wedging. Contour shifting allows clinicians to smooth or move regions of a contour. Wedging allows the clinicians to add or remove materials in areas using standard tools (e.g., wedges, abductors). Expert clinicians can also use patch editing, which allows individual nodes on the contour to be moved. Mirroring can also be used to visualize the person's seat rather than the cushion.

## References and Further Reading

Andersson G. B. J., Murphy R. W., Oertengren R., Nachemson A. L. (1979) The influence of backrest inclination and lumbar support on the lumbar lordosis in sitting. *Spine*, 4, 52–58.

Axelson P. W., Chesney D. A. (1995) Potential hazards of wheelchair lap belts. *Proceedings RESNA '95 Annual Conference*, 314–316.

Bergen A. F., Presperin J., Tallman T. (1990) *Position for Function: Wheelchairs and Other Assistive Technologies*. Valhalla, NY, Valhalla Rehabilitation Publications, Ltd.

Chaffin D. B., Andersson G. B. J. (1991) *Occupational Biomechanics*, 2nd ed. New York, NY, John Wiley & Sons.

Cook A. M., Hussey S. M. (1995) *Assistive Technologies: Principles and Practices*. St. Louis, MO, Mosby-Year Book.

Ferguson-Pell M., Cochran G. van B., Palmieri V. R., Brunski J. B. (1986) Development of a modular wheelchair cushion for spinal cord injured persons. *Journal of Rehabilitation Research and Development*, 23, 3, 63–76.

Ferguson-Pell M. W. (1980) Design criteria for the measurement of pressure at body/support interfaces. *Engineering in Medicine*, 9, 209–214.

Galvin J. C., Scherer M. J. (1996) *Evaluating, selecting, and using appropriate assistive technology*. Gaithersburg, MD: Aspen Publishers.

Gillette Children's Hospital. (1996) *Sure Fit Instruction Booklet*, St. Paul, MN.

Grieco A. (1986) Sitting posture: An old problem and a new one. *Ergonomics*, 29, 345–362.

Grady J. H., Kuipers I. (1993) Modular systems in wheelchairs: Purpose in relation to function. *Proceedings Second European Conference on Advancement of Rehabilitation Technology*, Stockholm, Sweden, 33.1.

Jacobs K., Bettencourt C. M. (1994) Newton, MA: Butterworth-Heinemann.

Katz R. T., Rymer W. Z. (1989) Spastic hypertonia: Mechanisms and measurement. *Archives of Physical Medicine and Rehabilitation*, 70, 2, 144–155.

Keegan J. J. (1953) Alterations of the lumbar spine related to posture and seating. *Journal of Bone and Joint Surgery*, 35-A, 589.

Laenger C. J., Lee J. H. (1991) Small improvements in seating hardware. *Proceedings RESNA 14th Annual Conference*, Kansas City, MO, 353–355.

Seelen H. A. M. (1993) Dynamic sitting posture and impaired postural control in seated spinal cord injured people. *Proceedings Second European Conference on Advancement of Rehabilitation Technology*, Stockholm, Sweden, 33.2.

Sengupta D., Sherwood A. M., McDermott M. (1974) Comparative evaluation of control surfaces for disabled patients. *27th ACEMB*, Philadelphia, PA, 356.

Shapcott N., Bar K. (1990) Seating simulation as an aid to assessment. *Proceedings RESNA 13th Annual Conference*, Washington, DC.

Shapcott N., VanNote D., Kelly C., Bouge T., Lenker J. (1991) A vinyl vacuum forming for covering FIP systems. *Proceedings RESNA 14th Annual Conference*, Kansas City, MO, 367–369.

Shaw G. (1985) Rigid pelvic restraint. *Proceedings RESNA 8th Annual Conference*, Memphis, TN, 409–411.

Shields R. K., Cook T. M. (1988) Effect of seat angle and lumbar support on seated buttock pressure. *Journal of the American Physical Therapy Association*, 68, 1682–1686.

Sopsato B. A., Chung K.-C., McLaurin C. A. (1990) Prescribing customized contoured seat cushions by computer-aided shape sensing. *Proceedings RESNA 13th Annual Conference*, Washington, DC, 103–104.

Trefler E., Hobson D. A., Taylor S. J., Monahan L. C., Shaw C. G. (1993) Tucson, AZ, Therapy Skill Builders.

van Eijk D., Bulsink D. (1993) Design of a series of positioning systems for handicapped children. *Proceedings Second European Conference on Advancement of Rehabilitation Technology*, Stockholm, Sweden, 9.2.

Zollars J. A., Axelson P. (1993) The back support shaping system: an alternative for persons using wheelchairs with sling back upholstery. *Proceedings RESNA 16th Annual Conference*, Las Vegas, NV, 274–276.

Webster J. G., ed. (1991) *Prevention of Pressure Sores: Engineering and Clinical Aspects*. Bristol, UK, Institute of Physics Publishing.

# CHAPTER 13

# Principles of Assessment and Intervention

*Chapter Goals*

☑ To know when to obtain an assessment of abilities in the areas of gross motor, fine motor, oral motor, sensory, cognitive, and psychosocial functions

☑ To understand advantages and disadvantages of different service delivery models

☑ To understand the roles, constraints, and perspectives of distributors, suppliers, and payers

☑ To know sequence of activities or functions required to deliver technologies

☑ To know what constitutes a functional assessment

## 13.1 Interview Techniques

One of the first steps in a wheelchair and seating assessment is to obtain some basic information about the client. In some cases information may be contained in a patient chart, when the person has recently been or is currently in a hospital or rehabilitation center. It is not unusual for seating and mobility clinics or specialists to receive referrals for people about whom they have no prior knowledge. This requires the clinical specialist to have some basic skills in interview techniques.

Appearances of the clinic and of the specialist are going to set the tone for a personal interview. This is where the client will gain a first impression and will judge what to expect. There are several differing opinions on how a clinic should appear. The views vary by the target client population (e.g., children versus seniors) and the atmosphere desired by the clinical staff. Clinics tend to fall under broad appearances, as either hospital or rehabilitation-type centers where they give a very medical appearance or seem more consumer/business oriented. Both models are effective and need to be evaluated for the target client population. Clinical staff may be required to wear a uniform (e.g., a white lab coat) or to dress in business attire. Many clinics suggest that their male physicians wear a tie to distinguish themselves from other clinic personnel. All people interacting with clients should dress professionally and present an orderly appearance.

Interviews must be conducted in a private setting to protect the privacy of the client. Clinicians should be attentive and considerate of the client's answers and provide guidance as necessary. Interviews may consist of a written questionnaire, a computer-administered questionnaire, or personal interviews. Some clients will require assistance with written or computer-administered questionnaires. Clinics should prepare questionnaires in a variety of formats (e.g., large type, bold type, audio tapes). Good questionnaires ask some questions in different ways during different portions of the questioning. This helps to validate the information received. During personal interviews questions can be asked in different ways as well. Personal interviews have the flexibility to probe further, based on the client's answers. However, it is important not to get sidetracked and miss information.

Interviewers should always introduce themselves prior to beginning the interview, and inform the client of the interviewer's credentials (e.g., a physical therapist or occupational therapist). Some clinics use telephone interviews to pre-screen clients. When conducting telephone interviews, people should always ask whether it is a convenient time for the interview, and inform the potential client of the length of time required to conduct the interview and if the interview is included as part of the client's assessment. The clinician must inform the client or potential client if the interview is going to be taped.

Interviews are used to collect a variety of sensitive information. Clinics require a thorough case history in order to make a proper assessment; most institutions require clinicians to obtain information about the client's preferred method of payment; and information is required to ascertain current health and mobility status. It is also helpful to obtain the client's experience with previous clinics, durable equipment dealers, and assistive technology. Some consumers will have a preferred physician, therapist, and assistive technology specialist. It is helpful to ascertain some of the client's desires prior to arranging a visit to the clinic.

## 13.2 Task Analysis

Cook and Hussey have proposed that the process of evaluating a person's assistive technology can be posed as a human performance question. They describe the human activity assistive technology (HAAT) model as a context for assessing an individual's needs. The HAAT model is described graphically in Figure 13.1. The HAAT model states that there must be a person performing a task in some envi-

FIGURE 13.1   Human activity assistive technology (HAAT) model

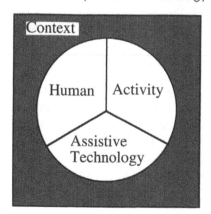

ronment using some form of assistive technology. Task analysis focuses on each of these components and their interactions. An improper task analysis can lead to abandonment of the wheelchair or costly modifications to the user's environment. The human is the person being assessed. The assessment typically consists of a physical assessment of the individual's motor skills, posture, and compensatory mechanisms. Client assessment also requires assessment of the person's cognitive skills, including problem solving, management of emotional stress, perseverance, and diligence. Physical and cognitive skills cannot be ascertained without information about the other components of the HAAT model. For example, a client may have difficulty remembering without the aid of a digital tape recorder to note key words.

Context is used to describe the environment in which the person is going to function, perhaps broad and varied. It is important to have the consumer or family member assist in defining this environment. Many consumers must operate their wheelchairs within their home, work/school, community, rehabilitation center, and in the homes of family and friends. Context also includes the social environment of the consumer. Socioeconomic status, religious preference, and profession all influence the selection of the appropriate wheelchair. For example, a physician will likely wish to have a wheelchair that reflects his/her professional status. Some religions encourage members to wear subdued colors, which will influence the choice of wheelchair.

Activity is used to describe how the wheelchair will be used. There are a wide variety of activities that must be considered. The most common activities include driving, shopping, food preparation, personal hygiene, child care, airline travel, and recreation. This list is by no means exhaustive. People have used wheelchairs to perform nearly every activity imaginable. Wheelchair manufacturers have worked to anticipate many of the activities that wheelchair users will participate in. The assistive technology selected influences how a person performs various activities under different circumstances. A good starting point is to use the person's current assistive technology in the initial assessment. If the person has never used assistive technology, the clinician must use his/her best judgment based on the physical and cognitive assessment information that can be obtained without assistive technology. Based on this information, surrogate assistive technology (i.e., a practice wheelchair from the clinic) can be used in the task assessment.

The task of driving a personal automobile is very important to some individuals. The ability to drive a personal automobile provides a greater degree of autonomy than using public transportation or relying on another person to drive. The choice of motor vehicle and the type of wheelchair are intertwined. For example, Judy has paraplegia due to spina bifida. She is the head of household with one adult child. She is employed in a management position in an office, and as part of her employment she is required to attend meetings throughout the city where she lives. Judy used braces and crutches to ambulate for years, but she started to use a manual wheelchair when she began college. She did not receive a formal assessment for her first manual wheelchair. She knew that the distances required to attend college were too great for her to negotiate effectively with crutches and braces, so she purchased an inexpensive wheelchair. She used this "depot" or "classic" type wheelchair for several years. Then she was exposed to ultralight wheelchairs. She decided to be assessed for a manual wheelchair. During college she lived near campus and used public transportation. After graduation, she found gainful employment and purchased a sedan. She was able to load her ultralight manual wheelchair into her sedan without assistance. She used her vehicle to drive to work and when attending meetings away from her workplace. Judy began to develop shoulder pain. At first she would rest periodically, and her shoulders would feel better. Eventually she went to see a physician. The physician worked with Judy on altering her manual wheelchair's setup. She did some exercises to improve her muscle balance, and was placed on anti-inflammatory medication. Unfortunately, her shoulders continued to deteriorate and her physician urged her to consider using an electric-powered wheelchair. Judy was faced with making the choice of changing her mobility for the second time. The manual wheelchair became too painful for her to push, but she could use her sedan to drive around. Switching to an electric-powered wheelchair would mean purchasing a new automobile or using public transportation. Moreover, an electric-powered wheelchair would require a change in her self-image and perceptions of her by others. Judy decided to use a lightweight electric-powered wheelchair. She no longer drove her automobile, and for the short term a motor vehicle suitable for an electric-powered wheelchair was too expensive. Judy began to use public transportation. The power chair allowed Judy to get around pain-free and made her more active around the office. She was also able to use her power chair to drive to some meetings. However, she had to rely on public transportation, which imposed greater structure on her life. She could not spontaneously go somewhere or attend meetings on short notice without great difficulty. Judy and her assistive technology team had to make decisions that accommodated Judy's paraplegia and her chronic severe shoulder pain. Although Judy became more mobile in some senses, her life became more structured in another sense.

### 13.2.1 Allocation of Functions

Assistance technology is used to help a person perform a set of activities. Each activity is composed of a set of tasks. Each task must be completed in order to perform a given activity. One aspect of task analysis is to determine the tasks required to perform a specific activity. Then the ability of the individual to perform each of the tasks, and the activity itself, must be assessed. In some cases people will be able to perform tasks and complete activities without the use of assistive technology. In other cases assistive technology is necessary to complete some tasks or to perform an entire activity. The choice of assistive technology is influenced by the allocation of functions. Functions are allocated to the person and to the assistive technology used to complete a task. Activities, tasks, and functions represent a hierarchical system (Figure 13.2).

The allocation of functions may be based on one of several philosophies. The most basic approach is called *comparison allocation*. The person's skills define the functions assigned to the human, and the device's characteristics determine the functions assigned to it. The task of driving an electric-powered wheelchair down a straight hallway with a manual joystick assigns some tasks to the driver and others to the wheelchair. The driver is assumed to be able to sit in the wheelchair, to operate the on/off switch, to operate the joystick, to sense the walls of the hallway, and to sense the speed of the wheelchair. If the driver is unable to perform these tasks, then the wheelchair must be altered. If the person has difficulty sitting in the wheelchair, then customized seating could be added to provide greater support. Driving straight down a hallway is only one simple task. If the context is changed

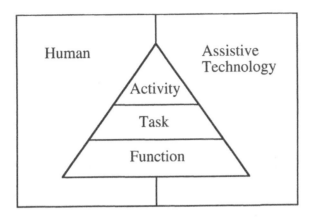

**FIGURE 13.2**  Hierarchy of activity, task, function

to driving over a lawn, then the joystick may need to be modified with a T-handle to improve the driver's ability to grasp it.

Another approach to function allocation is to use *leftover allocation.* Leftover allocation assumes that as many tasks as are feasible are assigned to the human, and the remainder are assigned to the technology. This approach is the most commonly used allocation among assistive technology clinicians. The basic philosophy is to provide the human as much control over his or her life and to use assistive technology only to augment functions where necessary. The definition of control or autonomy is an issue of considerable debate. For example, if an individual is capable of propelling a manual wheelchair with considerable effort and potential risk of wrist or shoulder injury, should he or she use a manual wheelchair or an electric-powered wheelchair? The problem lies in providing the person greatest self-direction, and how this is impacted by the choice of technology. Some wheelchairs can function as manual or electric-powered wheelchairs. Some products incorporate small electric motors directly into the hubs of the wheelchair's rear wheels. The wheels are easily removed and can be replaced with standard rear wheels. The motorized rear wheels are typically used when a person is going to go long distances or up steep hills. In this case, the person is responsible for providing the power for mobility during most activities, but the in-hub motors are assigned hills and long distances.

The decision to allocate functions between assistive devices and the individual can also be based on economic consequences. This process is called *economic allocation.* Economic allocation is mostly an issue when it comes to assistive technology that supplements or replaces the need for a personal assistant. For example, Cal has quadriplegia due to a traumatic spinal cord injury. He is able to drive an electric-powered wheelchair with a sip-&-puff access system. He has a specialized seating system and he uses a positive-flow respirator. Cal has a personal assistant with him at home and work. Cal has asked about obtaining a wheelchair-mounted robotic arm to allow him to feed himself, pick up objects from the floor and off shelves, open doors, and operate some appliances. The robotic arm costs about $50,000 and has an annual service contract that costs $2,000. Cal believes that the robotic arm would provide him with greater autonomy, and would allow him to work without a personal assistant for about four hours each day. An economic allocation would examine the cost of the robotic arm over its lifetime, and compare that to the cost of the personal assistant over the same time period. The decision as to whether Cal would get the robotic arm would be based on which was more cost effective.

*Flexible allocation* allows the balance between the allocations of functions and tasks to change. This is the preferred method of allocating tasks between people with disabilities and assistive technology. Flexible allocation recognizes that people learn and that disability is a dynamic process. The need for assistive technology varies with context and skill level. With flexible assistive technology, the configuration of the system or the manner in which tasks are performed can change as the person learns new skills. Multiple master multiple slave allows a person with a very severe disability to control multiple assistive devices. Lars has cerebral palsy, and uses an electric-powered wheelchair with an ultrasonic head control system. He has a college degree in computer science, and was offered a position as a computer programmer in a high technology company. Lars can effectively use the ultrasonic head control and a sip-&-puff switch. He was evaluated for an integrated control system that allows him to use the ultrasonic head control system and sip-&-puff switch to control his wheelchair, communication device, telephone, computer, and environmental control unit. These devices were added on to the system as Lars' skills improved. He is also able to program the system so that the controls are placed in layers and orders most accessible to him and his most commonly performed functions. This form of flexible allocation allowed Lars to maximize the use of his physical and cognitive abilities as he became more familiar with the assistive technology.

## 13.3 Performance Measurement

The effectiveness of assistive technology and the impact of training over time must be measured, and the measurement process must be integrated into the assessment process. The first step in measuring performance is to define the performance desired to be obtained, and a timeline for obtaining that performance. This is accomplished by working with an individual to define the activities desired to be performed and the context in which the activities will be performed. The clinical team and the consumer must set realistic and measurable performance and training goals. Without this process the probability of assistive technology abandonment or dissatisfaction is high.

### 13.3.1 Observation

Observation can be used to measure performance. Observation provides a measure of relative performance. By observing a person using an assistive device, notes can be made about the person's performance. Observation is useful for determining whether the activity is performed fluidly with little effort, or if the activity is performed awkwardly. Observations can be made with the knowledge of the individual, taking the form of passive or active observation. Passive observation consists of making notes describing performance of a specific activity or set of activities. Active observation is similar to coaching, intervening while the activity is in process and working to improve performance. Active observation involves interaction and communication with the consumer, taking notes about the performance of the activity as well as about the intervention strategy used. Two clinicians can be used to develop notes from both active and passive observation or a clinician can combine active and passive observation in sequential sessions.

### 13.3.2 Interviews

Interviews are useful for obtaining information about a person's satisfaction and frequency of use of assistive devices. Interviews can be formal with a set of targeted questions or more free-form where the consumer's answers direct the questioning. Interviews provide information about the use of the assistive technology or performance of activities when the clinician is not present. Interviewing family members, spouses, parents, and personal assistants can also be useful in determining the performance of activities with particular assistive devices and in changes in behavior of the client. Notes should be taken from interviews and used to develop strategies for improving task performance.

### 13.3.3 Measurement Instrumentation

Some aspects of performance can be measured directly. This often requires reducing activities to basic functions. The performance of each basic function is measured by time, distance, accuracy, and reliability. Performance is measured by obtaining a certain standard. Improvement is measured by comparing current data for an individual with past data from the same individual. Seating simulators are a form of performance measurement system. A seating simulator allows a clinical team and consumer to work together to establish a seating posture that allows the individual to sit comfortably with adequate postural support, and to be able to perform critical tasks (e.g., wheelchair driving). Seating simulators consist of a chair or wheelchair that has dimensions which can be adjusted in various directions and which mimic the dimensions that are adjustable or selectable on a wheelchair. The dimensions are adjusted for the individual and then the measurements of the simulator are recorded. This helps to provide functional seating for people with complex seating needs. Some seating simulators allow the wheelchair to be driven short distances, and to be used to experiment with various activities. This allows the function of the seating to be evaluated while various tasks are performed. Seating simulators can be used to modify the cushioning to provide pressure relief or postural support. This is especially important for people who require specialized seating to effectively drive an electric-powered wheelchair. The shape of the simulated seating surface is recorded and used to produce the individual's finished product.

The time required to perform a task or activity can be recorded. Time can be used to compare assistive devices or training programs, and as a metric of acceptable performance. For example, donning a pair of pants for someone with impaired arm and leg function can be quite difficult. The selection of the type of pants and pants closure (e.g., snap, button, drawstring) will affect the time required to don/doff the pants. Time can be used to select the type of pants needed in order to reduce the time for dressing to an acceptable level.

People can perform some tasks in one position easier than they can in another position. The space that a person can use may be divided into reachable space, workable space, and flexible space (see Figure 13.3). The *reachable space*

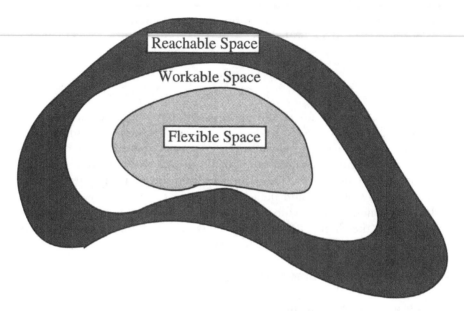

**FIGURE 13.3** Illustration of reachable, workable, and flexible space for performing tasks or activities

defines the entire area that a person can reach. At the extremes of the reachable space, one is able only to touch an object, but not to manipulate it. The *workable space* defines the area in which a given task or activity can be performed. Within the workable space there may be only one way to perform a given task or activity. The *flexible workspace* is the area in which a given task or activity can be performed in two or more ways. For example, if a glass of water is placed within the reachable space, but outside the workable space, then the person would be able to touch or grab the glass, but not be able to bring the glass to the mouth to take a drink. If the glass were in the workable space the person would be able to drink the water, but only by following a specific pattern of motion. For example, the person may only be able to reach the glass and drink from it with one hand. Within the flexible space, the person is provided options for performing the task. For example, the person can use either hand to grasp the glass and drink the water. Goniometers are used to measure joint angles and can be used to measure performance. This is typically accomplished by measuring whether a therapy or assistive device helps to increase joint range of motion. Reachable, workable, and flexible space can also be determined using a video camera while performing various tasks or activities.

Some tasks require accuracy or reliability. Accuracy is determined by the precision with which a task must be performed. For example, driving an electric-powered wheelchair through a crowded grocery store requires a certain degree of accuracy. If the grocery store were devoid of customers, then the degree of accuracy would be lessened. Speed and accuracy are often inversely proportional. When trying to type as fast as possible, the number of errors increases. Typing slower tends to increase accuracy. When evaluating the performance of a task with an assistive device, both speed and accuracy must be measured as part of the performance assessment. Reliability is used to determine how well a person working with an assistive device is able to perform a given task or activity repeatedly. For example, a wheelchair racer may set the world record in a 100-meter race with a time of 13.4 seconds. However, in all previous and following races, he is unable to finish in less than 18 seconds. This athlete would not be considered to be very reliable and would be unlikely to make the Paralympic team.

## 13.4 Team Assessment

Successful assessment requires matching the assistive technologies to the person's abilities and temperament. Scherer has proposed the Matching Person and Technology (MPT) model for assessing assistive technology for an individual. The MPT model advocates addressing the environment and psychosocial setting in which the assistive technology is to be used, the key features of the individual's personality and temperament, and the critical features of the assistive technology. The MPT model uses a checklist-type assessment instrument to obtain and record a person's goals and preferences. This information is used to determine the person's views on the potential benefit of technology, and to measure perceived outcome of assistive technology interventions. An example of the MPT model applied to the selection of a wheelchair is presented in Table 13.1.

The assessment team consists of people with various backgrounds. The center of the assessment team is the individual for whom the technology is being

**TABLE 13.1   Matching person and technology model for selecting a wheelchair**

| Environment | Personality | Technology |
|---|---|---|
| Expectations of family, friends, and employer | Self-motivation to use wheelchair | Assist in attaining goals without excessive pain, fatigue, or stress |
| Security and support provided by family, friends, and peers | Optimism toward use of wheelchair and disability | Compatible with other assistive devices that the person will use |
| Rewards for use of assistive technology | Skill and ability to use wheelchair | Is the wheelchair safe, reliable, simple to use, and easy to maintain? |
| Where does the rider want to drive the wheelchair? | Recognizes potential benefits to wheelchair use | Is the wheelchair affordable for this person? |
| Does the rider plan to travel? | Has realistic expectations for wheelchair use | Does the wheelchair allow for improvement in the skill of the user? |
| What are potential environmental barriers that the rider may encounter? | Does the wheelchair meet the user's desired mobility needs? | Is the driver satisfied with the appearance of the wheelchair? |
| How involved are modifications to the home, work, or school environment? | Does the person want a wheelchair? | Will the wheelchair require modification of the user's home, work, or school environment? |
| Are resources available to make environmental accommodations? | Are the rider's expectations for the wheelchair realistic? | Will the wheelchair necessitate modification of the user's motor vehicle? |
| | Are there other devices that will meet the user's mobility needs? | |

considered. An assessment implies a deliberate process designed to obtain the goals defined by the end user. Because assistive technology must interact closely with a person in order to be most effective, skills are contributed by different people. Physicians have the authority to prescribe assistive devices, including wheelchairs, and are most familiar with the medical aspects of disability. The physician often participates in the person's ongoing care, and can be an important advocate for the assistive device user. A physical or occupational therapist specializing in assistive technology provides insight into how devices interact with the user, and is most often the person providing training for the user. The therapist will often provide the necessary therapy to assist the user in obtaining maximum benefit from the assistive technology. A rehabilitation engineer has the greatest understanding of the assistive technology, and can make needed adjustments and modifications to the technology to accommodate the user. A knowledgeable durable medical equipment dealer or rehabilitation technology supplier can provide assistance with ordering the proper device, and contribute knowledge about current products and services. In many cases family members or personal service assistants should also participate in the assessment. They can provide information about the environment, the need for assistance required by the end user, and may benefit from the knowledge gained about the product.

The Rehabilitation Engineering and Assistive Technology Society of North America (RESNA) has developed a certification program for assistive technology service providers and rehabilitation technology suppliers. Certification requires professional experience and passing an examination. Certification is desirable to be recognized as a professional in assistive technology and to demonstrate competency. RESNA supports the position that people with disabilities and third-party payers should support professionals who have received RESNA certification. Certification requires knowledge of assessment and competency with a variety of assistive technologies.

## 13.5 Computerized Assessment

A large quantity of information is required to assess a person for the proper wheelchair. The process is further complicated by the impact the selection of the wheelchair has on the rider's home, work, and school environment. Personal transportation needs are also affected. There are few experts throughout the world who have the experience and knowledge to consistently provide the most appropriate wheelchair for an individual every time. Many people can provide wheelchairs to people who require only very simple assessments. Even the most experienced people occasionally make mistakes or overlook something during the assessment process. The use of a team approach helps to minimize this problem. However, many assistive technology users do not have access to multidisciplinary teams during the assessment.

Shapcott proposed that assessment could be improved through the use of an expert system that incorporated the knowledge obtained from cases presented by recognized experts in wheelchair prescription. The expert system would contain questions identified by the experts to be critical to the assessment process. These questions are posed in a form similar to the MPT model. Shapcott's expert system also includes QuickTime video to describe activities performed by wheelchair users, ANSI-RESNA standards information, and manufacturers' catalog information. This allows the output of the expert system to include recommendations for specific products as well as a description of the wheelchair's characteristics. The software developed by Shapcott et al. also allows for its database to be updated by collecting data from the software users. This should improve the robustness of the software as time goes on. The primary strengths of the computerized approach are that computers do not forget, the collective knowledge of large numbers of experts can be embedded into the software, and a computer can easily search thousands of product files to find the appropriate match. Computers are also well suited to optimizing the results from numerous factors.

## 13.6 Service Delivery Systems

When a person needs a wheelchair any number of things may happen. The process of obtaining the wheelchair depends primarily on the decision to use a wheelchair and the region in which the person lives. The process of selecting a wheelchair and then actually obtaining the wheelchair is called a channel. Table 13.2 shows various channels for obtaining a wheelchair. A channel path is illustrated in Figure 13.4. Several channel paths require minimal or no input from an assistive technology service delivery system. To appropriately select and configure assistive technology, three systems are suggested. They may be center-based, community-based,

**TABLE 13.2  Example channels for obtaining assistive technology**

| Initial Source of Information | Fitting and Ordering | Funding | Delivery |
|---|---|---|---|
| Durable Medical Equipment Dealer | Physician | Preferred Provider Insurance | Physician |
| Advertisement | Therapist | Health Maintenance Organization | Therapist |
| Friend/Family | Rehabilitation Engineer | Education Assistance Program | Rehabilitation Engineer |
| Salesperson | Rehabilitation Center | Vocational Rehabilitation Program | Rehabilitation Center |
| Therapist | Prosthetics Chief | | Prosthetics Chief |
| Physician | Rehabilitation Clinic | U.S. Department of Veterans Affairs | Rehabilitation Clinic |
| Sporting Event | Durable Medical Equipment Dealer | Medicare | Durable Medical Equipment Dealer |
| Conference or Congress | Nurse | Self-pay | Nurse |
| Clinic/Workshop | Product Distributor | Medicaid | Product Distributor |
| Social Event | Manufacturer | Financing | Manufacturer |
| Consumer Group | Service Center | Personal or Employer Tax Incentives | Service Center |
| Direct Mail | Individual | Employer ADA Accommodation Program | |
| Consumer or Clinical Report | | | |
| Rehabilitation Engineer | | | |

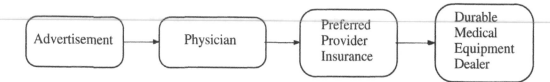

**FIGURE 13.4** Sample channel path for obtaining a wheelchair

or mobile. Center-based service delivery systems are the more traditional approach. Many of the concepts used to select, design, and configure assistive devices were developed in rehabilitation centers with teams specializing in assistive technology. Rehabilitation centers employ a variety of healthcare professionals. This access to physicians, therapists, social workers, and rehabilitation engineers provides the means for a multidisciplinary assessment. Center-based delivery has the advantage of having access to a variety of assistive devices, rehabilitation professionals, and, in some cases, larger numbers of people with disabilities. Centers tend to have high overhead and are working to reduce costs for provision of some services. Center-based systems are often used to provide assistive technology to people who progress to a rehabilitation center.

Community-based service delivery systems were developed to address the needs of people with disabilities in the community. This appears to be a fast-growing area of service delivery. Some durable medical equipment supplier chains have begun to provide in-store services to their customers. Persons can either bring a prescription from their physician or see a physician by appointment at the store. The store has therapists on staff who are familiar with assistive devices. These stores provide the technology, assessment, and assistance with obtaining funding. There is some concern among rehabilitation professionals that people will be directed toward the products that the store carries even when they are less than optimal. Some community-based systems are operated by rehabilitation centers or healthcare delivery systems. This is due to the realization that a broader base of assistive technology users can be served by reaching into the communities where the people live. This also helps the rehabilitation professionals better understand the local needs. Complex cases can be referred to a center-based service delivery system. The current trend tends to indicate that there will be fewer center-based service delivery systems, and those that remain will specialize in more complex assistive technology interventions.

In rural areas, community-based and center-based service delivery systems tend to become impractical. The people who require the assistive technology are dispersed over potentially large geographic regions. Transportation to a center-based delivery system may be impractical, and encouragement of this model may lead to people avoiding using specialists in assistive technology altogether. Community-based models are often impractical as well, because too many would be required to see people who are dispersed. This encouraged the concept of mobile service delivery systems, several of which receive funding through Tech Act grants to states. Mobile service delivery systems use self-contained workshops and assessment stations that are driven to scheduled locations throughout a region. The mobile units are usually staffed by a rehabilitation engineer and a therapist specializing in assistive technology. The mobile teams work with local physicians to provide service to the people within the local area. This approach has been very effective at providing services to people who were previously excluded from traditional service delivery models.

## 13.7 Funding Considerations

Funding for assistive technology can be a very complex maze, and many people with disabilities require assistance to obtain funding for a new wheelchair. Most wheelchairs are purchased by a third-party payer. Third-party payers consist of private, state, and federal insurance or assistance programs. Eligibility for third-party payment varies from state to state, and is highly dependent on the individual's status and the wheelchair characteristics (see Table 13.3). A common factor that

**TABLE 13.3   Examples of issues related to funding for a wheelchair**

| Individual's Status | Wheelchair Characteristics | Payment Options |
|---|---|---|
| Is the wheelchair medically necessary? | How much does the wheelchair cost? | Preferred Provider Insurance |
| How old is the current wheelchair? | How long should the wheelchair be usable? | Health Maintenance Organization |
| What is the condition of the current wheelchair? | How much will maintenance cost? | Education Assistance Program |
| Is the person of employment age? | What is availability? | Vocational Rehabilitation Program |
| Is the person of school age? | Will use of the wheelchair precipitate other expenses? | U.S. Department of Veterans Affairs |
| Is the person of retirement age? | Do other assistive devices exist that will better meet mobility needs? | Medicare |
| Is the person a military veteran? | | Self-pay |
| | | Medicaid |
| Is the person currently employed? | Will use of the wheelchair meet criteria specified by third-party payer? | Financing |
| Does the individual have medical insurance? | Will use of the wheelchair meet the user's mobility needs? | Personal or Employer Tax Incentives |
| Does the person's employer provide medical insurance? | Is there a trade-in market for the wheelchair? | Employer ADA Accommodation Program |
| Can the person afford to purchase the wheelchair? | | |
| Can the person afford to maintain the wheelchair? | | |
| Are there tax incentives for the employer or individual? | | |
| How convenient is the payment plan for the wheelchair user? | | |

unites all third-party payers is the concept of "medical necessity." Medical necessity is used to determine eligibility. The concept implies that the wheelchair or other assistive device is necessary for the individual to perform some activity of daily living. Third-party payers often use medical necessity as a means of denying payment for items that they may consider convenience items. Most third-party payers require a medical justification prior to authorization for payment. An assessment team may be required to provide very detailed justification for why a specific wheelchair is necessary.

Proper documentation is required to obtain payment for a wheelchair or other complex assistive device. Documentation must include a medical assessment of the individual's impairment and the individual's prognosis. A plan for documenting the assessment process should be developed prior to seeing the individual in a clinic for an assessment. Documentation must include the need for the assessment, a detailed description of what was performed during the assessment, and justification for the assessment components. The funding documentation should provide a clear picture of the assessment process, including goals for the assessment, results of the assessment, and follow-up if funding for the technology is approved. The funding documentation must support the decision to select a specific product or set of products to ameliorate a functional deficit or to facilitate return to some activity (e.g., work, school). Most funding agencies want to see that thought was given to the assessment process, that tests were conducted to determine functional deficits, that technologies were tested to ameliorate those functional deficits, that selection of technology considered cost-benefit ratios, that there is a plan to provide adequate training, and that there is a plan to follow up with the individual to ensure that the technology truly met the individual's needs. Developing a strong approach to assessment and funding documentation builds trust between the third-party payer and the assessment team. This trust benefits the individual with a disability, because the third-party payer will be more apt to authorize funding for the most appropriate technology rather than the least costly technology.

A specific wheelchair for an individual requires a *justification report.* For example, simply stating that a person requires a manual wheelchair because of paraplegia as a result of a traumatic spinal cord injury will likely result in that person's receiving authorization for the least expensive wheelchair available. This is because there was little information provided in the justification. In order to receive authorization for a more specific wheelchair type, greater information must be provided. This information must be gathered and organized in an orderly fashion. During the assessment the team should gather information about the support structure available to the individual, the community in which the person lives, employment and educational status, transportation needs, and proposed activity level. Other factors must be considered as well. A more thorough justification for the same person may say that a titanium ultralight manual wheelchair with a rigid frame and quick-release rear wheels is required. The wheelchair is to be equipped with a lumbar support and air flotation cushion. The titanium frame is required because of shoulder pain developed as a result of chronic wheelchair use over a period of 20 years. The individual has been diagnosed with mild rotator cuff tendinitis. The reduced weight and strength of the titanium will ease the burden placed on the arms during transfers (e.g., loading into an individual's motor vehicle) and reduce energy required for propulsion. The individual prefers a rigid frame due to increased durability and improved handling on common surfaces encountered during his normal activities of daily living. Quick-release rear wheels are necessary to facilitate travel related to employment and transport of the wheelchair in a private motor vehicle. The lumbar support is necessary to prevent further spinal deformity and to maintain proper sitting posture. The air flotation cushion is necessary for pressure relief to prevent decubitus ulcers. Pressure-mapping readings indicate that an air flotation cushion is most appropriate for this individual.

The time is approaching when greater justification is going to be required. Currently there are very few studies that support claims that a specific type of assistive device is effective in meeting the needs of the individuals for whom they are prescribed. It is currently an issue of personal experience, with a few cross-sectional studies performed on small convenience samples. As the research base builds for the application of assistive devices, tests will result that will need to be included in justifications. This should help to obtain authorization for appropriate technology and minimize technology abandonment by consumers.

Not all funding decisions are favorable to the clinic or individual. Third-party payers may request additional justification or simply deny a claim. Denials are typically based on the perception of the claims reviewer that the request falls outside the norm of the claims reviewed by that individual or within the region. This may necessitate an appeal. It is important to solicit the assistance of the individual's physician during the claims appeal process. However, there is no substitute for strong documentation that the requested wheelchair or assistive device is most appropriate for a specific individual. Appeals often end favorably if the assessment team is convinced that the technology is most appropriate and they can provide evidence of such. Some third-party payers require co-payments by the individual. It is not unusual for people requiring complex assistive technology systems to acquire funding from several sources. Co-payments are often required to purchase assistive technologies above insurance spending caps. Some insurance companies require deductibles prior to payment. Deductibles are typically sums of money that must be expended by the individual in a given year or for a given incident prior to the individual's insurance taking effect. For example, it is common for people to have insurance that requires the individual to pay the first $1500 in medical expenses each year prior to being eligible for insurance payments.

Some larger healthcare systems purchase assistive technology or negotiate pricing for assistive technology using bid systems. Bid systems are used when the healthcare system (e.g., HMO, VA) knows that it will buy 25,000 wheelchairs in a typical year. This will make the healthcare system a large purchaser and as such it can negotiate a discounted rate on the products it purchases. This allows the insurer to provide the most appropriate technology to an individual at a reduced rate due to the volume of products that it purchases. For example, it is not unusual for the U.S. Department of Veterans Affairs to insist on a 20% discount on wheelchairs.

## 13.8 Documentation

Documentation is important so that effort is not duplicated and so that there is an institutional memory. There are two types of records typically stored: archival records and legal records. Archival records are used to reconstruct the process of applying for assistive technology. Archival records are useful in determining the types of assistive technology that work well for various people. In some cases archival records can be used to determine trends or patterns. This can help to provide reference for a person assessing a new patient or a new product. Archival records typically address how something was done.

Legal records address why something was done. Legal records are necessary for the purposes of financial audits, audits by third-party payers, and litigation. In all three of these types of cases, records are necessary to demonstrate that a process was followed, that all necessary implications were considered, and that there is adequate justification for the end result. Legal records address each individual case, as well as trends. The rights and needs of each individual must be considered in all legal records. Legal records are used to demonstrate that any reasonable person with the appropriate credentials would draw the same conclusion, and that the fees generated would be similar. If there is disagreement, legal records are used to support the conclusions drawn by the clinic or assistive technology professional.

Many states have laws governing access to records and the length of time that they must be stored. In most cases access to records is based on a need-to-know basis. Need-to-know is determined by the job descriptions of the individuals who have access to the records. It is important to safeguard confidentiality and the personal nature of patient records.

Photographs and videotapes can be important tools for saving records. They can be used to record information in compact form that cannot be described adequately in text. Text is necessary to justify why something was done. Photographs and videotapes must be treated as confidential patient information. A written release is often required if images are to be used in publications. Some agencies require that images be destroyed after a specified number of years to protect the privacy of the individual.

All clinics should develop policies that address access to records, storage of records, methods for retrieval, and the minimum information to be contained in each record. Using a consistent format aids in information retrieval and in interpreting previous cases. Many institutions store data in electronic formats. There are many simple database programs that operate on personal computers, and there are many forms of electronic media that can store large amounts of data.

## 13.9 Quality Assurance

The provision of assistive technology demands communication between rehabilitation professionals, third-party payers, and the individual with a disability. Communication must continue throughout the assessment process and into the training and tracking process. Because people have such diverse backgrounds and, possibly, expectations, it is important to ensure that all parties understand one another. Communication with the end user is most critical. The person with a disability must clearly understand the capabilities of the wheelchair, why it is most appropriate for him or her, and the necessity to remain in contact with the other members of the assessment team. A tool for facilitating ongoing communication is to schedule periodic maintenance and training with the rehabilitation team. Some larger rehabilitation centers organize recreational and sports activities for their patients. This helps to maintain contact and provide ongoing communication. People with disabilities must establish long-term relationships with their rehabilitation professionals in order to remain healthy and to benefit the most from their assistive technology.

Rehabilitation professionals must remain open and responsive to the needs and interests of their patients with disabilities. It is unacceptable to treat people with disabilities as consumers who have short-term needs that must be met, and then to have the person return to the community on his/her own accord. In order to be responsive to the people with disabilities, there needs to be a fundamental understanding of disability and its impact on the individual, family, peers, community, and society. With this understanding a relationship can be built that benefits both the person with a disability and the rehabilitation professional. It is important for rehabilitation professionals to be aware of the concerns of the disability community and to advocate for the rights of their patients.

Assistive technology is all too often abandoned or misused because people did not receive adequate training. Even the simplest wheelchair requires training to be of maximum benefit to the user, and it is for this reason that people have specialized in assistive technology service provision. People often neglect or downplay training in their haste to leave rehabilitation or to return to other activities. It is understandable that rehabilitation professionals and people with disabilities have busy schedules that may not permit them to do everything the way they would like, but training is a critical component of the assessment process and is necessary to ensure maximal appropriate use of the assistive technology. Rehabilitation professionals also require ongoing training. Assistive technology, clinical practice, and issues concerning people with disabilities are constantly evolving. This necessitates continuing training for rehabilitation professionals.

Quality is a continuous evolving process. Deming outlined the plan-do-act cycle as a means of implementing continuous quality improvement (see Figure 13.5). The plan-do-act cycle supposes that the team develops a plan to assess the individual's abilities and goals, a plan to evaluate the capabilities of the assistive technology, and a plan to evaluate the effectiveness of the person working in concert with the assistive technology. The next phase of the model moves from plan-

**FIGURE 13.5** Plan-do-act cycle for continuous quality improvement

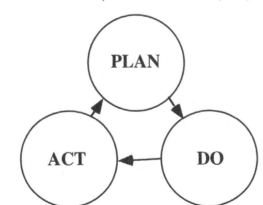

ning to implementation. The plan is implemented, and the person is provided with the selected assistive technology. The person receives training and if successful uses the assistive technology. The final step in the process is to evaluate the effectiveness of the person and assistive technology working in concert to attain the goals set out by the rehabilitation team during the planning process. Shortcomings in meeting the goals set out in the planning process are identified, and the planning process is repeated. The process is repeated continuously. The concept of continuous quality improvement recognizes that technology and disability are dynamic processes that constantly change and evolve. By accepting the concept that assistive technology provision is a dynamic process, planning and evaluation logically follow as continuous processes. This does not imply that a person will require a new wheelchair every three months, but it does mean that the rehabilitation team should develop a long-term partnership with the person with a disability. *Continuous quality improvement* can simply mean that the team works with the individual to learn more skills with the wheelchair, makes adjustments, and attempts to prevent injuries. Through continuous relationships, the need for a new wheelchair evolves from recognizing when the wheelchair no longer meets the individual's needs or goals.

Continuous quality improvement requires that people give the rehabilitation process considerable thought, and that the process is directed toward meeting specific goals. A common flaw in current rehabilitation approaches is that the goals of the individual are often overshadowed by the goals set by rehabilitation professionals. Rehabilitation is the process of establishing or returning to a lifestyle desirable to the individual. The focus must be on the individual's goals. The consequences of ignoring the individual's goals can be as severe as suicide. It is not simple to assess or obtain the individual's goals. This is because a number of factors influence the individual's expectations and perspective. An individual's perspective, goals, and objectives are best considered to be evolving and must be regularly reassessed. An example process for integrating a person's goals into the rehabilitation process is presented in Figure 13.6.

Assistive technology is not the panacea for overcoming disability. Even when CQI is implemented perfectly, there are factors that remain beyond the control of the individual. Disability extends beyond the physical impairment and is a function of society and the physical environment (see Figure 13.7). If there were no societal misconceptions or impositions based on appearance or ability, many forms of assistive technology would be unnecessary. Moreover, disability is partially defined by the physical environment. If products and facilities were all designed with broader concepts about their users, many assistive technologies would simply become mainstream products. Also, many tasks could be accomplished without assistance. For example, automatic door openers are quite common in commercial buildings. Automatic door openers are installed to provide uninterrupted flow of pedestrian traffic and to increase safety. However, they have the unexpected added benefit of allowing people in wheelchairs to easily pass through doorways. Disability can be seen as emanating from a physical or sensory impairment. This impairment can be ameliorated by assistive technology in appropriate instances.

The effectiveness of the assistive technology, when helpful, influences the person's perceived disability. Family, peer, and employer support augment the function of a person's assistive technology. The augmentation can take many forms. For some people, personal assistance services are a very effective means of

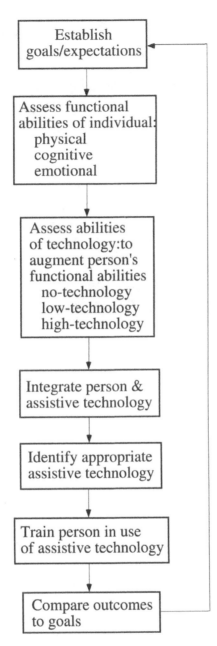

**FIGURE 13.6** Decision-making process for implementing CQI

augmenting their functional abilities. For most people with disabilities, family members provide personal assistance services. Family, peer, and employer/school support can encourage greater function and integration into society. For example, wheelchair racing was a novelty in many running road races during the early 1980s. As athletes trained harder and better racing wheelchairs were developed, the wheelchair racers began to move from being inspiring participants who were courageous for completing the race to becoming respected elite athletes deserving

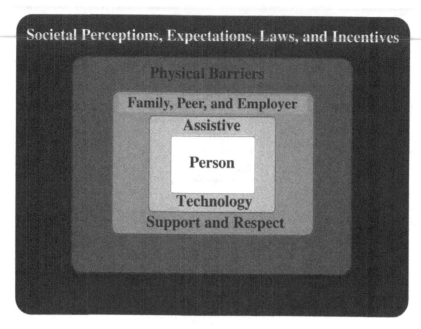

**FIGURE 13.7** A framework for disability: an individual and societal relationship

of prize money for leading the pack. Runners changed their attitude from sympathy to respect as wheelchair racers improved from 45 minutes to 20 minutes for a 10-kilometer race.

A person also defines his or her own disability. It is surprising how two people will react to the same physical impairment. There is as great a diversity among the community of people with disabilities as there is among all people. One person will see physical impairment as a redirection of life goals, another as a stumbling block in the way of his or her previous lifestyle, and still others as a catastrophic event that cannot be overcome. Many other variations exist. Disability begins with the person and expands outward toward society.

Success is a very personal issue, and it varies greatly among individuals. Rehabilitation success may define how well a person becomes integrated into society or measure how well a person meets his or her personal expectations. These definitions represent external and internal views of rehabilitation success. External rehabilitation success is typically defined by the rehabilitation team and society. Internal rehabilitation success is defined by the individual. Sometimes the two coincide; other times they are in direct opposition. A simple example of the dichotomy that can occur between internally and externally defined rehabilitation success centers around the issue of walking post–spinal cord injury. Twenty years ago nearly all people with paraplegia were given a pair of long leg braces, and they spent many hours in vigorous physical therapy working their way to hobbling 400 meters. Most people realized very quickly that the wheelchair was a far more effective means of mobility, and that it was far more flexible. People with disabilities defined success as being mobile—with the wheelchair they could leave rehabilitation and go about their business. Rehabilitation professionals defined success as being able to ambulate on long leg braces. This was partially due to the perception that walking was more desirable than wheeling. Many people with spinal cord injury took a more pragmatic and less societal approach, and opted for the wheel-chair because it was quicker, easier, and safer. This did not deter some scientists and clinicians. They interpreted the rejection of the leg braces to mean that more efficient forms of walking needed to be developed. For years millions of dollars were invested in functional electrical stimulation (FES) walking systems. However, the efficiency, ease of use, convenience, and mobility of FES ambulation could not compete with the continuously improving wheelchair. Recently, FES research has been largely redirected toward other more promising applications.

Quality of life is also interpreted by the individual and by society. An individual with a disability may consider himself or herself as very successful: have a good job, be respected by peers, have a family, and participate in many enjoyable activities. Yet another person may look at himself with pity because of the disability. It is fascinating that a person in a wheelchair who is the president of a $100 million-a-year business can be greeted by people with positions of much less responsibility and authority as a poor pathetic person. A model for defining rehabilitation success is presented in Figure 13.8. The concept of this model is that the individual represents the center of the process. Assistive technology may interact with the person to provide greater function and autonomy. Professional, peer, and family support can augment or replace assistive technology where necessary or preferable. The support provided by other individuals depends on the ability of the assistive technology to augment function, the personal preference of the individual with a disability, and the resources available to provide this type of support.

Some people prefer the human contact provided by another person. Autonomy may not be as important as self-direction. If persons can accomplish everything they desire by working *with* other people, they do not need to be able to accomplish everything independently. Self-direction may lead to greater accomplishment and a higher quality of life than independence. This leads to the concept of the person with a disability's perceived life experiences. All people assess

**FIGURE 13.8**   Model of factors related to rehabilitation success

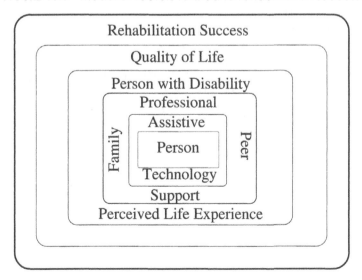

their life experiences periodically. Some life experiences are pleasant; others are not. We tend to rely on hope and past experience to overcome bad experiences. We tend to try to prolong pleasant experiences. The quality of life for persons with a disability depends on their perception of life experiences. If persons perceive all life experiences as unpleasant, their quality of life will be perceived as low, even though others may perceive those persons as having a high quality of life. It is very important to consider the individual's perception of his or her own situation.

## References and Further Reading

Axelson P. (1993) Power chairs. *Paraplegia News*, April, 14–31.

Cook A. M., Hussey S. M. (1995) *Assistive Technologies: Principles and Practice*. St. Louis, MO, Mosby.

Cron L., Sprigle S. (1993) Clinical evaluation of the hemi wheelchair cushion. *American Journal of Occupational Therapy*, 47, 2, 141–144.

Enders A. (1996) Service delivery intensity: a key variable in AT outcome measurement. *RESNA News*, May-June, 1,6.

Flippo K. F., Inge K. J., Barcus J. M. (1995) *Assistive Technology: A Resource for School, Work, and Community*. Baltimore, MD, Paul H. Brookes Publishing.

Galvin J. C., Scherer M. J. (1996) *Evaluating, Selecting, and Using Appropriate Assistive Technology*. Gaithersburg, MD, Aspen Publishers.

Gyorki J. R. (1991) Enabling the disabled. *Machine Design*, November, 108–113.

Lipskin R. (1970) An evaluation program for powered wheelchair control systems. *Bulletin of Prosthetics Research*, Fall, 121–129.

Mattingly D., Wheelchair selection. *Orthopaedic Nursing*, 12, 4, 11–17.

Park L. D. (1975) Barriers to normality for the handicapped adult in the United States. *Rehabilitation Literature*, 36, 4, 108–111.

Richards E. P. (1993) Medical device reporting: new rules, new concerns. *IEEE Engineering in Medicine and Biology Magazine*, September, 103–105.

Thacker J. G., Sprigle S. H., Morris B.O. (1994) *Understanding the Technology When Selecting Wheelchairs*. Arlington, VA, RESNA Press.

Thompson D. L., Thomas K. R., Fernandez M. S. (1994) The Americans with Disabilities Act: Social policy and worldwide implications for practice. *International Journal of Rehabilitation Research*, 17, 109–121.

Trefler E., Hobson D. A., Taylor S. J., Monahan L. C., Shaw C. G. (1993) *Seating and Mobility for Persons with Disabilities*. Tucson, AZ, Therapy Skill Builders.

Warren C. G., Minkel J. (1996) Policies proposed by the professional standards board. *RESNA News*, January–February, 1, 6–7.

Zola I. K. (1982) Denial of emotional needs to people with handicaps. *Archives of Physical Medicine and Rehabilitation*, 63, 63–67.

# Wheelchair Adjustment and Maintenance

*Chapter Goals*

☑ To understand the need for maintenance and repairs for wheelchairs
☑ To know how to assemble, adjust, or program wheelchairs for optimal consumer use
☑ To know how to implement training into a delivery plan

## 14.1 Wheelchair Adjustments

Many wheelchair users never experience the full performance of their wheelchairs. This is partially because many wheelchairs are not adjusted from the factory setting, which in most cases is the most conservative and least functional position for the wheelchair's components. It is important for the wheelchair users, clinicians, and rehabilitation engineers/technicians to experiment with the adjustments on the wheelchair to provide each rider maximum mobility. Adjustments should be made in a controlled manner in order to ensure the rider's safety. Wheelchair riders should always exercise caution after having made adjustments to their wheelchairs.

### 14.1.1 Adjusting Camber

Some wheelchairs allow for the adjustment of camber (the outward tilting of the bottom of the wheels). Camber allows the wheelchair to turn easily, provides greater lateral stability, and helps to protect the hands and fingers from objects like doorways. Excessive camber in a wheelchair can wear tires more rapidly and can make pushing the wheelchair more difficult. Pushing the wheelchair is more difficult because the side walls are not loaded as designed, so the tire deforms to increase rolling friction.

Camber is adjusted by changing the angle made by the rear wheels with respect to a vertical line. Several mechanisms exist to adjust camber. The most common systems are illustrated in Figure 14.1. Camber is added to or subtracted from a camber plate–type wheelchair by inserting or removing washers between the axle plate and the frame. The wheel spacing can be adjusted by adding or subtracting washers in equal numbers at the top and bottom of the axle plate. Some

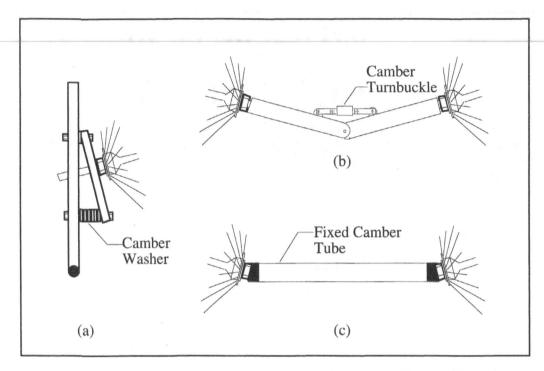

**FIGURE 14.1** Common mechanisms for adjusting wheel camber: (a) an axle plate with camber washers, (b) an axle tube with a turnbuckle mechanism to adjust wheel camber, (c) a camber tube with fixed camber angle

wheelchairs connect the rear wheels via an axle tube. If the axle tube is hinged in the middle, a turnbuckle mechanism can be used to adjust wheel camber. In the example shown in Figure 14.1, if the turnbuckle is lengthened the camber is reduced; if the turnbuckle is shortened the camber increases. Some axle tubes have a fixed camber angle when manufactured. The only way to adjust camber is to replace the tube with another tube with a different preset camber angle. Adjusting camber affects the distance between the tops of the rear wheels. Care must be taken not to create or order a camber angle that makes the wheelchair dysfunctional. Excessive camber can make it difficult to maneuver indoors. Sports wheelchairs use a high degree of camber in order to enhance turning and lateral stability for sports like tennis or basketball. Racing wheelchairs use camber to increase stability and so that the arms can reach all of the way around the pushrim without hitting the wheel, which can be a painful experience.

### 14.1.2 Adjusting Wheel Alignment

Wheel alignment describes the degree to which the rear wheels are parallel to each other and parallel with the centerline of the wheelchair (see Figure 14.2). Wheelchairs perform best when the wheels are perfectly parallel to each other and to the centerline of the wheelchair. Even very small differences can affect the performance of the wheelchair. Users have reported that they can feel an increase in rolling resistance with as little as 1/8 inch difference between the front and rear of the tires. Misalignment of the rear wheels with respect to the centerline of the wheelchair is not

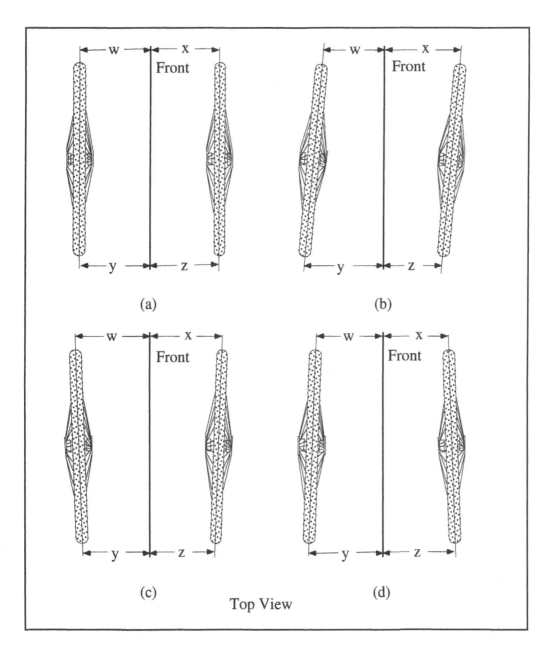

**FIGURE 14.2** Diagram depicting the definitions of alignment: (a) shows the wheels are in proper alignment, and in such cases w = x = y = z; (b) shows the wheels when they are parallel to each another (w = z and x = y), but the wheels are not parallel with the wheelchair's centerline; (c) shows the definition of toe-out—in such case, the wheels are farther apart in the front than they are in the rear (w = x > y = z); (d) shows the definition of toe-in—in such case, the wheels are farther apart in the rear than they are in the front (y = z > w = x).

quite so critical. If the rear wheels do not run parallel to the centerline of the wheelchair, then the wheelchair will have a tendency to veer to one side. This means that the user will need to expend more energy to keep driving the wheelchair straight.

Alignment is adjusted similar to camber, and in fact the two variables are often related. If the camber is adjusted, the height of the axle from the ground will change. The change in height causes the alignment to change. Therefore, most wheelchair manuals suggest adjusting the camber to the desired angle and then setting the misalignment to zero. There are two common means of adjusting wheel alignment (see Figure 14.3).

Camber plates use washers to adjust the wheel alignment. Using camber plates allows for a wide range of adjustment for camber and wheel alignment, but at the cost of increased complexity. Camber tubes are twisted until the proper alignment is achieved. If the wheels are not properly aligned they will scuff. Scuffing can cause excessive wear on tires and rolling surfaces (e.g., carpet). Proper alignment makes driving the wheelchair easier and less stressful to the wheelchair components.

### 14.1.3 Adjusting the Center of Gravity

Seat position with respect to the wheels alters the center of gravity for the person and the wheelchair. Some manual and power wheelchairs adjust the center of gravity by moving the seat forward and backward with respect to the wheels (see

**FIGURE 14.3** Drawings showing wheel mounting mechanisms: (a) wheel alignment for axle plates are adjusted by adding thin washers to the front or back of the camber plate; (b) and (c) wheel alignment is adjusted by twisting the axle tube until the alignment is correct.

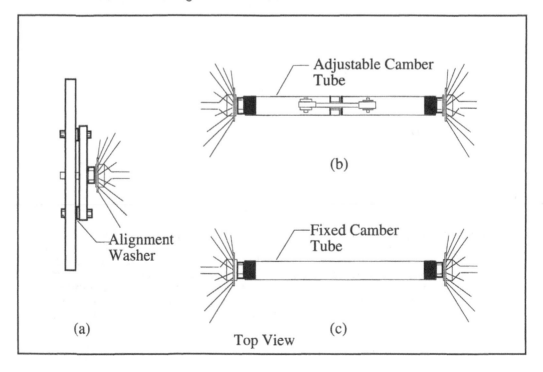

Figure 14.4). Typically, the wheels are not adjustable in these cases. Some wheelchairs have the legrests attached to the seat. When the seat is moved fore and aft to adjust the center of gravity, the legrests follow and the person's body position is unaltered. However, some wheelchairs adjust the seat independently of the legrests or the legrests may not be adjustable. This makes adjusting the center of gravity more complex as the center of gravity, position to the drive wheels, and seat depth may all vary simultaneously. Typically, seat depth is adjusted first, and fine adjustments are made around the proper seat depth to tune the center of gravity and position to the drive wheels. The seat is commonly adjusted by using clamps that attach between the seat and the wheelchair frame. As the clamps are loosened, the seat can slide. Other wheelchairs use brackets and a series of holes. Bolts are removed from the brackets, and the seat is moved to the desired hole position where the bolts are replaced.

The center of gravity of a wheelchair can also be adjusted by moving the position of the wheels with respect to the seat (see Figure 14.5). When changing the position of the wheels, the wheel base is also affected. A shorter wheelbase may make the wheelchair more maneuverable, and but also may make it more difficult to negotiate obstacles.

For manual wheelchairs, the ability to reach the pushrims is also affected by moving the seat or wheel position. Therefore, it is important to consider both center of gravity position and the effect of seating on pushing. The rolling resistance of the drive wheels is typically much lower than that of the caster wheels. Therefore, most riders can benefit by having most of their weight placed on the rear (drive) wheels. This makes the chair roll easier, but it also predisposes the wheelchair to tipping backwards more easily. An accomplished wheelchair rider can adjust to the wheelchair's having little weight on the front casters, and can learn to take advantage of the increased maneuverability. Other wheelchair riders need a more conservative center of gravity position to provide the additional stability. Power wheelchairs tend to have the center of gravity close to the midpoint of the wheelchair. This helps to provide stability while negotiating obstacles,

**FIGURE 14.4**  Side view illustrating how seat position is used to adjust the center of gravity position with respect to the wheels and casters: (a) shows the seat in the mid-position, (b) shows the seat in the aft-most position, and (c) shows the seat in the forward-most position.

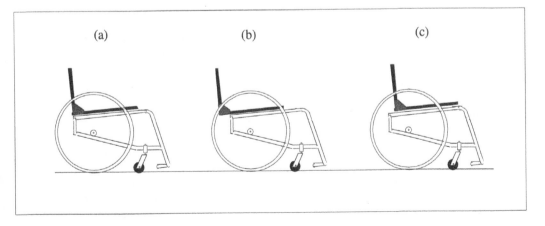

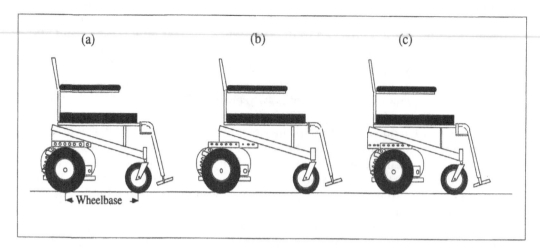

**FIGURE 14.5** Center of gravity adjustment by changing position of the rear wheels: (a) shows the wheels in the mid-position, (b) shows the wheels in the rear-most position, and (c) shows the wheels in the front-most position.

slopes, and slippery surfaces. Some adjustment of the center of gravity can help improve the performance of power wheelchairs to suit an individual's driving habits. For example, if a power wheelchair driver spends much of the time driving indoors, adjusting the seat to have less weight over the casters can improve turning. If a driver spends more time outdoors negotiating grass or unimproved surfaces, a more central center of gravity position can improve obstacle-climbing ability. The best position for the center of gravity depends on the driver, driving habits, and design of the wheelchair.

## 14.2 Seating System Adjustments

### 14.2.1 Seat Angle

Seat angle can be adjusted by changing axle position, wheel size, or frame tube location. When the rear axles are moved upward without changing the caster stem length or caster wheel size, the seat angle is significantly shifted toward the rear. The rear seat height can also be altered by changing the diameter of the rear wheels, whereas the front seat height can be adjusted by changing the size of the front casters or the length of the caster stem (see Figure 14.6). When the seat angle is adjusted using these methods, it is likely that the rear wheel alignment will be altered. After adjusting the seat angle, the caster housing should be adjusted to vertical. This will allow the wheelchair to turn properly. Once this is completed, the alignment of the rear wheels should be checked and corrected as necessary.

Some rigid-frame wheelchairs are constructed with custom-fixed angles or with adjustable seat frame tubes (see Figure 14.7). By adjusting the seat tubes, the seat angle can be tuned for the user without the need to adjust the caster housings or the rear wheel alignment. This is preferred by many rigid-frame wheelchair users. Adjusting the seat angle of a wheelchair will also influence the position of the

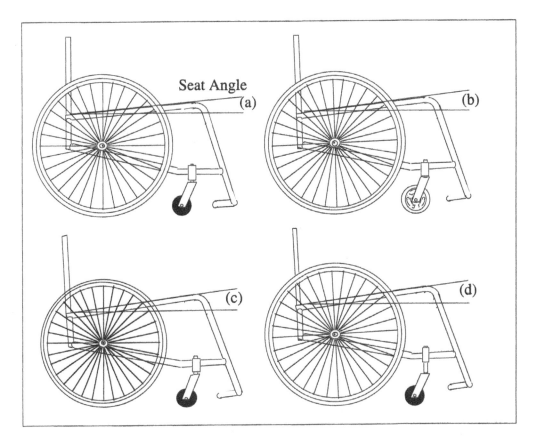

**FIGURE 14.6**  The wheelchair will come with a seat angle set by the factory as specified in the order (a). The seat angle may be altered by using larger caster wheels (b), using smaller rear wheels (c), or using a longer caster stem (d).

center of gravity, and hence the performance of the wheelchair. Experimentation is often required to find the ideal position.

The seat angle for the wheelchair illustrated in Figure 14.7 is adjusted by removing the bolts that attach the lateral seat tubes to the backrest. Typically, a series of holes is available to select different seat angles. Some wheelchairs take advantage of the hinges in the lateral seat tubes to use them as swing-arms for suspension. In such cases an elastomer spring/dampener is integrated into the joint with the backrest. The elastomer dampeners act to reduce the shock when traversing rough terrain or going over curbs.

### 14.2.2 Specialized Seating Hardware

Some people require specialized seating hardware in order to gain the maximum benefit from their wheelchair. Wheelchair manufacturers often make specialized seating hardware to accommodate users who require additional support for orthopaedic malformations or injuries. Other people need positioning belts and systems to provide them control over their wheelchair, and to ensure safe operation of their wheelchair. It is important to understand that attachment of specialized seating hardware does not negatively impact the integrity of the wheelchair.

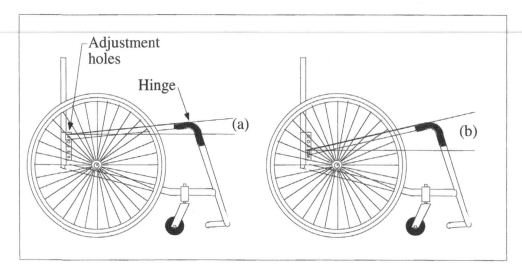

**FIGURE 14.7**   Illustration of seat angle adjustment by placing hinges in the lateral seat tubes and a set of adjustment holes at the seat-to-backrest intersection.

Drilling holes in some portions of wheelchair frames can cause the wheelchair to fail prematurely. In some cases wheelchair manufacturers will void the warranty for their products if seating hardware from another manufacturer is added to their products. However, some riders require seating hardware not produced by a wheelchair manufacturer.

Some specialized seating hardware is clamped to the wheelchair frame. This does not require modification to the wheelchair frame, but it may alter the way in which forces are applied to the wheelchair. If forces are applied differently from what the original manufacturer intended, then the wheelchair may not behave as designed. While specialized seating hardware is extremely valuable for some wheelchair riders, assistive technology providers must be aware that attaching such systems to the wheelchair may affect the wheelchair's safety and performance. For example, many specialized seating systems use metal seat pans and backrest frames. These additional metal components along with the foam, upholstery, and attachment hardware may alter the location of the center of gravity of the wheelchair. It is important to verify that the wheelchair remains safe to operate after making modifications. The simple static stability tests described in the ANSI/RESNA wheelchair standards can provide some useful clinical information in this regard.

### 14.2.3 Backrest

The back height of the wheelchair varies according to the individual's comfort and need for support. Low back heights tend to improve mobility, but they require greater balance and strength. Tall backs offer greater support, but they can limit mobility. Adjustable back heights allow for changing needs and some experimentation. The thickness of the cushion is going to influence the effectiveness of the back height. Backrest height is commonly adjusted using one of two mechanisms (see Figure 14.8).

The backrest supports are made of a smaller diameter tubing and slide within the rear section of the frame or a larger tube, forming the lower section of the

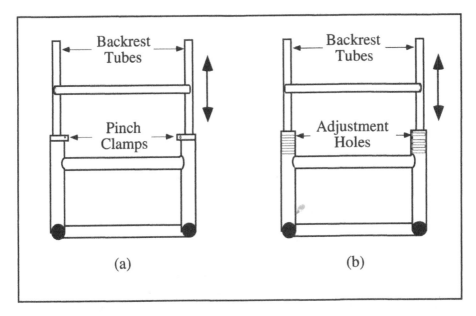

**FIGURE 14.8** The backrest height is commonly adjusted using either a pinch clamp (a) or a bolt with a series of holes (b).

backrest supports. The smaller diameter tube is adjusted up and down to meet the needs of the user. A pinch clamp or adjustment holes with a retaining bolt are used to hold the backrest in place.

Backrest angle is also adjustable on some wheelchairs. This is accomplished in a variety of ways, the most common being to hinge the backrest to the lateral supports of the seat (see Figure 14.9). The hinge is often used to allow the backrest to fold forward during transport. The rearward travel of the backrest is limited by an adjustable stop that determines the backrest angle. Adjusting the backrest

**FIGURE 14.9** Adjustment of backrest angle. The angle of the backrest is adjusted by screwing the adjustable stop into the seat tube, effectively shortening it. This causes the backrest angle to increase. Lengthening the adjustable stop decreases the backrest angle.

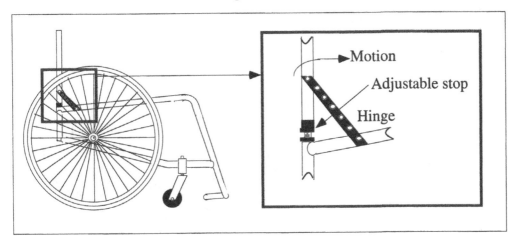

angle allows the person's seating position to be adjusted for optimum wheeling and appropriate balance. A slight recline can help to compensate for a weakened trunk or reduced hip range of motion. An adjustable backrest angle also helps to make changes for increases in strength and range of motion. In order to maintain proper balance, the backrest angle may require adjustment whenever the seat angle is changed.

### 14.2.4 Legrests

*Legrests* is a term used to describe a number of components. Legrests include the footrests, footplates on which the rider's feet sit, the assembly connecting the footrests to the wheelchair frame, and any mechanisms that may change the elevation of the footrests and their attachment to the wheelchair frame. Footrests are available in a variety of materials, styles, and sizes. Footrests provide support for the feet and lower legs. They also help to determine seating position and influence the weight distribution on the seat. Wheelchair riders also use footrests to assist in pushing doors open, in moving objects, and as protection for their feet. Footrests can be classified as flip-up or rigid. Flip-up footrests make transferring forward easier for some individuals. Some active wheelchair users prefer a rigid one-piece footrest. A rigid one-piece footrest adds strength to the wheelchair and is more durable than other models. Footplates are made of either composite materials or tubing. Tubular footplates tend to lighter weight, but do not offer as much support. Composite footplates provide a flat surface for good foot contact. Some users can use enlarged footrests to provide extra protection to their feet during a collision. Composite footplates are available with angle and rotation adjustments to accommodate orthopaedic restrictions (see Figure 14.10).

**FIGURE 14.10**    Illustration of footrest adjustment for a wheelchair. Footrest rotation and footrest angle can be adjusted on some wheelchairs in order to accommodate the rider's anatomy.

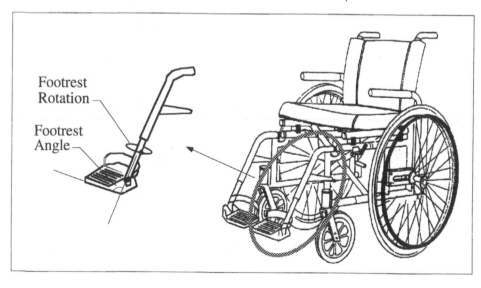

Legrests can be fixed or removable. Removable legrests commonly incorporate a swing-away feature that simplifies transfers for some people. Removable legrests reduce the component weight of the wheelchair during stowage. This helps to make it easier to lift and smaller. Some users swing the legrests to the side in order to get closer to counters, beds, and toilets. Removable legrests can be lost and are more susceptible to damage than rigid legrests. It is very important to properly adjust the length of the legrests (see Figure 14.11). When legrests are too short, excessive pressure may be placed under the ischial tuberosities. When legrests are positioned too high, circulation may be reduced to the legs, and the users will typically have poor seated balance.

As a wheelchair becomes more compact, it becomes easier to maneuver. If the wheelchair becomes too short, it becomes difficult to climb obstacles. The angle the front of the legrests makes helps to determine the compactness of the wheelchair. The greater the legrest angle, the more compact the wheelchair will be (see Figure 14.12). The degree of the front angle is determined by the range of motion of the user, the type and size of the front caster, the postural needs of the user, and the type of activities the user performs. Legrests on some wheelchairs are ordered with fixed angles, whereas others are adjustable. Adjustability adds weight, so many wheelchair users prefer a fixed legrest angle. Most manufacturers provide a range of standard legrest angles to select from and offer custom angles for additional cost.

## 14.3 Wheelchair Manufacturing and Modifications

People do not fit neatly into categories. Some wheelchairs are manufactured for mass production. These wheelchairs often limit choices, options, and mobility. Most high-performance manual and powered wheelchairs are built for each indi-

**FIGURE 14.11**   The length of the legrest is adjustable on many wheelchairs. This helps to properly set sitting posture and to accommodate the rider's anatomy.

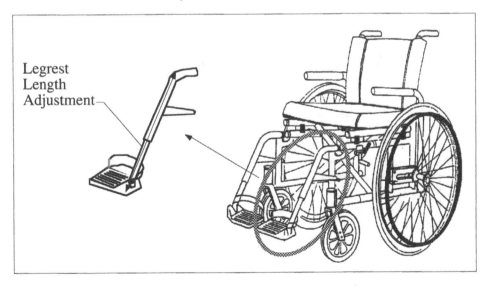

Legrest
Length
Adjustment

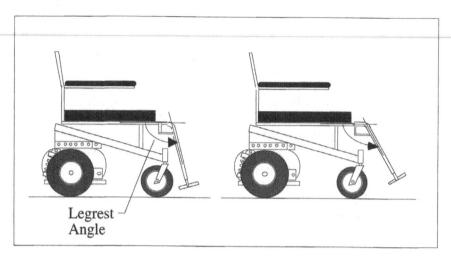

**FIGURE 14.12**   Legrest angle is defined with respect to the seat plane. Legrest
angle is chosen or adjusted to match the rider's anatomy, range
of motion, peripheral circulation, comfort, and desired mobility. As
shown in this figure, the greater the legrest angle, the longer the
wheelchair becomes. This decreases maneuverability.

vidual. When manufacturers make a wheelchair, they are working to make it fit the
individual. The large manufacturers literally offer thousands of customized permutations. While the task of selecting and adjusting a wheelchair from thousands
of permutations may seem daunting, there are some basic rules that when followed
will lead to the correct wheelchair for each person.

Manufacturers take the body dimensions recorded from each individual and
the type of wheelchair requested, and enter this data into their computers. Programs are used that translate the users' dimensions to the drawings required to
produce the type of wheelchair selected for that individual. The program specifies the exact location of every hole that must be drilled and the precise angle at
which to bend each piece of tubing.

### 14.3.1 Drilling

Drilling is a fundamental process used in the manufacture and customization of
wheelchairs. Drilling is the process of creating a hole in a material by using a spinning tool. The tool used in drilling is a drill bit. Drill bits are fluted pieces of round
metal bar. Flutes are cut to cause the bit to remove material as it spins and pressure is applied by the drill bit to the part. As the drill bit spins, it cuts chips from
the material in which the hole is being drilled. Drill bits come in a wide variety of
sizes—number sizes, metric sizes, and fractional (inch) sizes. Drill bits may be
coated with titanium or cobalt in order to increases their hardness. This helps the
bits cut hard or tough materials.

When using a drill, the operator must choose the spindle speed and feed rate
of the drill bit. Spindle speed is usually determined in revolutions per minute. The
feed rate is defined as the speed with which the drill bit enters the part. Feed rate
is usually controlled by a lever that is turned by the operator. The rate at which the
part can be drilled is dependent on the linear speed of the cutting surface of the

drill bit. The linear speed is determined by the spindle speed and feed rate. Faster drilling can be achieved by using a high spindle speed and high feed rate. With a slower speed, a slower feed rate must be used. High-speed drilling presents a problem with cooling the part and drill bit and often requires coolant. Drilling at high speeds can also cause rapid tool wear.

Wheelchair manufacturers drill numerous holes in their wheelchair frames and in components. The holes are used to attach parts and accessories. Hole tolerances are important to ensure proper fit and alignment. In manufacturing a computer numerically controlled (CNC) drill press can be used to drill holes in very precise positions repeatedly. This is useful in production where thousands of the same part must be made. In most rehabilitation engineering shops a hand-operated drill press is sufficient (see Figure 14.13).

**FIGURE 14.13** Photograph of a bench-top drill press used in a rehabilitation engineering shop (Photograph courtesy of Rory Cooper)

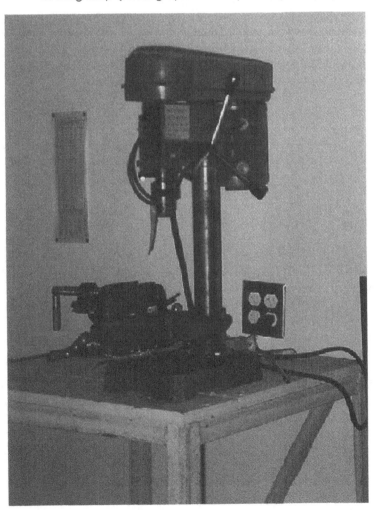

### 14.3.2 Milling

Milling is very much like drilling and a mill can be used as a drill press. However, a mill is more versatile than a drill press. A mill or milling machine is used to cut slots, cut shapes, and cut contours. A mill is made from an x-y table, a knee, and a spindle. The spindle rotates and moves up-down. The cutting tool is placed in the spindle. The part is clamped to the x-y table. The x-y table may move in-out and side-to-side. Both motions are possible simultaneously. This provides very powerful diversity. By carefully controlling the motion of the x-y table, milling machines can be used to cut complex shapes. The knee is used to move the part up-down. The knee has greater travel than the spindle and it is much stiffer. The spindle is provided with finer control. Therefore, the knee is used to bring the part close to the final position of the tool, and the spindle is used for fine adjustments.

Cutting tools for milling machines come in a very wide variety. Cutting tools are used to make a number of different types of slots. Cutting tools are also used to ensure that the part is square. Milling machines are also governed by feed and speed rate like drilling machines, but the relationship is more complex. Milling machines use a spinning tool whose rotational speed is determined by the spindle speed. Milling machines have three different feed rates for the x, y, and z directions. The x and y feed rates are determined by the x-y table. They are often controlled by electric motors, which can be adjusted by the operator or a computer. The z feed rate is determined by the spindle feed. Typically, the spindle feed is controlled by hand. However, for computer numerically controlled (CNC) milling machines spindle feed rate is determined by an electric motor and computer. CNC milling machines are used to make many wheelchair parts. This is because they allow manufacturers to maintain very high quality parts at reasonable costs in large quantities. CNC milling machines have allowed wheelchair manufacturers to produce unusually shaped parts that help make wheelchairs lighter and more functional. A rehabilitation engineering service or small manufacturer will typically have a milling machine (see Figure 14.14), but the additional cost of a CNC milling machine is often not warranted.

### 14.3.3 Turning

Turning is unique in that the part turns and the cutter remains stationary. Turning is done on a lathe. A lathe is a simple but very versatile machine (see Figure 14.15). A lathe uses a motor, a chuck (a clamp to hold the part), a tail-stock, and a tool-post holder. The part is held in a chuck connected to the motor through a gear box. The tail-stock is used to hold the other end of the part or to hold a tool. For example, a drill bit can be placed in the tail-stock in order to drill a hole along the center axis of the part. Lathes are used to make round parts, axles, caster spindles, and some caster wheels. Wheelchair manufacturers use computer numerically controlled lathes to make numerous round and circular parts. Rehabilitation engineering shops may also have a lathe to make or repair round parts (e.g., axles, shafts, bushings).

### 14.3.4 Welding

Most high-performance wheelchairs are made of aircraft-grade aluminum or aircraft-grade steel. Most wheelchair frames are made of round drawn tubing. This type of tubing is formed while the metal is still in its molten state and creates a

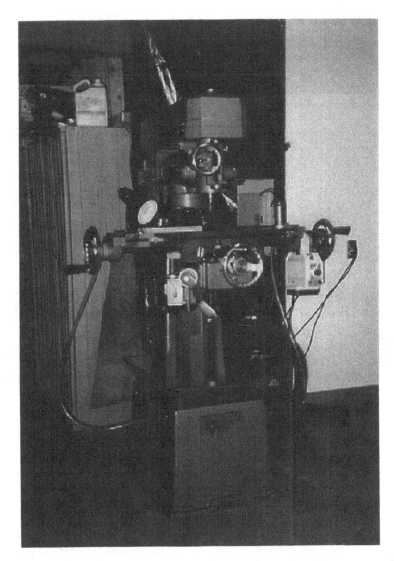

**FIGURE 14.14** Photograph of a vertical milling machine used in a rehabilitation engineering shop (Photograph courtesy of Rory Cooper)

seamless tube. This makes the tubing stronger for its size and weight. Wheelchairs are typically hand-welded on specially constructed jigs. There is a jig, or holding fixture, for each weld. This helps to ensure that the complete wheelchair frame is correctly built and aligned. After welding, parts are placed in a test jig to ensure that they were properly aligned. Manufacturers often use a tolerance of less than 0.060 inches to determine if joint alignment is acceptable.

Welding requires specialized training to look good and to provide adequate strength. Wheelchairs are either brass-welded or electrically welded in an inert gas. Depot-type metal wheelchairs are typically brass-welded by placing small amounts of brass on one piece of metal forming the welded joint; then the two pieces of metal to be welded are held together and placed in a furnace. The furnace heats the metal and melts the brass forming a bond when cooled. This is an inexpensive

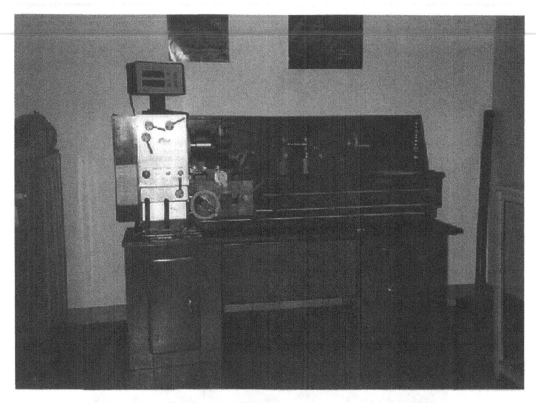

**FIGURE 14.15**  Photograph of a metal turning lathe used in a rehabilitation engineering shop (Photograph courtesy of Rory Cooper)

process that can be used with most common steels. To get higher strength or to use lighter weight materials, more complex welding methods are used. The most common method in called TIG (tungsten inert gas) welding. This type of welding is used to make aluminum and chromolly wheelchairs. An alternating current electric arc is passed through a tungsten electrode to the metal being welded. The electrode is shrouded in a cloud of inert gas, usually argon. The gas help to prevent corrosion, which happens very rapidly in aluminum and alloy steels. Electric arc welding localizes the heat to a very small area around the weld. This makes it possible to weld materials like aluminum, which transitions from a solid to a liquid very rapidly (i.e., over a small change in temperature).

The strength of a weld depends on the skills of the welder, the welding process, and the materials being welded. To test the strength of their welds, most manufacturers perform periodic test welds. This is done by measuring the strength required to destroy a weld. For example, every hundredth part is destroyed and the process is determined to be acceptable if all parts tested have a strength above a predefined threshold.

### 14.3.5 Cutting

Materials for wheelchairs come in the form of raw stock. Stock usually consists of round and square tubing, extruded tubing, round and square bar stock, and plate. Extruded tubing is used when a similar complex shape is used often. Many caster forks are made of an extrusion. When looking at a caster fork from the front, there is a common shape used on many wheelchairs. Therefore, it is simplest and most cost effective to make an extruded piece and cut it to make individual forks. Axle plates are made from plate, which is cut and then milled to the proper shape and tolerances.

Wheelchair manufacturers use two type of cutting. Abrasive cutting is used to rapidly cut tubing or bar stock to roughly the correct shape (see Figure 14.16). A metal-bladed band saw can be used to cut tubing, extrusions, bar stock, and plate (see Figure 14.17). Abrasive cutting is mostly used with steel and titanium. Aluminum has a tendency to melt with an abrasive cutter. Cutting is used to create the rough shape of the part and/or to make its length appropriate for turning or milling.

## 14.3.6 Painting

Once the frame is completed, the color coating is added. There are three common processes used. Plating is used on most depot-type wheelchairs. These wheelchairs are cleaned and etched to remove oil and dirt. Then an electrode is placed on the frame. The frame is then dipped in a charged vat of chrome. The amount of charge and the length of time in the vat determines the thickness of the plating. The exact process varies slightly with the type of material being plated.

Other wheelchairs are painted using enamel or lacquer paints. These paints are sprayed on in a dust-free room. Most are sprayed by hand. Several layers are typically

**FIGURE 14.16** Photograph of an abrasive cut-off saw used in a rehabilitation engineering shop (Photograph courtesy of Rory Cooper)

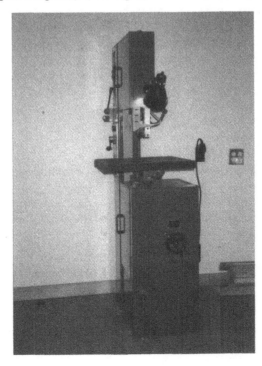

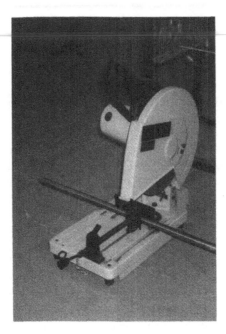

**FIGURE 14.17**   Photograph of band saw used in a rehabilitation engineering shop (Photograph courtesy of Rory Cooper)

required. Once a color is completed, the frame is placed in an oven to cure the paint. This process allows for a wide variety of colors and individualized paint schemes. The most durable form of painting is called powder coating. Powder coating is somewhere between plating and painting. With powder coating, the frame is etched and cleaned, then sprayed with a base coat. After this the frame is electrically charged, and then sprayed with a charged powder. The powder is attracted to the charged frame and sticks. Then the frame is placed in an oven to cure. The powder and metal form a very strong bond. The finish of a powder coat is very durable. The number of colors is more limited than normal painting, but the number of colors is constantly increasing. It is difficult to use multiple colors on a single part with color coating.

## 14.4 User Maintenance

Few items on a wheelchair are designed to be maintained by the user. This is primarily because wheelchairs are typically designed for low maintenance. When maintenance is required, a person with specialized training can do the best job. It is important for the wheelchair user to see that the wheelchair remains properly maintained.

### 14.4.1 Cleaning and Inspection

Wheelchair users should keep their wheelchairs clean and free from debris. Since wheelchairs are used daily by many people, their proper maintenance will enhance function and reliability. The user has the greatest contact with the wheelchair and is often the first to notice problems or changes in driving performance. It is important for the wheelchair rider to ensure that the wheelchair is properly maintained. A properly maintained wheelchair will provide several years of reliable service.

Wheelchair users should check to see that the wheelchair folds easily and smoothly, and check components for bending or excessive wear. Armrests should be easily removable or flip-up easily. Quick-release axles should operate smoothly. Figure 14.18 provides a checklist for items that wheelchair users should monitor

**FIGURE 14.18** Checklist for basic wheelchair maintenance

| Upon Receipt | Weekly | Monthly | Periodically | Item |
|:---:|:---:|:---:|:---:|---|
| | | | | **General** |
| ● | | | ● | Wheelchair opens and folds easily |
| ● | ● | | | Wheelchair rolls straight with no excess drag or pull |
| ● | | | ● | Footrests flip up/down easily |
| ● | | | ● | Legrests swing away and latch easily |
| ● | | | ● | Backrest folds and latches easily |
| ● | | | ● | Armrests easy to move and latch |
| ● | | | ● | All nuts and bolts are snug |
| | | | | **Wheels** |
| ● | | | ● | Axle threads in easily or slides in and latches properly |
| ● | ● | | | No squeaking, binding, or excessive side motion while turning |
| ● | | | ● | All spokes and nipples are tight and not bent or nicked |
| ● | ● | | | Tire pressure is correct and equal on both sides |
| ● | | ● | | No cracks, looseness, bulges in tires |
| | | | | **Casters** |
| ● | | | ● | No cracks, looseness, or bulges in caster tires |
| ● | ● | | | No wobbling of caster wheel |
| ● | ● | | | No excessive play in the caster spindle |
| ● | ● | | | Caster housing is aligned vertically |
| | | | | **Wheel Locks** |
| ● | | | ● | Do not interfere with tire when rolling |
| ● | ● | | | Easily activated and released by operator |
| ● | ● | | | Hold tires firmly in place while activated |
| | | | | **Electrical System** |
| ● | | | ● | Wires show no crackes, splits, or breaks |
| ● | ● | | | Indicators and horn work properly |
| ● | ● | | | Controls work smoothly and repeatably |
| ● | | ● | | Battery cases are clean and free from fluids |
| ● | | | ● | Motor runs smoothly and quietly |
| | | | | **Upholstery** |
| ● | | | ● | No tears, rips, burn marks, or excessive fraying |
| ● | | ● | | No excessive stretching (e.g., hammocking) |
| ● | ● | | | Upholstery is clean |

or have monitored regularly. Wheelchair users should also schedule periodic maintenance with an authorized service center, as prescribed in the user manual for their wheelchair.

### 14.4.2 Tires and Tubes

Wheelchair users, a friend, family member, or local bicycle shop should be able to replace tires and repair tubes. Many bicycle shops can order manual wheelchair tires. A bicycle shop may be more convenient for many wheelchair users than a durable medical equipment (DME) dealer. If tires are not properly inflated, they will wear prematurely. The proper tire pressure is typically cast into the sidewall of the tire. Wheelchair tires are nearly standard throughout the world. For this reason, wheelchair tire manufacturers usually cast the proper tire pressure in pounds per square inch (PSI), kilopascals (kPa), and atmospheres (BAR). A common 24-inch rear wheelchair tire is commonly properly inflated at 65 PSI or 450 kPa or 45 BAR. Pneumatic tires typically last between six months and one year depending on the level of use. Caster tires may last longer. Caster tires do not carry as much weight as rear tires, and do not experience as much scuffing; this helps them last longer.

Tires can be changed using simple tire tools (available from a durable medical equipment dealer or bicycle shop). Changing a tire requires strength and dexterity. Some users may require assistance. There are several common types of wheelchair tires and casters. The most common type of tire is a pneumatic (air filled) tire with a separate tube. With the tube deflated, the tire can be readily removed. Care should be taken not to puncture the tube when removing or replacing the tire. Solid or semi-pneumatic tire inserts can be used instead of tubes. The options are a bit heavier, but they do not puncture. Solid or semi-pneumatic inserts make changing tires more difficult. They are fairly stiff and cannot be deflated. Wheelchairs also use solid tires. Solid tires also require periodic replacement. It is often best to go to a durable medical equipment dealer to replace solid tires. DME dealers have the solid tire replacements and experience in changing the tires.

## 14.5 Service Center Maintenance

### 14.5.1 Service Center Models

Wheelchairs are typically serviced by a network of durable medical equipment dealerships. DME dealerships are commonly independent businesses. There are no regulations governing the requirements for service personnel within DME dealerships. However, there are some industry standards. The most prominent of industry standards for DME dealerships is the National Registry of Rehabilitation Technology Suppliers (NRRTS). NRRTS is a voluntary industry organization that promotes education, advocacy for small business, and professional certification through RESNA. NRRTS members agree to provide quality service and to participate in continuing education. Service personnel within DME dealerships may participate in service and maintenance training offered by assistive technology manufacturers. Most major manufacturers require participation in formal training prior to becoming an authorized service representative. This helps to ensure some degree of product knowledge by local service personnel.

DME dealerships vary widely in quality. Some are very conscientious and remain abreast of new developments. DME dealerships may be involved in the assessment process. Some clinics and/or clinicians integrate the DME dealer into the assessment and delivery process for wheelchairs. This is because the DME dealer may be the most knowledgeable person on the team about existing products and the product's capabilities. DME dealers are also likely to service the assistive device once it has been delivered to the client. Good DME dealers provide added value to the product, and contribute to the mobility of the consumer. Poor DME dealers increase the cost of the product without adding value.

DME dealerships can provide pick-up and delivery of wheelchairs. This provides a very useful service to people who do not have personal means of transportation or who cannot move or transport a broken electric-powered wheelchair. Repair and maintenance of wheelchairs is an important service provided by DME dealers. Service is a factor that often defines the consumer's view of the DME dealer's quality. Wheelchair users will tolerate very few repairs due to the impact repairs have on mobility. Consumers want periodic maintenance at reasonable cost and rapid repairs. Maintenance costs can make an otherwise acceptable wheelchair intolerable. Most companies only provide very limited warranties on their products. Therefore, maintenance costs are passed directly on to the consumer. However, consumers and DME dealers are burdened with paperwork to get reimbursement for maintenance. Some DME dealers include maintenance for a limited term, typically one year, with the purchase of the wheelchair. This is typically best for the consumer because the maintenance for the first year is embedded in the purchase price. The cost for the maintenance helps the payer because the dealer can amortize expenses over all customers and the dealer has less overhead associated with payment.

Some wheelchair manufacturers have begun to work more closely with DME dealerships to ensure a higher level of service to customers. This is taking place through developing a service network affiliated with a particular manufacturer. These service networks receive technical training, guidance in setting up maintenance programs, and access to a computer service network. Some manufacturers also provide assistance with reimbursement for service, and will delay billing for replacement parts until the DME dealer receives payment. This helps the consumer get maintenance performed more rapidly, and helps improve quality. Some of these services are embedded into the cost of the wheelchair. Wheelchair users are demanding warranties to protect themselves against the proverbial "lemon." A "lemon" is a wheelchair with substantial continuing defects that are not the fault of the consumer. Thirteen states across the United States have enacted consumer protection laws that specifically provide minimum warranties for assistive devices. Assistive technology "lemon laws" typically demand a one-year warranty on equipment beginning on the date of delivery. The date of delivery removes the time often required to obtain the product once an order has been placed. The stipulations of the laws vary from state to state.

Some dealerships maintain computer profiles of their clients. This helps them to understand and anticipate their customers' service needs. For example, computer profiles can be used to target a stock of loaner wheelchairs to the needs of customers who are going to need them most often, or to choose a selection of loaner chairs.

Computer profiles and records can be used to maintain inventory for the most commonly replaced parts and components. Computer profiles can contain wheelchair settings so that when a new wheelchair arrives or when a replacement part is installed, it can be tuned to the rider's preferred setting. From a rider's consumer profile, the dealer will know whether to arrange pick-up or delivery of the wheelchair or whether the rider prefers to come to the dealership. Computer profiles and inventories allow for virtual service centers to exist. Virtual service centers are organizations that do not operate out of a local storefront. Commonly, a service representative works from a service vehicle (e.g., a truck or van). The service representative is available by phone. The service representative makes an appointment and meets the consumer at a designated location (e.g., home, rehabilitation center, senior center). The service representative carries a set of common parts in the vehicle, and has access to other parts within a few hours (e.g., 24 to 48 hours). Once the problem is diagnosed, the service representative will either fix the problem immediately or order the parts and set up another appointment. In some cases, virtual dealers supply loaner wheelchairs. Currently, virtual dealers are used mostly in rural areas. The concept was started by several of the Tech Act projects to provide better service to assistive technology users who did not have ready access to DME dealerships. The concept of the virtual dealership is used extensively in the computer industry. It has been successful in reducing maintenance costs. However, good storefront dealers provide valuable service, which some riders prefer to direct sales.

### 14.5.2 Maintenance

All wheelchairs require periodic maintenance for them to operate properly. Most periodic maintenance consists of ensuring that nuts and bolts are properly adjusted, and that parts are properly lubricated. The bolts used on wheelchairs are of various grades. Bolts are graded for strength and hardness. The specific grade is selected by the manufacturer for the part where the bolt is to be used. Bolts used on wheelchairs must be replaced with the proper size and type bolt. Nuts and bolts on wheelchairs are also tightened to a specific torque. Service centers use torque wrenches to measure the torque as they tighten or retighten nuts and bolts. Nut and bolts that are too loose will loosen further or not hold the part properly. Over-tightening nuts and bolts can cause damage to the part and/or bolt.

Wheelchair wheels also require periodic maintenance. Through use spokes can become loosened, damaged, or broken, and rims can bend or go out of true. Spokes must be tensioned to a specific torque range. This helps prevent them or their nipples from breaking, and helps keep the wheel true. Three terms are used to describe the alignment of a wheel with respect to its axle: true, roundness, and dish (see Figure 14.19). The true of the wheel determines how much it wobbles from side to side. Roundness determines how much the wheel moves up and down, while looking from the side, as the wheel spins. Dish determines how close the center of the tire lines up with the center of the hub. Wheelchair wheels are set up from the factory to be true (i.e., no wobble), round (i.e., no up-down motion while turning), and without dish (i.e., centered over the hub). A special stand is used to ensure that a wheel has these three properties properly adjusted. If a spoke or rim is damaged it must be replaced and the wheels need to be readjusted. This requires a specialist. When a spoke becomes loose, the wheel will begin to go out of true, and the wheel will require adjustment.

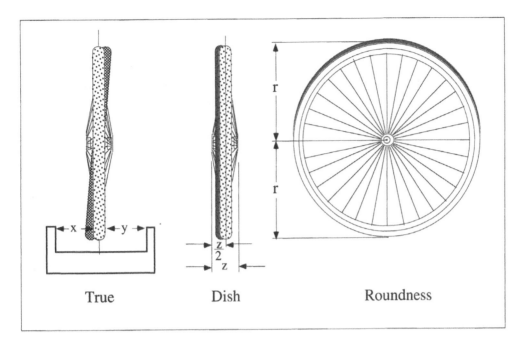

**FIGURE 14.19**  Definitions for true, dish, and roundness of a wheel. The shadowed parts illustrate deviations from ideal.

Moving parts on wheelchairs require periodic lubrication. The frequency of lubrication and proper lubricant are listed in service or owners' manuals. People living in humid or wet climates will need to have maintenance performed more often on their wheelchairs. Caster housings, ball bearings, and folding mechanisms require lubrication. Bearings require special care so that they are not destroyed. Many wheelchair bearings have seals or wipers to discourage water and dirt from entering them. Special skill is required to remove and replace the seals without damaging them. Wheelchair bearings use a variety of lightweight greases. Most folding mechanisms and exposed hinges can be lubricated with simple Teflon®-based spray lubricants.

### 14.5.3 Repair and Replacement

Some wheelchair parts require periodic repair and replacement. Repair and replacement of components can extend the life of the wheelchair and make using it much easier. Once a wheelchair falls behind in maintenance it becomes more difficult to operate, and it will not perform as well as when it was new. Some components will wear with use and need to be replaced periodically. Bearings and bushings will wear out on a wheelchair during normal use. Their life can be extended through cleaning and lubrication, but eventually they need to be replaced. Upholstery also tends to wear with age. Upholstery may need to be replaced even when it looks fine, because the upholstery may have stretched to the point that it is no longer providing proper postural support or a proper foundation for the cushion. The wheelchair user should have posture monitored by a professional to help determine when upholstery should be changed. Some users may need to change their upholstery as often as every year. When the upholstery is changed it is best to replace the bolts or screws that hold it in place. This will ensure that they are properly maintained as well.

Some components tend to wear out or become damaged during use. Legrests are used to open doors, act as bumpers, and support the feet and legs. Legrests are also often scraped along the ground when the wheelchair is loaded into a motor vehicle. This type of use tends to make them wear out with time. Most legrests are simply replaced by trained personnel. Armrests, anti-tip casters, and other removable components may wear out or become damaged with time. Cross-braces also receive a substantial amount of wear and tear during normal use. Therefore, wheelchair users should have their wheelchairs thoroughly serviced at least once each year. In areas where winters can be harsh, it may be best to have wheelchairs serviced just before winter and again in the spring. This will help to ensure safe operation throughout the year.

Electric-powered wheelchairs may require greater maintenance than manual wheelchairs. This is because electric-powered wheelchairs are more complex, and complexity increases the probability of failure. Most electric-powered wheelchairs are designed to be highly reliable, and wheelchairs are among the most reliable devices ever produced when properly maintained. Electric-powered wheelchairs must have a properly operating electrical system to be functional. This requires periodic inspection of cables, connectors, interfaces, the battery charger, and all electrical components. Minor damage to battery cables, motor connectors, or interface connectors can lead to severe problems if not addressed. Corrosion can render connectors useless, resulting in motors that will not drive or batteries that will not charge. Specialized personnel are required to make electrical system inspections and repairs. With time, wires will fray or break, connectors will corrode or break, and electrical components will fail. Most motors on electric-powered wheelchairs use brushes. These brushes occasionally need to be replaced.

Drive belts should be checked regularly for wear and stretching. Worn or improperly adjusted belts can break or slip. Irregular noises or slipping should immediately be eliminated. Some electric-powered wheelchairs use direct drives or transmissions. Repairs on these types of systems can be expensive. Direct drives and transmissions require lubrication, which may be indicated by changes in the sound they produce or in the performance of the wheelchair. Drivers should also look for loss of lubricant. Any symptoms of problems with direct drives or transmissions should be brought to the attention of a service technician. Most electrical wheelchair components will last many years with proper maintenance. Some electric-powered wheelchair users get 15 years of active life out of their wheelchairs with proper maintenance. At some time the wheelchair will wear out and replacement will become less costly than repair.

### 14.5.4 Replacing Batteries

Batteries are the fuel system for electric-powered wheelchairs. If the batteries do not work properly, the wheelchair will not work properly. Choosing the proper battery and maintaining it is vital to the performance of the wheelchair. Battery technology has changed considerably over the past few years. Wheelchair batteries offer more power in the same size package and provide more consistent performance than previously. Wheelchairs use deep cycle batteries. Deep cycle batteries are those designed to be regularly charged and recharged. Automotive and many marine batteries are designed for rapid bursts of power after which they are quickly recharged by an alternator. Wheelchairs may use gel/sealed batteries or wet lead acid batteries. Wet lead acid batteries are less costly than gel/sealed and can provide about 10% more running time, given equal size. However, wet lead acid batteries require much more maintenance than gel/sealed batteries. Wet lead acid batteries also present more of a risk of explosion due to hydrogen gas build-up or exposure to battery acid. Gel/sealed lead acid batteries are safer and are approved for all forms of transport (e.g., airline, bus, motor vehicle). Gel/sealed and wet lead acid batteries have about the same life span if properly maintained. To maximize the life of wheelchair batteries, only the charger provided with the wheelchair should be used. Do not use automotive chargers on gel/sealed batteries. Batteries last longer if they are never run completely flat. However, charging too frequently when the batteries have only been used a little will also decrease the battery's life. For most wheelchairs, the ideal charging point is when the "fuel gage" indicates 50%. Batteries should be stored fully charged. If stored for longer periods, the batteries should be disconnected from the wheelchair. A well-maintained battery should last from one to one and a half years.

All wheelchair batteries contain lead and sulfuric acid. Both are toxic and sulfuric acid is highly corrosive. When a lead acid battery is charged it generates hydrogen gas, which is highly flammable and can cause explosion. Wheelchair batteries need to be treated with a healthy degree of respect. If a battery is mishandled several problems can occur. Improper charging, poor maintenance, or battery failure can result in low acid/electrolyte levels. This may allow for high concentrations of hydrogen gas. This condition is possible with all types of lead acid batteries. It is less likely to occur in gel/sealed type batteries. Overfilled or excessively charged wet batteries can result in acid being forced into the wheelchair's battery box. This can result in corrosion and, in some cases, burns. Battery acid will cause damage to clothing. Batteries can provide a devastating shock. Dropping a wrench or screwdriver across the terminals can result in a large spark, a brilliant flash, smoke, and sometimes an explosion. Batteries are required to be recycled by an approved source. Batteries must be installed and maintained by a properly trained wheelchair or scooter technician.

## References and Further Reading

Axelson P. (1983) Power chairs. *Paraplegia News*, April 14–31.

Brattgard S. O., Lindstrom I., Severinsson K., Wihk L. (1984) Wheelchair design and quality. *Scandinavian Journal of Rehabilitation Medicine*, 9, 15–19.

*Built for Life: 1996 Custom Manual Wheelchairs*. Invacare Corporation, 899 Cleveland Street, Elyria, OH, 44036–4028.

*Champion 3000 Owner's Manual*. Kuschall of America, 708 Via Alondra, Camarillo, CA, 93012.

*Champion 1000 Owner's Manual*. Kuschall of America, 708 Via Alondra, Camarillo, CA, 93012.

(1991) Evaluation: Rechargeable, deep-cycle, lead acid batteries for powered wheelchair and scooter Uusers. *Health Devices*, 20,12, 474–492.

Roberts J., Stilson R. (1992) Preventative maintenance for power drive chairs. *Action Digest*, May/June, 14.

*Quickie 2 Owner's Manual*, No. 930302-A. Sunrise Medical Incorporated, Quickie Designs Inc., 2842 Business Park Avenue, Fresno, CA 93727.

*Quickie GP/GPV Owner's Manual*, No. 930301-B. Sunrise Medical Incorporated, Quickie Designs Inc., 2842 Business Park Avenue, Fresno, CA 93727.

Shepard M. (1992) Tuning your lightweight chair. *Action Digest*, July/August, 6–7.

Sullivan M. (1992) Over, under, round-a-bout: Light weight wheelchairs and you. *Action Digest*, July/August, 10–12.

Thacker J. G., Sprigle S. H., Morris B. O. (1994) Understanding the technology when selecting wheelchairs. *RESNA Press*, Arlington, VA.

*The HME Battery Guide.* MK Battery Incorporated, Los Angeles, CA.

Whitt R., Wilson D. G. (1982) *Bicycling Science*, 2nd ed. Cambridge, MA, The MIT Press.

# Appendixes

## *Appendix A.   A Partial List of Consumer and Professional Organizations and Services*

AbleData

American Society of Biomechanics

American Occupational Therapy Association

American Physical Therapy Association

American Spinal Cord Injury Association

Association of Academic Physiatrists

IEEE-Engineering in Medicine and Biology Society (IEEE-EMBS)

Paralyzed Veterans of America

Rehabilitation Engineering and Assistive Technology Society of North America (RESNA)

United Cerebral Palsy Association

Wheelchair Sports USA

World Institute on Disability (WID)

## *Appendix B.   United States Research and Training Funding Agencies*

Bioengineering and Technical Aids for People with Disabilities Program, National Science Foundation

National Center for Medical Rehabilitation Research, National Institute for Child and Human Development, National Institutes of Health

National Institute on Disability and Rehabilitation Research, U.S. Department of Education

Rehabilitation Research and Development Services, U.S. Department of Veterans Affairs

Rehabilitation Services Administration, U.S. Department of Education

Spinal Cord Research Foundation, Paralyzed Veterans of America

Education and Training Foundation, Paralyzed Veterans of America

## *Appendix C.   Journals and Periodicals Related to Wheelchairs and Seating*

*Adapted Physical Activity Quarterly*

*American Journal of Physical Medicine and Rehabilitation*

*Archives of Physical Medicine and Rehabilitation*

*Assistive Technology*

*Bulletin of Prosthetics Research*

*Ergonomics*

*Human Factors*

*IEEE Transactions on Rehabilitation Engineering*

*IEEE Transactions on Biomedical Engineering*

*IEEE Transactions on Systems, Man, and Cybernetics*

*Journal of Biomechanics*

*Journal of Bone and Joint Surgery*

*Journal of the Orthopaedic Research Society*

*Journal of Rehabilitation Research and Development*

*Medicine and Science in Sports and Exercise*

*Orthotics and Prosthetics*

*Palaestra*

*Paraplegia*

*Paraplegia News*

*Team Rehab Report*

*Technology and Disability*

*Sports 'N Spokes*

# Index

*Page numbers followed by* f *indicate figures; page numbers followed by* t *indicate tables.*